SO-AZL-951

Childhood Diseases and Disorders

SOURCEBOOK

FIFTH EDITION

Health Reference Series

Childhood Diseases and Disorders

SOURCEBOOK

FIFTH EDITION

Basic Consumer Health Information about the Physical, Mental, and Developmental Health of Preadolescent Children, Including Facts about Infectious Diseases, Asthma and Allergies, Cancer, Diabetes, Growth Disorders. The Medical Conditions Appearing in Childhood Are Explained along with Developmental and Pediatric Mental-Health Concerns

Along with Information about Vaccines, Medications, Promotion, a Glossary of Related Terms, and a List of Resources for Parents and Caregivers

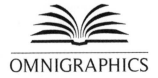

OMNIGRAPHICS

615 Griswold St., Ste. 520, Detroit, MI 48226

Bibliographic Note
Because this page cannot legibly accommodate all the copyright notices, the Bibliographic Note portion of the Preface constitutes an extension of the copyright notice.

* * *

OMNIGRAPHICS
Angela L. Williams, *Managing Editor*
* * *

Copyright © 2020 Omnigraphics
ISBN 978-0-7808-1729-6
E-ISBN 978-0-7808-1730-2

Library of Congress Cataloging-in-Publication Data

Names: Williams, Angela, 1963- editor.

Title: Childhood diseases and disorders sourcebook : basic consumer health information about the physical, mental, and developmental health of pre-adolescent children, including facts about infectious diseases, asthma and allergies, cancer, diabetes, growth disorders, and conditions affecting the blood, heart, ear, nose, throat, gastrointestinal tract, kidney, liver, bones, muscles, brain, lungs, skin, and eyes; along with information about vaccines, medications, wellness promotion, a glossary of related terms, and a list of resources for parents and caregivers / Angela L. Williams.

Description: Fifth edition. | Detroit : Omnigraphics, Inc., [2019] | Series: Health reference series | Includes bibliographical references and index. | Summary: "Provides basic consumer health information about the physical and mental health of preadolescent children including common illnesses and injuries, disease prevention and screening, and wellness promotion. Includes index, glossary of related terms, and other resources"--Provided by publisher.

Identifiers: LCCN 2019029139 (print) | LCCN 2019029140 (ebook) | ISBN 9780780817296 (library binding) | ISBN 9780780817302 (ebook)

Subjects: LCSH: Pediatrics. | Children--Health and hygiene. | Children--Diseases.

Classification: LCC RJ61.C5427 2019 (print) | LCC RJ61 (ebook) | DDC 618.92--dc23

LC record available at https://lccn.loc.gov/2019029139

LC ebook record available at https://lccn.loc.gov/2019029140

Electronic or mechanical reproduction, including photography, recording, or any other information storage and retrieval system for the purpose of resale is strictly prohibited without permission in writing from the publisher.

The information in this publication was compiled from the sources cited and from other sources considered reliable. While every possible effort has been made to ensure reliability, the publisher will not assume liability for damages caused by inaccuracies in the data, and makes no warranty, express or implied, on the accuracy of the information contained herein.

This book is printed on acid-free paper meeting the ANSI Z39.48 Standard. The infinity symbol that appears above indicates that the paper in this book meets that standard.

Printed in the United States

Table of Contents

NOV 2 6 2019

Part III: Medical Conditions Appearing in Childhood

ix

Part IV: Developmental and Pediatric Mental-Health Concerns

Part V: Additional Help and Information

Preface

About This Book

According to the Centers for Disease Control and Prevention (CDC), about 13.9 percent of children aged 2 to 5 have obesity and 18.4 percent of children aged 6 to 11 do. The number rises to 20.6 percent for adolescents aged 12 to 19. Every 1 in 4 U.S. student has a chronic health condition such as asthma, diabetes, or epilepsy. These matters, along with environmental hazards, lack of physical activity, poor diet, and other dangers, create concern for the well-being of our nation's children.

Childhood Diseases and Disorders Sourcebook, Fifth Edition provides information about children's health and safety and how to prevent your child from injuries, seizures, and fever. It also discusses infections caused by bacteria, viruses, fungus, and parasites. The medical conditions of children, such as cancer, cardiovascular disorders, allergies, and other disorders, including endocrine and growth disorder, gastrointestinal disorder, kidney and urological disorder, liver, and neurological disorders, are also explained. Information about developmental and pediatric mental-health concerns are included, along with a glossary of related terms and a list of organizations providing further information.

How to Use This Book

This book is divided into parts and chapters. Parts focus on broad areas of interest. Chapters are devoted to single topics within a part.

Part One: Introduction to Children's Health and Safety provides basic information on routine and emergency medical care for children, as well as guidelines for childhood vaccination and medication. It also discusses childhood obesity, secondhand smoke, and other health problems.

Part Two: Childhood Infections and Related Concerns focuses on food-borne, bacterial, viral, parasitic, and fungal infections that can occur in childhood as well as other diseases associated with infections.

Part Three: Medical Conditions Appearing in Childhood describes conditions and disorders that are generally diagnosed during childhood. This part provides facts about allergies, cancer, diabetes, growth disorders, and disorders affecting the blood and heart, ear, nose, and throat, gastrointestinal tract, endocrine system, kidneys, liver, muscles and bones, brain, lungs, skin, and eyes.

Part Four: Developmental and Pediatric Mental-Health Concerns details mental-health disorders than can affect children, as well as developmental and learning disabilities.

Part Five: Additional Help and Information provides a glossary of terms related to childhood diseases and disorders and concludes with a list of resources for parents and caregivers.

Bibliographic Note

This volume contains documents and excerpts from publications issued by the following U.S. government agencies: Centers for Disease Control and Prevention (CDC); *Eunice Kennedy Shriver* National Institute of Child Health and Human Development (NICHD); Food Safety and Inspection Service (FSIS); Genetic and Rare Diseases Information Center (GARD); Genetics Home Reference (GHR); National Cancer Institute (NCI); National Eye Institute (NEI); National Heart, Lung, and Blood Institute (NHLBI); National Institute of Allergy and Infectious Diseases (NIAID); National Institute of Arthritis and Musculoskeletal and Skin Diseases (NIAMS); National Institute of Diabetes and Digestive and Kidney Diseases (NIDDK); National Institute of Mental Health (NIMH); National Institute of Neurological Disorders and Stroke (NINDS); National Institute on Deafness and Other Communication Disorders (NIDCD); National Institutes of Health (NIH); Office of Disease Prevention and Health Promotion (ODPHP); Office on Women's Health (OWH); U.S. Department of

Health and Human Services (HHS); and U.S. Food and Drug Administration (FDA).

It may also contain original material produced by Omnigraphics and reviewed by medical consultants.

About the Health Reference Series

The *Health Reference Series* is designed to provide basic medical information for patients, families, caregivers, and the general public. Each volume takes a particular topic and provides comprehensive coverage. This is especially important for people who may be dealing with a newly diagnosed disease or a chronic disorder in themselves or in a family member. People looking for preventive guidance, information about disease warning signs, medical statistics, and risk factors for health problems will also find answers to their questions in the *Health Reference Series*. The *Series*, however, is not intended to serve as a tool for diagnosing illness, in prescribing treatments, or as a substitute for the physician/patient relationship. All people concerned about medical symptoms or the possibility of disease are encouraged to seek professional care from an appropriate healthcare provider.

A Note about Spelling and Style

Health Reference Series editors use *Stedman's Medical Dictionary* as an authority for questions related to the spelling of medical terms and *The Chicago Manual of Style* for questions related to grammatical structures, punctuation, and other editorial concerns. Consistent adherence is not always possible, however, because the individual volumes within the *Series* include many documents from a wide variety of different producers, and the editor's primary goal is to present material from each source as accurately as is possible. This sometimes means that information in different chapters or sections may follow other guidelines and alternate spelling authorities. For example, occasionally a copyright holder may require that eponymous terms be shown in possessive forms (Crohn's disease vs. Crohn disease) or that British spelling norms be retained (leukaemia vs. leukemia).

Medical Review

Omnigraphics contracts with a team of qualified, senior medical professionals who serve as medical consultants for the *Health Reference*

Series. As necessary, medical consultants review reprinted and originally written material for currency and accuracy. Citations including the phrase "Reviewed (month, year)" indicate material reviewed by this team. Medical consultation services are provided to the *Health Reference Series* editors by:

Dr. Vijayalakshmi, MBBS, DGO, MD

Dr. Senthil Selvan, MBBS, DCH, MD

Dr. K. Sivanandham, MBBS, DCH, MS (Research), PhD

Our Advisory Board

We would like to thank the following board members for providing initial guidance on the development of this series:

- Dr. Lynda Baker, Associate Professor of Library and Information Science, Wayne State University, Detroit, MI

- Nancy Bulgarelli, William Beaumont Hospital Library, Royal Oak, MI

- Karen Imarisio, Bloomfield Township Public Library, Bloomfield Township, MI

- Karen Morgan, Mardigian Library, University of Michigan-Dearborn, Dearborn, MI

- Rosemary Orlando, St. Clair Shores Public Library, St. Clair Shores, MI

Health Reference Series *Update Policy*

The inaugural book in the *Health Reference Series* was the first edition of *Cancer Sourcebook* published in 1989. Since then, the *Series* has been enthusiastically received by librarians and in the medical community. In order to maintain the standard of providing high-quality health information for the layperson the editorial staff at Omnigraphics felt it was necessary to implement a policy of updating volumes when warranted.

Medical researchers have been making tremendous strides, and it is the purpose of the *Health Reference Series* to stay current with the most recent advances. Each decision to update a volume is made on an individual basis. Some of the considerations include how much new information is available and the feedback we receive from people who use the books. If there is a topic you would like to see added to the update list, or an area of medical concern you feel has not been adequately addressed, please write to:

Managing Editor
Health Reference Series
Omnigraphics
615 Griswold St., Ste. 520
Detroit, MI 48226

Part One

Introduction to Children's Health and Safety

Chapter 1

Child Health Statistics

Your child's health includes physical, mental, and social well-being. Most parents know the basics of keeping children healthy, such as offering them healthy foods, making sure they get enough sleep and exercise, and ensuring their safety.

It is also important for children to get regular checkups with their healthcare provider. These visits are a chance to check your child's development. They are also a good time to catch or prevent problems.

Other than checkups, school-age children should be seen for:

- Significant weight gain or loss

- Sleep problems or changes in behavior

- Fever higher than 102°C

- Rashes or skin infections

- Frequent sore throats

- Breathing problems

This chapter contains text excerpted from the following sources: Text in this chapter begins with excerpts from "Children's Health," MedlinePlus, National Institutes of Health (NIH), March 25, 2015. Reviewed September 2019; Text under the heading "Fact and Statistics on Children's Health" is excerpted from "Facts and Statistics," President's Council on Sports, Fitness & Nutrition (PCSFN), U.S. Department of Health and Human Services (HHS), January 26, 2017.

Fact and Statistics on Children's Health
Physical Activity

- Only one in three children are physically active every day.

- Children now spend more than seven and a half hours a day in front of a screen (e.g., TV, videogames, computer).

- Nationwide, 25.6 percent of persons with a disability reported being physically inactive during a usual week, compared to 12.8 percent of those without a disability.

- Only about one in five homes have parks within a half-mile, and about the same number have a fitness or recreation center within that distance.

- Only six states (Illinois, Hawaii, Massachusetts, Mississippi, New York, and Vermont) require physical education in every grade, K–12.

- 28.0 percent of Americans or 80.2 million people, ages 6 and older are physically inactive.

- Nearly one-third of high-school students play video or computer games for three or more hours on an average school day.

Nutrition

- Typical American diets exceed the recommended intake levels or limits in four categories: calories from solid fats and added sugars, refined grains, sodium, and saturated fat.

- Americans eat less than the recommended amounts of vegetables, fruits, whole grains, dairy products, and oils.

- About 90 percent of Americans eat more sodium than is recommended for a healthy diet.

- Reducing the sodium Americans eat by 1,200 mg per day could save up to $20 billion a year in medical costs.

- Food available for consumption increased in all major food categories from 1970 to 2008. The average daily calories per person in the Marketplace increased by approximately 600 calories.

- Since the 1970s, the number of fast-food restaurants has more than doubled.

- More than 23 million Americans, including 6.5 million children, live in food deserts—areas that are more than a mile away from a supermarket.

- In 2008, an estimated 49.1 million people, including 16.7 million children, experienced food insecurity (limited access to safe and nutritionally adequate foods) multiple times throughout the year.

- In 2013, residents of the following states were most likely to report eating at least five servings of vegetables four or more days per week: Vermont (68.7%), Montana (63.0%) and Washington (61.8%). The least likely were Oklahoma (52.3%), Louisiana (53.3%) and Missouri (53.8%). The national average for regular produce consumption is 57.7 percent.

- Empty calories from added sugars and solid fats contribute to 40 percent of total daily calories for 2- to 18-year olds and half of these empty calories come from six sources: soda, fruit drinks, dairy desserts, grain desserts, pizza, and whole milk.

- Food safety awareness goes hand-in-hand with nutrition education. In the United States, food-borne agents affect 1 out of 6 individuals and cause approximately 48 million illnesses, 128,000 hospitalizations, and 3,000 deaths each year.

- The U.S. per capita consumption of total fat increased from approximately 57 pounds in 1980 to 78 pounds in 2009 with the highest consumption being 85 pounds in 2005.

- The U.S. percentage of food-insecure households, those with limited or uncertain ability to acquire acceptable foods in socially acceptable ways, rose from 11 percent to 15 percent between 2005 and 2009.

Obesity

- Data from 2009 to 2010 indicates that over 78 million U.S. adults and about 12.5 million (16.9%) children and adolescents are obese.

- For children with disabilities, obesity rates are approximately 38 percent higher than for children without disabilities.

- Obesity then and now:
  - Prevalence of obesity for children ages 2 to 5 years doubled

- Early 1970s: 5 percent

- 2007 to 2008: 10 percent

- Prevalence of obesity for children ages 6 to 11 years—quadrupled

  - Early 1970s: 4 percent

  - 2007 to 2008: 20 percent

- Prevalence of obesity for children ages 12 to 19 years—tripled

  - Early 1970s: 6 percent

  - 2007 to 2008: 18 percent

- Nearly 45 percent of children living in poverty are overweight or obese compared with 22 percent of children living in households with incomes 4 times the poverty level.

- Almost 40 percent of Black and Latinx youth ages 2 to 19 are overweight or obese compared with only 29 percent of White youth.

- Obesity among children in the United States has remained flat— at around 17 percent—in 2003 to 2004 and 2011 to 2012.

- Between 2003 and 2012, obesity among children between 2 and 5 years of age has declined from 14 to 8 percent—a 43 percent decrease in just under a decade.

- Obesity rates in children 6 to 11 years old have decreased from 18.8 percent in 2003 to 2004 to 17.7 percent in 2011 to 2012; obesity rates for children 12 to 19 years of age have increased from 17.4 to 20.5 percent in the same time period.

Human and Financial Costs of Obesity

- Obesity-related illness, including chronic disease, disability, and death, is estimated to carry an annual cost of $190.2 billion.

- Projections estimate that by 2018, obesity will cost the U.S. 21 percent of the total healthcare costs—$344 billion annually.

- Those who are obese have medical costs that are $1,429 more than those of normal weight on average (roughly 42% higher).

- The medical-care costs of obesity in the United States are staggering. In 2008, these costs totaled about $147 billion.

Chapter 2

Doctor Visits and Your Child

Young children need to go to the doctor or nurse for a "well-child visit" seven times between the ages of one and four.

A well-child visit is when you take your child to the doctor for a full checkup to make sure she or he is healthy and developing normally. This is different from other visits for sickness or injury.

At a well-child visit, the doctor or nurse can help catch any problems early, when they may be easier to treat. You will also have a chance to ask questions about things such as your child's behavior, eating habits, and sleeping habits.

To make the most of your child's visit:

- Gather important information

- Make a list of questions for the doctor

- Know what to expect from the visit

This chapter contains text excerpted from the following sources: Text in this chapter begins with excerpts from "Make the Most of Your Child's Visit to the Doctor (Ages 1 to 4)," Office of Disease Prevention and Health Promotion (ODPHP), U.S. Department of Health and Human Services (HHS), March 29, 2019; Text beginning with the heading "Make the Most of Your Child's Visit to the Doctor" is excerpted from "Make the Most of Your Child's Visit to the Doctor (Ages 5 to 10)," Office of Disease Prevention and Health Promotion (ODPHP), U.S. Department of Health and Human Services (HHS), March 29, 2019.

How Often Do You Need to Take Your Child for Well-Child Visits?

Young children grow quickly, so they need to visit the doctor or nurse regularly to make sure they are healthy and developing normally.

Children ages one to four need to see a doctor or nurse when they are:

- 12 months old

- 15 months old (1 year and 3 months)

- 18 months old (1 year and 6 months)

- 24 months old (2 years)

- 30 months old (2 years and 6 months)

- 3 years old

- 4 years old

If you are worried about your child's health, do not wait until the next scheduled visit—call the doctor or nurse right away.

How Do You Determine That Your Child Is Growing and Developing on Schedule?

Your child's doctor or nurse can help you identify "developmental milestones," the new skills that children usually develop by a certain age. These include physical, mental, language, and social skills.

Each child grows and develops differently. For example, some children will take longer to start talking than others.

At each visit, the doctor or nurse will look for some basic developmental milestones to see if your child is developing on schedule. This is an important part of the well-child visit.

By age 12 months, most kids:

- Have at least one tooth

- Stand up by pulling on a table or chair

- Walk (either with help or on their own)

- Try to copy animal sounds

- Say "mama" and "dada," plus one or two other words

- Follow simple directions, such as "Pick up the toy"

By age 15 months, most kids:

- Bend to reach the floor without falling
- Put blocks in a cup
- Make scribbles with crayons
- Take toys over to show a parent
- Listen to a story and look at pictures

By age 18 months, most kids:

- Walk up steps
- Try to run
- Climb onto small chairs without help
- Build towers of two to four blocks
- Use a spoon to eat and a cup to drink (with help)
- Take off simple pieces of clothing (such as socks and hats)
- Point to show someone what they want
- Play simple pretend games, such as feeding a doll

By age 24 months (two years), most kids:

- Stand on their tiptoes
- Kick a ball without losing their balance
- Have at least 16 teeth
- Can tell someone when they are hungry, thirsty, or need to use the bathroom
- Understand instructions with two steps, such as "Put on your shoes and then get your ball"
- Copy others, especially adults and older children
- Can name items in a picture book (such as a cat or dog)

By age 30 months, most kids:

- Point to different body parts when asked ("Point to your nose.")
- Play simple games with other kids, such as tag
- Brush their teeth with assistance

- Jump up and down in one place
- Put on their clothes with assistance

By age 3 years, most kids:

- Have all 20 "baby" teeth
- Use the toilet during the day (may still need a diaper overnight)
- Copy a circle when drawing
- Put one foot on each step when walking up and down stairs
- Speak in sentences of three to four words
- Ask questions
- Know their first name, age, and sex

By age four years, most kids:

- Hop on one foot and balance on one foot for a short time
- Use child-safe scissors
- Count to at least four
- Ask lots of questions
- Play with imaginary (pretend) friends
- Can name some colors and numbers
- Play simple board games and card games

Steps to Help You and Your 1- to 4-year old Child Get the Most out of Well-Child Visits

Take these steps to help you and your child get the most out of well-child visits.

Gather Important Information

Take any medical records you have to the appointment, including a record of shots your child has received.

Make a list of any important changes in your child's life since the last doctor's visit, such as:

- A serious illness or death in the family

- A separation or divorce

- A change in childcare

Ask Other Caregivers about Your Child

Before you visit the doctor, talk with others who care of your child, such as a grandparent, daycare provider, or babysitter. They may be able to help you think of questions to ask the doctor or nurse.

Take a List of Questions You Want to Ask the Doctor

Before the well-child visit, write down three to five questions you have. This visit is a great time to ask the doctor or nurse any questions about:

- A health condition your child has (such as asthma or an allergy)

- Changes in sleeping or eating habits

- How to help kids in the family get along

Some Questions You May Want to Ask

- Is my child up to date on shots?

- How can I make sure my child is getting enough physical activity?

- Is my child at a healthy weight?

- How can I help my child try different foods?

- What are the appropriate ways to discipline my child?

- How much TV time and computer time is okay for young children?

Take a notepad and write down the answers so that you can review them later.

Ask What to Do If Your Child Gets Sick

Make sure you know how to get in touch with a doctor or nurse when the office is closed. Ask how to reach the doctor on call—or if there is a nurse information service you can call at night or during the weekend.

Know What to Expect

During each well-child visit, the doctor or nurse will ask you questions about your child, do a physical exam, and update your child's medical history. You will also be able to ask your questions and discuss any problems you may be having.

The doctor or nurse may ask about:

- **Behavior**—Does your child have trouble following directions?

- **Health**—Does your child often complain of stomach aches or other kinds of pain?

- **Safety**—Does your child always ride in a car seat in the back seat of the car?

- **Activities**—What types of pretend play does your child like?

- **Eating habits**—What does your child eat on a normal day?

- **Family**—Have there been any changes in your family since your last visit?

Your answers to questions such as these will help the doctor or nurse make sure your child is healthy and developing normally.

The Doctor or Nurse Will Also Check Your Child's Body

To check your child's body, the doctor or nurse will:

- Measure your child's height and weight
- Check your child's blood pressure
- Check your child's vision
- Check your child's body parts (this is called a "physical exam")
- Give shots your child needs

Make the Most of Your 5- to 10-year-old Child's Visit to the Doctor

Children who are 5 to 10 years of age need to go to the doctor or nurse for a "well-child visit" once a year.

How Do I Know If My Child Is Growing and Developing on Schedule?

Your child's doctor or nurse can help you identify "developmental milestones," the new skills that children usually develop by a certain age. This is an important part of the well-child visit.

Developmental milestones for children ages 5 to 10 include physical, learning, and social skills—things such as:

- Developing skills for success in school, (such as listening, paying attention, reading, and math)

- Taking care of their bodies without help, (such as bathing, brushing teeth, and getting dressed)

- Learning from mistakes or failures and trying again

- Helping with simple chores

- Following family rules

- Developing friendships and getting along with other children

- Participating in activities, such as school clubs, sports teams, or music lessons

Steps to Help You and Your 5- to 10-year-old Child Get the Most out of Well-Child Visits

Take these steps to help you and your child get the most out of well-child visits.

Gather Important Information

Take any medical records you have to the appointment, including a record of shots your child has received. If your child gets special services at school because of a health condition or disability, bring that paperwork, too.

Make a list of any important changes in your child's life since the last doctor's visit, such as:

- A new sibling

- A serious illness or death of a friend or family member

- A new school or a move to a new neighborhood

Help Your Child Get More Involved in Doctor Visits

When children are age seven or older, most doctors will spend a few minutes alone with them if the child feels comfortable. This helps your child develop a relationship with the doctor.

You can also help your child get involved by:

- Letting her or him know what to expect at a doctor's visit

- Encouraging her or him to ask questions during the visit

Make a List of Questions You Want to Ask the Doctor

Before the well-child visit, write down three to five questions you have. This visit is a great time to ask the doctor or nurse any questions about:

- A health condition your child has (such as asthma, allergies, or a speech problem)

- Changes in behavior or mood

- Problems in school—with learning or with other children

Here are some important questions to ask:

- Is my child up to date on shots?

- How can I make sure my child is getting enough physical activity?

- How can I help my child eat healthy?

- Is my child at a healthy weight?

- How can I teach my child to use the Internet safely?

- How can I talk with my child about bullying?

- How can I help my child know what to expect during puberty?

Take a notepad and write down the answers so you can remember them later.

Ask What to Do If Your Child Gets Sick

Make sure you know how to get in touch with a doctor or nurse when the office is closed. Ask how to contact the doctor on call, or if there is a nurse information service you can call at night or on the weekend.

Know What to Expect

During each well-child visit, the doctor or nurse will ask you questions about your child, do a physical exam, and update your child's medical history. You will also be able to ask your questions and discuss any problems.

The doctor or nurse will ask you and your child questions.

The doctor or nurse may ask about:

- **Behavior**—Does your child have trouble following directions at home or at school?

- **Health**—Does your child often complain of headaches or other pain?

- **School**—Does your child look forward to going to school?

- **Activities**—What does your child like to do after school and on weekends?

- **Eating habits**—What does your child eat on a normal day?

- **Family**—Have there been any changes in your family since your last visit?

Your answers to questions like these will help the doctor or nurse make sure your child is healthy and developing normally.

The Doctor or Nurse Will Also Check Your Child's Body

To check your child's body, the doctor or nurse will:

- Measure your child's height and weight

- Check your child's blood pressure

- Check your child's vision and hearing

- Check your child's body parts (this is called a "physical exam")

- Give shots your child needs

Chapter 3

How to Give Medicine to Children

Children are not just small adults. It is especially important to remember this when giving medicines to children. Giving a child the wrong dose or a medicine that is not for children can have serious side effects.

The drug labels for prescription medicines have a section on "Pediatric Use." It says whether the medicine has been studied for its effects on children. It also tells you which age groups were studied. Some over-the-counter (OTC) medicines, such as those that treat fever and pain, have been studied for effectiveness, safety, or dosing in children. But, many other OTC medicines have not. It is important to read the labels carefully, to make sure that the medicine is right for your child.

Here are some other tips for giving medicine safely to your child:

- **Read and follow the label directions every time.** Pay special attention to usage directions and warnings.

This chapter contains text excerpted from the following sources: Text in this chapter begins with excerpts from "Medicines and Children," MedlinePlus, National Institutes of Health (NIH), December 2, 2014. Reviewed September 2019; Text under the heading "Daily Medicine Record for Your Child" is excerpted from "Daily Medicine Record for Your Child," U.S. Food and Drug Administration (FDA), February 26, 2018; Text under the heading "Teaching Your Children How to Use Medicines Safely as They Grow" is excerpted from "As They Grow: Teaching Your Children How to Use Medicines Safely," U.S. Food and Drug Administration (FDA), September 25, 2013. Reviewed September 2019.

- **Watch out for problems.** Contact your healthcare provider or pharmacist right away if:
  - You notice any new symptoms or unexpected side effects in your child
  - The medicine does not appear to be working when you expect it to. For example, antibiotics may take a few days to start working, but a pain reliever usually starts working soon after your child takes it.

- **Know the abbreviations for the amounts of medicines.**
  - Tablespoon (Tbsp.)
  - Teaspoon (tsp.)
  - Milligram (mg.)
  - Milliliter (mL.)
  - Ounce (oz.)

- **Use the correct dosing device.** If the label says two teaspoons and you are using a dosing cup with ounces only, do not try to guess how many teaspoons it would be. Get the proper measuring device. Do not substitute another item, such as a kitchen spoon.

- **Check with your healthcare provider or pharmacist before giving two medicines at the same time.** That way, you can avoid a possible overdose or an unwanted interaction.

- **Follow age and weight-limit recommendations.** If the label says not to give the drug to children under a certain age or weight, then do not do it.

- **Always use the child-resistant cap and relock the cap after each use.** Also, keep all medicines out of the reach of children.

- **Ask your healthcare provider or pharmacist** if you have any questions.

Daily Medicine Record for Your Child
Why Should I Keep a Daily Medicine Record for My Child?

- To keep your child safe, a daily record will help you keep track of the amount of medicine your child takes so you or someone else will not accidentally give too much.

- To have a way of sharing this information with others who may be caring for your children, such as a spouse, grandparent, babysitter, and your child's healthcare professional.

How Do I Keep a Daily Medicine Record?

Make your own record and write down the following:

- Name of the child
- Child's age and weight. (It is always best to use your child's weight to decide how much medicine to give. Use age if you do not know your child's weight.)
- The day's date
- Time of day you give the medicine
- Symptom or problem the medicine is used for
- Medicine's name
- Medicine's active ingredient(s)
- The medicine's formula (infant, children, junior, or other)
- The amount of medicine you give

Where Should I Keep a Daily Medicine Record?

You should keep it where all of your child's caregivers can easily find it. The information you write will help you and others remember the last time a dose was given and how much your child has taken.

Always keep medicines where they cannot be seen or reached by children and pets. A locked box, cabinet, or closet is best.

How Often Should I Fill Out a Daily Medicine Record?

You should fill out a Daily Medicine Record each time your child takes medicine. Start a new Daily Medicine Record each day until your child is no longer taking medicine.

Teaching Your Children How to Use Medicines Safely as They Grow

As parents and guardians, you have the important jobs of protecting your children from harm and teaching them to make good choices as they grow and become adults. At a young age, start talking to your children about medicines and how you make medical decisions for yourself and for them. This teaches children how to use medicines safely and correctly and to avoid harm from the misuse of medicines. It also encourages them to ask questions about medicines and medicine decisions.

Sometimes your child may ask you a question for which you have no answer. This is a great chance to show your child that it is okay to ask health professionals for advice about medicines—health professionals, such as doctors and pharmacists, are there to help you and your family make smart medicine and health choices.

Table 3.1 suggests the kinds of information you should share with your children about medicines at different ages. Every child is different, so your child may be ready for some of these ideas a little earlier or a little later than the age suggested here.

Table 3.1. What Your Child Should Know about Medicine Safety

Three-Year-Olds	• If you find a pill or a piece of candy, give it to a grown-up. Do not taste it. • Take medicines and vitamins only when your parent or guardian says you should. • Tell a grown-up right away if other children are getting into medicines.
Five-Year-Olds	• Ask your parents to put your name or a sticker on the medicine bottle so everyone knows which medicine is yours. • Keep all medicines (and dietary supplements) out of the reach of young children. Tell guests to do the same. • If you take medicine and feel worse, tell your parent or another grown-up.

Six-Year-Olds	• Remind the person giving you medicine to read the label and check how much you should use. Read the label together.
	• Remind the person giving you the medicine when you are supposed to take it next. Read the label together if you do not remember.
	• At the doctor's office, ask the doctor to tell you:
	  • What medicine you will be using
	  • Why you need to use it
	  • What the medicine does

Table 3.1. Continued

Seven-Year-Olds	• Know the steps for taking medicine. Ask your parents which steps they should do alone, which steps you can do with them. • Know the rules for taking medicines at school and follow them. • Read the label before taking medicine. Is it what the doctor or your parent said? If not, tell them. Check how much medicine to use and how to use it. Use it as directed. • Do not put medicines in pockets, and keep medicines away from young children. • Do not take medicines in front of children younger than four years old. They may try to copy your behavior.
Eight-Year-Olds	• Know how much you weigh. Tell your parents how much you weigh when they check the medicine label to see how much you should use. If you have a bathroom scale, learn how to weigh yourself. • If you use medicine every day, write down the day and time you take it. Ask your parents to help you make a chart to fill in when you take your medicines. Tell them you will help fill the chart in. • Ask questions about drug ads. Discuss drug ads you see on TV and what you read on the Internet with your doctor, nurse, pharmacist, or parents. • Ask an adult what side effects can happen when you use a medicine. Watch for side effects and tell a grown-up if they happen. • Write down questions to ask a doctor, nurse, or pharmacist about your medicines.
Nine-Year-Olds	• Keep purses and backpacks with medicines in them out of the reach of young children at home and when visiting other people's homes.
Ten-Year-Olds	• Talk with your parents about taking more responsibility for using medicines. • Tell adults why it is important not to stop taking antibiotics until the prescribed amount is all gone. • Ask which side effects are dangerous and which are likely to go away. Decide with a parent what to do if you have a side effect. • Keep medicines with their package and in the original container with child-proof caps. Do not use pillboxes; they do not have all the important information about your medicine.

Table 3.1. Continued

Eleven-Year-Olds	• Know how to read dosage charts on over-the-counter medicine labels.
Twelve-Year-Olds	• Only keep medicines you will use. Throw away expired medicines at a home hazardous waste disposal site or in a garbage can away from small children and pets.

Chapter 4

Childhood Vaccinations

Chapter Contents

Section 4.1

Making the Vaccine Decision

This section includes text excerpted from "Making the Vaccine
Decision," Centers for Disease Control and
Prevention (CDC), March 18, 2019.

How Vaccines Prevent Diseases

The diseases vaccines prevent can be dangerous, or even deadly.
Vaccines reduce your child's risk of infection by working with their
body's natural defenses to help them safely develop immunity to
disease.

When germs such as bacteria or viruses, invade the body, they
attack and multiply. This invasion is called an "infection," and the
infection is what causes illness. The immune system then has to fight
the infection. Once it fights off the infection, the body has a supply of
cells that help recognize and fight that disease in the future. These
supplies of cells are called "antibodies."

Vaccines help develop immunity by imitating an infection, but
this "imitation" infection does not cause illness. Instead, it causes
the immune system to develop the same response as it does to a real
infection so the body can recognize and fight the vaccine-preventable
disease in the future. Sometimes, after getting a vaccine, an imitation
infection can cause minor symptoms, such as fever. Such minor symptoms are normal and should be expected as the body builds immunity.

As children get older, they require additional doses of some vaccines for the best protection. Older kids also need protection against
additional diseases they may encounter.

Vaccines and Your Child's Immune System

As a parent, you may get upset or concerned when you watch your
baby get 3 or 4 shots during a doctor's visit. But, all of those shots add
up to protection for your baby against 14 infectious diseases. Young
babies can get very ill from vaccine-preventable diseases.

The Advisory Committee on Immunization Practices (ACIP), a
group of medical and public-health experts that develops recommendations on how to use vaccines to control diseases in the United States,
designs the vaccination schedule. The ACIP designs the vaccination
schedule to protect young children before they are likely to be exposed
to potentially serious diseases and when they are most vulnerable to

serious infections. This is the schedule the Centers for Disease Control and Prevention (CDC) recommends.

Although children continue to receive several vaccines up to their second birthday, these vaccines do not overload the immune system. Every day, your healthy child's immune system successfully fights off thousands of antigens—the parts of germs that cause their immune system to respond. The antigens in vaccines come from weakened or killed germs and so cannot cause serious illness. Even if your child receives several vaccines in one day, vaccines contain only a tiny amount of antigens compared to the antigens your baby encounters every day.

This is the case even if your child receives combination vaccines. Combination vaccines take two or more vaccines that could be given individually and put them into one shot. Children get the same protection as they do from individual vaccines given separately—but with fewer shots.

Vaccine Side Effects or Risks

Like any medication, vaccines can cause side effects. The most common side effects are mild. On the other hand, many vaccine-preventable disease symptoms can be serious, or even deadly. Even though many of these diseases are rare in the United States, they still occur around the world. Unvaccinated U.S. citizens who travel abroad can bring these diseases to the United States and put unvaccinated children at risk.

The side effects of vaccines (such as redness and swelling where the shot was given) are almost always minor and go away within a few days. If your child experiences a reaction at the injection site, use a cool, wet cloth to reduce redness, soreness, and swelling.

Serious side effects after vaccination, such as severe allergic reaction, are very rare and doctors and clinic staff are trained to deal with them. Pay extra attention to your child for a few days after vaccination. If you see something that concerns you, call your child's doctor.

Vaccine Ingredients

Vaccines contain ingredients, called "antigens," which cause the body to develop immunity. Vaccines also contain very small amounts of other ingredients. All ingredients either help make the vaccine or ensure the vaccine is safe and effective. These types of ingredients are listed in Table 4.1.

Table 4.1. Ingredients of Vaccines

Type of Ingredient	Examples	Purpose
Preservatives	Thimerosal (only in multidose vials of flu vaccine)*	To prevent contamination
Adjuvants	Aluminum salts	To help stimulate the body's response to the antigens
Stabilizers	Sugars, gelatin	To keep the vaccine potent during transportation and storage
Residual cell culture materials	Egg protein	To grow enough of the virus or bacteria to make the vaccine
Residual inactivating ingredients	Formaldehyde	To kill viruses or inactivate toxins during the manufacturing process
Residual antibiotics	Neomycin	To prevent contamination by bacteria during the vaccine manufacturing process

Today, the only childhood vaccines used routinely in the United States that contain thimerosal (mercury) are flu vaccines in multi-dose vials. These vials have very tiny amounts of thimerosal as a preservative. This is necessary because each time an individual dose is drawn from a multi-dose vial with a new needle and syringe, there is the potential to contaminate the vial with harmful microbes (toxins).

There is no evidence that the small amounts of thimerosal in flu vaccines cause any harm, except for minor reactions, such as redness and swelling at the injection site. Although no evidence suggests that there are safety concerns with thimerosal, vaccine manufacturers have stopped using it as a precautionary measure. Flu vaccines that do not contain thimerosal are available (in single-dose vials).

Ensuring Vaccine Safety

The United States' long-standing vaccine safety system ensures vaccines are as safe as possible. In fact, as of now, the United States has the safest vaccine supply in its history.

Safety monitoring begins with the U.S. Food and Drug Administration (FDA), which ensures the safety, effectiveness, and availability of vaccines for the United States. Before the FDA approves a vaccine for use by the public, highly trained FDA scientists and doctors evaluate the results of studies on the safety and effectiveness of the vaccine.

The FDA also inspects the sites where vaccines are made to make sure they follow strict-manufacturing guidelines.

Although scientists identify the most common side effects of a vaccine in studies before the vaccine is licensed, they may not detect rare adverse events in these studies. Therefore, the U.S. vaccine safety system continuously monitors for possible side effects after the FDA licenses a vaccine. When millions of people receive a vaccine, less common side effects that studies did not identify earlier may occur.

If the CDC and FDA find a link between a possible side effect and a vaccine, public-health officials take appropriate action. They will weigh the benefits of the vaccine against its risks to determine if recommendations for using the vaccine should change.

The Vaccine Adverse Event Reporting System (VAERS) is a national system used by scientists at the FDA and CDC to collect reports of adverse events (possible side effects) that happen after vaccination.

Section 4.2

Types of Routinely Administered Vaccines Children

This section includes text excerpted from "Vaccines for Children—A Guide for Parents and Caregivers," U.S. Food and Drug Administration (FDA), September 5, 2018.

Vaccines work by preparing the body's immune system for future exposure to disease-causing viruses or bacteria. Vaccines contain antigens, which are weakened bacteria or viruses, or parts of bacteria or viruses, which mimic the disease-causing agents. As a result of vaccination, the body's immune system thinks the antigens from the vaccine are foreign and should not be in the body, but the antigens do not cause disease in the person receiving the vaccine. After receiving the vaccine, if the virus or bacteria that cause the real disease then enters the body in the future, the immune system is prepared and responds quickly and forcefully to attack the disease-causing agent to prevent the person from getting sick with the disease. Vaccines are frequently given by injection (a shot), but some are given by mouth and one is sprayed into the nose.

Attenuated (weakened) live viruses: These vaccines contain a live virus that has been weakened during the manufacturing process so that they do not cause the actual disease in the person being vaccinated. However, because they contain a small amount of the weakened live virus, people with weakened immune systems should talk to their healthcare provider before receiving them. Examples include vaccines that prevent chickenpox and rotavirus and measles, mumps, and rubella.

Inactivated (killed) viruses: These vaccines contain a virus that has been killed so as not to cause disease, but the body still recognizes it and stimulates the production of antibodies against the virus. They can be given to individuals with weakened immune systems. Examples include vaccines to prevent polio and hepatitis A.

Subunits: In some cases, the entire virus or bacteria is not required for an immune response to prevent disease; just the important parts, a portion or a "subunit" of the disease-causing bacteria or virus, is needed to provide protection. The vaccine to prevent influenza (the flu) that is given as a shot is an example of a subunit vaccine, because it is made with parts of the influenza virus.

Toxoids: Some bacteria cause illness in people by secreting a poison (a toxin). Scientists discovered that weakening the toxins so that they are "detoxified" does not cause illness. Examples of vaccines that contain toxoids include those to prevent tetanus and diphtheria disease.

Recombinant: These vaccines are made by genetic engineering—the process and method of manipulating the genetic material of an organism. An example of this type of vaccine is those that prevent certain diseases, such as cervical cancer, that are caused by human papillomavirus (HPV). In this case, the genes that code for a specific protein from each of the virus types of HPV included in the vaccine are expressed in yeast to create large quantities of the protein. The protein that is produced is purified and then used to make the vaccine. Because the vaccine only contains a protein and not the entire virus, the vaccine cannot cause the HPV infection. It is the body's immune response to the recombinant protein(s) that then protect against diseases caused by the naturally occurring virus.

Polysaccharides: To protect against certain disease-causing bacteria, the main antigens in a vaccine are sugarlike substances called "polysaccharides;" these are purified from the bacteria to make polysaccharide vaccines. However, vaccines composed solely of purified polysaccharides are only effective in older children and adults. Pneumovax 23, a vaccine for the prevention of pneumococcal disease caused by 23 different strains, is an example of a polysaccharide vaccine.

Conjugates: Vaccines made only with polysaccharides do not work very well in young children because their immune system has not fully developed. To make vaccines that protect young children against diseases caused by certain bacteria, the polysaccharides are connected to a protein so that the immune system can recognize and respond to the polysaccharide. The protein acts as a "carrier" for the part of the vaccine that will make protective antibodies in the body. Examples of conjugate vaccines include those to prevent invasive disease caused by *Haemophilus influenzae type b* (Hib).

Routinely Administered Vaccines for Children

Some of the most commonly administered vaccines are briefly discussed below. A complete list of licensed vaccines in the United States.

Diphtheria and Tetanus Toxoids and Acellular Pertussis Adsorbed

Brand names: Daptacel® and Infanrix®

- **What it is for:** Prevents the bacterial diseases diphtheria, tetanus (lockjaw), and pertussis (whooping cough). This combination vaccine is given as a series in infants and children six weeks through six years of age, prior to their seventh birthday. The bacteria that cause diphtheria can infect the throat, causing a thick covering that can lead to problems with breathing, paralysis, or heart failure. Tetanus can cause painful tightening (spasms) of the muscles, seizures, paralysis, and death. Pertussis, also known as "whooping cough," has the initial symptoms of runny nose, sneezing, and a mild cough, which may seem like a typical cold. Usually, the cough slowly becomes more severe. Eventually, the patient may experience bouts of rapid coughing followed by the "whooping" sound that gives the disease its common name as they try to inhale. While the coughing fit is occurring, the patient may vomit or turn blue from lack of air. Patients gradually recover over weeks to months.

- **Common side effects may include:** Fever, drowsiness, fussiness or irritability, and redness, soreness, or swelling at the injection site.

- **Tell your healthcare provider beforehand if:** The child is moderately or severely ill, has had swelling of the brain within seven days after a previous dose of vaccine, has a neurologic disorder, such as epilepsy, or has had a severe allergic reaction to a previous shot.

Tetanus Toxoid, Reduced Diphtheria Toxoid, and Acellular Pertussis Vaccine Adsorbed

Brand names: Adacel® and Boostrix®

- **What it is for:** Booster shot for kids at 10 or 11 years of age to prevent the bacterial infections diphtheria, tetanus (lockjaw), and pertussis (whooping cough). In addition, Boostrix is approved for all individuals 10 years of age and older, (including the elderly). Adacel is approved for use in people ages 10 through 64 years.

- **Common side effects may include:** Pain, redness and swelling at the injection site, headache, and tiredness.

- **Tell your healthcare provider beforehand if:** The child is moderately or severely ill, has had swelling of the brain within seven days after a previous dose of pertussis vaccine, or any allergic reaction to any vaccine that protects against diphtheria, tetanus or pertussis diseases.

Haemophilus B Conjugate Vaccine

Brand names: ActHIB®, Hiberix®, PedvaxHIB®

- **What it is for:** Prevents *Haemophilus influenzae type b* (Hib) invasive disease. Before the availability of Hib vaccines, Hib disease was the leading cause of bacterial meningitis among children under 5 years of age in the United States. Meningitis is an infection of the tissue covering the brain and spinal cord, which can lead to lasting brain damage and deafness. Hib disease can also cause pneumonia, severe swelling in the throat, infections of the blood, joints, bones, and tissue covering of the heart, as well as death. Both ActHIB® and PedvaxHIB® are approved for infants and children beginning at 2 months. ActHIB® can be given through 5 years of age and PedvaxHIB® can be given through 71 months of age; Hiberix is approved for children 6 weeks through the age of 4 (prior to their 5th birthday).

- **Common side effects may include:** Fussiness, sleepiness, and soreness, swelling and redness at the injection site.

- **Tell your healthcare provider beforehand if:** The child is moderately or severely ill, or has ever had an allergic reaction to a previous dose of the Hib vaccine.

Hepatitis A Vaccine

Brand names: Havrix® and Vaqta®

- **What it is for:** Prevents disease caused by hepatitis A virus. People infected with hepatitis A may not have any symptoms; and if they do have symptoms, they may feel like they have a mild "flu-like" illness; or they may have jaundice (yellow skin or eyes), tiredness, stomachache, nausea, and diarrhea. Young children may not have any symptoms, so when a child's caregiver becomes sick, that is when it is recognized that the child is infected. Hepatitis A is most often spread by an object contaminated with the feces of a person with hepatitis A, such as when a parent or caregiver does not properly wash her or his hands after changing diapers or cleaning up the stool of an infected person. Both vaccines are approved for use in people 12 months of age and older.

- **Common side effects may include:** Soreness and redness at the injection site, and loss of appetite.

- **Tell your healthcare provider beforehand if:** The child is moderately to severely ill, or has ever had an allergic reaction to a previous dose of the vaccine.

Hepatitis B Vaccine

Brand names: Engerix-B® and Recombivax HB®

- **What it is for:** Prevents infection caused by hepatitis B virus. Hepatitis B is spread when body fluid infected with hepatitis B enters the body of a person who is not infected. Hepatitis B can lead to chronic hepatitis (liver inflammation), liver cancer, and death. The vaccines are approved for individuals of all ages, including newborns. It is particularly important for those at increased risk of exposure to hepatitis B virus, such as a baby born to mom who is infected with the virus, to be vaccinated.

- **Common side effects may include:** Soreness, redness, swelling at the injection site, irritability, fever, diarrhea, fatigue or weakness, loss of appetite, and headache.

- **Tell your healthcare provider beforehand if:** The child is moderately or severely ill, or has ever had a life-threatening allergic reaction to yeast or to a previous dose of the vaccine.

Human Papillomavirus Vaccine

Brand name: Gardasil 9®

- **What it is for:** Gardasil 9® is for use in females and males ages 9 through 45 years. It prevents cervical, vulvar, vaginal, and anal cancers caused by any of the following human papillomavirus (HPV) types 16, 18, 31, 33, 45, 52, and 58. Overall, Gardasil 9® has the potential to prevent approximately 90 percent of cervical, vulvar, vaginal, and anal cancers. Gardasil 9® is also approved for the prevention of genital warts caused by types 6 and 11 in both males and females.

- **Common side effects may include:** Headache, fever, nausea, dizziness, fainting, and pain, swelling, redness, itchiness or bruising at the injection site.

- **Tell your healthcare provider beforehand if:** The individual has had an allergic reaction to yeast or to a previous dose of the vaccine.

Influenza Vaccine (Administered with a Needle)

Brand names: Afluria®, Afluria Quadrivalent®, Fluarix Quadrivalent®, Flucelvax Quadrivalent®, FluLaval Quadrivalent®, and Fluzone Quadrivalent®

- **What it is for:** Different vaccines are approved for different age groups to prevent influenza disease, caused by the strains of influenza virus that are included in the vaccine. Influenza, commonly called "flu," is a contagious respiratory virus that can cause mild to severe illness. The elderly, young children, and people with certain health conditions (such as asthma, diabetes, or heart disease) are at high risk for serious influenza-related complications. Complications may include pneumonia, ear infections, sinus infections, dehydration, and worsening of certain medical conditions, such as congestive heart failure, asthma, or diabetes. The strains of influenza virus that cause disease in people frequently change, so yearly vaccination is needed to provide protection against the influenza viruses likely to cause illness each winter.

- **Common side effects may include:** Pain, redness and swelling at the injection site, low-grade fever, and muscle aches, headache, fatigue, and a general feeling of being unwell.

- **Tell your healthcare provider beforehand if:** The child is moderately or severely ill, has a weakened immune system, has asthma or recurrent wheezing, or has a history of GBS, a neurological disorder that causes severe muscle weakness. Also, tell your healthcare provider about any allergies, including severe allergies to eggs and any allergic reaction to a previous dose of any influenza vaccine. In addition, because of the association of Reye syndrome with aspirin and wild-type influenza infection, the healthcare provider should be made aware if the child is currently receiving aspirin or aspirin-containing therapy.

Influenza Vaccine, Intranasal (Nasal Spray)

Brand name: FluMist Quadrivalent®

- **What it is for:** Protects against four different strains of influenza virus included in the vaccine; for children and adults ages 2 through 49 years of age.

- **Common side effects may include:** Runny or stuffy nose and cough.

- **Tell your healthcare provider beforehand if:** The child is moderately or severely ill, has a weakened immune system, has asthma or recurrent wheezing, or has a history of GBS, a neurological disorder that causes severe muscle weakness. Also, tell your healthcare provider about any allergies, including severe allergies to eggs and any allergic reaction to a previous dose of any influenza vaccine. In addition, because of the association of Reye syndrome with aspirin and wild-type influenza infection, the healthcare provider should be made aware if the child is currently receiving aspirin or aspirin-containing therapy.

Measles, Mumps, and Rubella Vaccine

Brand name: M-M-R II®

- **What it is for:** Prevents measles, mumps, and rubella in those 12 months of age and older. Measles is a respiratory disease that causes a skin rash all over the body, and fever, cough, and runny nose. Measles can be severe, causing ear infections, pneumonia, seizures, and swelling of the brain. Mumps causes fever, headache, loss of appetite and the well-known sign of swollen cheeks and jaw which is from the swelling of the salivary glands. Rare complications include deafness, meningitis (infection of the lining that surrounds the brain and spinal cord), and painful swelling of the testicles or ovaries. Rubella, also called "German measles," causes fever, a rash, and—mainly in women—can also cause arthritis. Rubella infection during pregnancy can lead to birth defects.

- **Common side effects may include:** Fever, mild rash, fainting, headache, dizziness, irritability, and burning or stinging, redness, swelling, and tenderness at the injection site.

- **Tell your healthcare provider beforehand if:** The child is ill and has a fever or has ever had an allergic reaction to gelatin, the antibiotic neomycin, or a previous dose of the vaccine, has immune system problems, or cancer, or problems with the blood or lymph system.

Meningococcal Vaccine

There are two different types of meningococcal vaccines. One type protects against four groups of meningococcal bacteria called groups "A," "C," "W-135," and "Y." The FDA has approved two vaccines of this type. The other type protects against a meningococcal bacterium called "group B." The FDA has also approved two meningococcal group B vaccines, but they are only recommended for routine use in certain high-risk groups.

Brand names: Bexsero®, Menactra®, Menveo®, and Trumenba®

- **What it is for:** Prevents certain types of meningococcal disease, a life-threatening illness caused by the bacteria *Neisseria meningitidis (N. meningitidis)* that infects the bloodstream and the lining that surrounds the brain and spinal cord (meningitis). *Neisseria meningitidis* is a leading cause of meningitis in young children. Even with appropriate antibiotics and intensive care, between 10 and 15 percent of people who develop meningococcal disease die from the infection. Another 10 to 20 percent suffer complications, such as brain damage or loss of limb or hearing. Bexsero and Trumenba are approved for use in those 10 through 25 years of age to prevent invasive meningococcal disease caused by *N. meningitidis* serogroup B. Menactra® and Menveo® prevent meningococcal disease caused by *N. meningitidis* serogroups A, C, Y and W-135. Menactra® is approved for use in those 9 months through 55 years of age. Menveo® is approved for use in those 2 months through 55 years of age.

- **Common side effects may include:** Tenderness, pain, redness and swelling at the injection site, irritability, headache, fever, tiredness, chills, diarrhea, and loss of appetite for a short while.

- **Tell your healthcare provider beforehand if:** The child is moderately or severely ill, has had a severe allergic reaction to a previous dose of meningococcal vaccine, or has a known sensitivity to vaccine components.

Pneumococcal 13-Valent Conjugate Vaccine

Brand name: Prevnar 13®

- **What it is for:** Prevents invasive disease caused by 13 different types of the bacterium Streptococcus pneumoniae in infants, children and adolescents ages 6 weeks through 17 years. In infants and children 6 weeks through 5 years of age, it is also approved for the prevention of otitis media (ear infection) caused by 7 different types of the bacterium. *Streptococcus pneumoniae* can cause infections of the blood, middle ear, and the covering of the brain and spinal cord, as well as pneumonia. Prevnar 13 is also approved for adults 18 years of age and older.

- **Common side effects may include:** Pain, redness and swelling at the injection site, irritability, decreased appetite and fever.

- **Tell your healthcare provider beforehand if:** The child is moderately or severely ill, has ever had an allergic reaction to a previous dose or component of the vaccine, including diphtheria toxoid (for example, DTaP vaccine).

Poliovirus Vaccine

Brand name: Ipol®

- **What it is for:** Prevents polio in infants as young as six weeks of age. Polio is a disease that can cause paralysis or death.

- **Common side effects may include:** Redness, hardening, and pain at the injection site, fever, irritability, sleepiness, fussiness, and crying.

- **Tell your healthcare provider beforehand if:** The child is moderately or severely ill, including illness with a fever, has ever had a severe allergic reaction to a previous dose of the polio vaccine, any component of the vaccine, or an allergic reaction to the antibiotics neomycin, streptomycin, or polymyxin B.

Rotavirus Vaccine

Brand names: Rotarix® and RotaTeq®

- **What it is for:** Prevents gastroenteritis caused by rotavirus infection in infants as young as 6 weeks of age. Rotavirus disease is the leading cause of severe diarrhea and dehydration in infants worldwide. In the United States, the disease occurs more often during the winter. Before rotavirus vaccines were available, most children in the United States were infected with rotavirus before the age of 2. In addition, rotavirus resulted in about 55,000 to 70,000 hospitalizations and 20 to 60 infant deaths in the United States each year.

- **Common side effects may include:** Fussiness or irritability, cough or runny nose, fever, and loss of appetite.

- **Tell your healthcare provider beforehand if:** The child has illness with a fever, a weakened immune system because of a disease, has a blood disorder, any type of cancer, has gastrointestinal problems, has had stomach surgery or ever had intussusception, which is a form of blockage of the intestines, is allergic to any of the ingredients of the vaccine, or has ever had an allergic reaction to a previous dose of the vaccine, or has regular close contact with a member of a family or household who has a weak immune system.

Varicella Virus Vaccine

Brand name: Varivax®

- **What it is for:** Prevents Vaccine-Preventable Diseases (chickenpox) in children 12 months of age and older. Chickenpox usually causes a blister-like itchy rash, tiredness, headache, and fever. It can be serious, particularly in babies, adolescents, adults and people with weak immune systems, causing less common, but more serious complications, such as skin infection, scarring, pneumonia, brain swelling, Reye syndrome, (which affects the liver and brain), and death.

- **Common side effects may include:** Soreness, pain, redness or swelling at the injection site, fever, irritability, and chickenpox like rash on the body or at the site of the shot.

- **Tell your healthcare provider beforehand if:** The child is moderately or severely ill, including a fever, has a weak immune system, has received a blood or plasma transfusion or immune globulin within the last five months, takes any medicines, has allergies including any life-threatening allergic reaction to gelatin, the antibiotic neomycin, or a previous dose of chickenpox or any other vaccine.

Section 4.3

Your Child's Vaccine Visit

This section includes text excerpted from "Your Child's Vaccine Visit," Centers for Disease Control and Prevention (CDC), April 15, 2016. Reviewed September 2019.

There are things that parents can do before, during, and after vaccine visits to make them easier and less stressful.

Before the Visit

Arrive prepared! Take these steps before your child gets a shot to help make the immunization visit less stressful for you both.

- Read any vaccine materials you received from your child's healthcare professional and write down any questions you may have.

- You can request vaccine information statements (VIS) at the doctor's office.

- Find your child's personal immunization record and bring it to your appointment. An up-to-date record tells your doctor exactly what shots your child has already received.

- Pack a favorite toy or book or a blanket that your child uses regularly to comfort your child.

- A mild illness is usually not a reason to reschedule a vaccination visit.

For Older Children

- Be honest with your child. Explain that shots can pinch or sting, but that it will not hurt for long.

- Engage other family members, especially older siblings, to support your child.

- Avoid telling scary stories or making threats about shots.

- Remind children that vaccines can keep them healthy.

At the Doctor's Office

If you have questions about immunizations, ask your child's doctor or nurse. Your child's doctor will give you VIS for the shots that your child will be getting that day. VIS includes information about the risks and benefits of each vaccine. If your doctor does not give you one you can request one.

For Babies and Younger Children

Try these ideas for making the shots easier on your child.

- Distract and comfort your child by cuddling, singing, or talking softly.

- Smile and make eye contact with your child. Let your child know that everything is okay.

- Comfort your child with a favorite toy or book. A blanket that smells familiar will help your child feel more comfortable.

- Hold your child firmly on your lap, whenever possible.

Once your child has received all of the shots, be especially supportive. Hold, cuddle, and for infants, breastfeed or offer a bottle. A soothing voice combined with praise and hugs will help reassure the child that everything is okay.

For Older Children and Adolescents

- Take deep breaths with your child to help "blow out" the pain.

- Point out interesting things in the room to help create distractions.

- Tell or read stories.

- Support your child if she or he cries. Never scold a child for not "being brave."

Fainting (syncope) can be common among adolescents immediately after getting shots. To help prevent any injuries that could occur from a fall while fainting, your preteen or teen should stay seated for 15 minutes after the shot.

Before you leave the appointment, ask your child's doctor for advice on using nonaspirin pain reliever and other steps you can take at home to comfort your child.

After the Shots

Sometimes children experience mild reactions from vaccines, such as pain at the injection site, a rash or a fever. These reactions are normal and will soon go away. The following tips will help you identify and minimize mild side effects.

- Review any information your doctor gives you about the shots, especially the Vaccine Information Statements or other sheets that outline which side effects might be expected.

- Use a cool, wet cloth to reduce redness, soreness, and swelling in the place where the shot was given.

- Reduce any fever with a cool sponge bath. If your doctor approves, give nonaspirin pain reliever.

- Give your child lots of liquid. It is normal for some children to eat less during the 24 hours after getting vaccines.

- Pay extra attention to your child for a few days. If you see something that concerns you, call your doctor.

Finding and Paying for Vaccines

Most health-insurance plans cover the cost of vaccines, but you may want to check with your insurance provider before going to the doctor to see what is covered under your plan.

If you do not have health insurance, or your plan does not cover vaccines, the Vaccines for Children (VFC) program may be able to help. This program provides vaccines at no cost to over 42,000 healthcare professionals who serve eligible children. Children younger than 19 years of age are eligible for VFC vaccines if they are Medicaid-eligible, American Indian or Alaska Native, or have no health insurance.

Parents of uninsured children who receive vaccines at no cost through the VFC Program should check with their doctor about possible vaccine administration fees that might apply. The administration fees help providers cover the costs that result from important services, such as storing the vaccines and paying staff members to give vaccines to patients.

Section 4.4

Vaccine Records

This section includes text excerpted from "Finding and Updating Vaccine Records," Centers for Disease Control and Prevention (CDC), May 17, 2019.

It is extremely important for you to track your child's vaccination records, especially if your state requires certain vaccines for childcare or school.

Saving Your Child's Vaccination Records

Good record-keeping begins with good record-taking. Start tracking your child's vaccination records as soon as your child gets her or his first shot when she or he is born. You can keep track of your child's records by:

- Getting a vaccination tracking card from your child's doctor or your state health department.

- Asking your doctor to enter the vaccines your child has received in your state's immunization information system (IIS). An IIS is a statewide immunization registry doctors and public-health clinics use to save and update vaccination records.

When you maintain a copy of your child's vaccination record:

- Keep the record in a safe place where you can easily locate it.

- Bring it to each of your child's doctor visits.

- Ask the doctor or nurse to jot down the vaccine given, date, and dosage on your child's vaccination record.

- Write down the name of the doctor's office or clinic where your child got the shot so you know where to get official records when you need them.

It is important for you to save and update your child's vaccine records since you will likely be required to provide them when you register your child for school, childcare, summer camp, or an athletic team. You may also need up-to-date records when your child travels internationally.

Finding Official Vaccination Records

If you do not have a copy of your child's vaccine records or cannot find them, you may be able to retrieve an official copy by contacting your:

- Child's doctor or clinic:

  - Doctors and public-health clinics usually track any shots they give to your child.

  - If your child has had more than one doctor or clinic give her or him shots, call or visit each one to get the records.

- Keep in mind doctors and clinics may only save vaccination records for a few years.
- States' immunization registry:
  - Your state's immunization registry may have most, if not all, of your child's records.
  - Contact your state's registry to request an official copy.
  - Please be aware that the process for requesting records can vary greatly across states and can take some time to complete.
  - Additionally, if your state does not automatically opt-in its residents or you requested to opt-out your child from the registry, then the vaccination records will not be available.
- Child's school:
  - Most K–12 schools, colleges, and universities keep on file the vaccination records of its students.
  - Take into account that schools generally keep these records for only a year or two after the student graduates, transfers to another school, or leaves the school system.
- If you need records from a college or university, contact the corresponding medical services or student-health department.

What If You Cannot Find Your Child's Records

Your child should be considered susceptible to disease and should be vaccinated (or revaccinated) if you cannot find her or his records or their records are incomplete. It is safe for your child to receive a vaccine, even if she or he may have already received it. Alternatively, your child could also have their blood tested for antibodies to determine her or his immunity to certain diseases. However, these tests may not always be accurate and doctors may prefer to revaccinate your child for the best protection. Talk to your child's doctor to determine what vaccines your child needs for protection against vaccine-preventable diseases.

Section 4.5

Vaccination FAQs

This section includes text excerpted from "Vaccination FAQs,"
Centers for Disease Control and Prevention (CDC), May 14, 2019.

Vaccine Safety
Are Vaccines Safe?

Yes. Vaccines are very safe. The United States' long-standing vaccine safety system ensures that vaccines are as safe as possible. As of now, the United States has the safest vaccine supply in its history. Millions of children safely receive vaccines each year. The most common side effects are typically very mild, such as pain or swelling at the injection site.

What Are the Risks and Benefits of Vaccines?

Vaccines can prevent infectious diseases that once killed or harmed many infants, children, and adults. Without vaccines, your child is at risk for getting seriously ill and suffering pain, disability, and even death from diseases, such as measles and whooping cough. The main risks associated with getting vaccines are side effects, which are almost always mild (redness and swelling at the injection site) and go away within a few days. Serious side effects after vaccination, such as a severe allergic reaction, are very rare and doctors and clinic staff are trained to deal with them.

The disease-prevention benefits of getting vaccines are much greater than the possible side effects for almost all children. The only exceptions to this are cases in which a child has a serious chronic medical condition, such as cancer or a disease that weakens the immune system, or has had a severe allergic reaction to a previous vaccine dose.

Is There a Link between Vaccines and Autism?

No. Scientific studies and reviews continue to show no relationship between vaccines and autism. Some people have suggested that thimerosal (a compound that contains mercury) in vaccines given to infants and young children might be a cause of autism. Others have suggested that the measles-mumps-rubella (MMR) vaccine may be linked to autism. However, numerous scientists and researchers have studied and continue to study the MMR vaccine and thimerosal, and reach the same conclusion: there is no link between MMR vaccine or thimerosal and autism.

Side Effects
What Are the Side Effects of Vaccines?

Vaccines, like any medication, may cause some side effects. Most of these side effects are very minor, such as soreness where the shot was given, fussiness, or a low-grade fever. These side effects typically only last a couple of days and are treatable. For example, you can apply a cool, wet washcloth on the sore area to ease discomfort.

Serious reactions are very rare. However, if your child experiences any reactions that concern you, call the doctor's office.

Can Vaccines Overload My Baby's Immune System?

Vaccines do not overload the immune system. Every day, a healthy baby's immune system successfully fights off thousands of germs. Antigens are parts of germs that cause the body's immune system to go to work to build antibodies, which fight off diseases.

The antigens in vaccines come from the germs themselves, but the germs are weakened or killed so they cannot cause serious illness. Even if babies receive several vaccinations in one day, vaccines contain only a tiny fraction of the antigens they encounter every day in their environment. Vaccines give your child the antibodies they need to fight off serious vaccine-preventable diseases.

Why Do Vaccines Start so Early?

The recommended schedule protects infants and children by providing immunity early in life before they come into contact with life-threatening diseases. Children receive immunization early because they are susceptible to diseases at a young age. The consequences of these diseases can be very serious, and even life-threatening, for infants and young children.

Should My Child Get Shots If She or He Is Sick?

Talk with your child's doctor, but children can usually get vaccinated even if they have a mild illness, such as a cold, earache, mild fever, or diarrhea. If the doctor says it is okay, your child can still get vaccinated.

Should I Delay Some Vaccines or Follow a Nonstandard Schedule?

Children do not receive any known benefits from following schedules that delay vaccines. Infants and young children who follow immunization schedules that spread out or leave out shots are at risk of developing diseases during the time you delay their shots. Some vaccine-preventable diseases remain common in the United States and children may be exposed to these diseases during the time they are not protected by vaccines, placing them at risk for a serious case of the disease that might cause hospitalization or death.

Why Can I Not Delay Some Vaccines If I Am Planning for My Baby to Get Them All Eventually?

Young children have the highest risk of having a serious case of disease that could cause hospitalization or death. Delaying or spreading out vaccine doses leaves your child unprotected during the time when they need vaccine protection the most. For example, diseases such as Hib or pneumococcus almost always occur in the first two years of a baby's life. And some diseases, such as Hepatitis B and whooping cough (pertussis), are more serious when babies get them at a younger age. Vaccinating your child according to the Centers for Disease Control and Prevention (CDC)'s recommended immunization schedule means you can help protect him at a young age.

If I Am Breastfeeding, Do I Vaccinate My Baby on Schedule?

Yes, even breastfed babies need to be protected with vaccines at the recommended ages. The immune system is not fully developed at birth, which puts newborns at greater risk for infections.

Breast milk provides important protection from some infections as your baby's immune system is developing. For example, babies who are breastfed have a lower risk of ear infections, respiratory tract infections, and diarrhea. However, breast milk does not protect children against all diseases. Even in breastfed infants, vaccines are the most effective way to prevent many diseases. Your baby needs the long-term protection that can only come from making sure he receives all his vaccines according to the CDC's recommended schedule.

Can I Wait to Vaccinate My Baby Who Is Not in Childcare?

No, even young children who are cared for at home can be exposed to vaccine-preventable diseases, so it is important for them to get all their vaccines at the recommended ages. Children can catch these illnesses from any number of people or places, including from parents, brothers or sisters, visitors to their home, on playgrounds or even at the grocery store. Regardless of whether or not your baby is cared for outside the home, she comes in contact with people throughout the day, some of whom may be sick but not know it yet.

If someone has a vaccine-preventable disease, they may not have symptoms or the symptoms may be mild, and they can end up spreading disease to babies or young children. Remember, many of these diseases can be especially dangerous to young children so it is safest to vaccinate your child at the recommended ages to protect her, whether or not she is in childcare.

Can I Wait until My Child Goes to School to Catch up on Immunizations?

Before entering school, young children can be exposed to vaccine-preventable diseases from parents and other adults, brothers, and sisters, on a plane, at childcare, or even at the grocery store. Children under age five are especially susceptible to diseases because their immune systems have not built up the necessary defenses to fight infection. Do not wait to protect your baby and risk getting these diseases when she or he needs protection now.

Why Do Adolescents Need Vaccines?

Vaccines are recommended throughout our lives to protect against serious diseases. As protection from childhood vaccines wears off, adolescents need vaccines that will extend protection. Adolescents need protection from additional infections as well, before the risk of exposure increases.

Vaccine Types, Doses, and Ingredients
Why Are There So Many Doses Needed for Each Vaccine?

Getting every recommended dose of each vaccine provides your child with the best protection possible. Depending on the vaccine, your child will need more than one dose to build high enough immunity to prevent disease or to boost immunity that fades over time. Your child may also receive more than one dose to make sure they are protected if they did not get immunity from a first dose, or to protect them against germs that change over time, such as flu. Every dose is important because each protects against infectious diseases that can be especially serious for infants and very young children.

What Are Combination Vaccines and Why Are They Used?

Combination vaccines protect your child against more than one disease with a single shot. They reduce the number of shots and office visits your child would need, which not only saves you time and money but also is easier on your child. Some common combination vaccines are Pediarix® which combines DTap, Hep B, and IPV (polio) and Pro-Quad® which combines MMR and varicella (chickenpox).

What Are the Ingredients in Vaccines and What Do They Do?

Vaccines contain ingredients that cause the body to develop immunity. Vaccines also contain very small amounts of other ingredients. All ingredients play necessary roles either in making the vaccine or in ensuring that the final product is safe and effective.

Protection from Diseases
Is the Natural Immunity of Infants Better Than the Kind from Vaccines?

Babies may get some temporary immunity (protection) from mom during the last few weeks of pregnancy, but only for diseases to which mom is immune. Breastfeeding may also protect your baby temporarily from minor infections, such as colds. These antibodies do not last long, leaving your baby vulnerable to disease.

Do We Still Have These Diseases in the United States?

Some vaccine-preventable diseases such as pertussis (whooping cough) and chickenpox, remain common in the United States. On the other hand, other diseases vaccines prevent are no longer common in this country because of vaccines. However, if we stopped vaccinating, the few cases we have in the United States could very quickly become tens or hundreds of thousands of cases. Even though many serious vaccine-preventable diseases are uncommon in the United States, some are common in other parts of the world. Even if your family does not travel internationally, you could come into contact with international travelers anywhere in your community. Children who do not receive all vaccinations and are exposed to a disease can become seriously sick and spread it through a community.

Why Does My Child Need a Chickenpox Shot? Is It Not a Mild Disease?

Your child needs a chickenpox vaccine because chickenpox can actually be a serious disease. In many cases, children experience a mild case of chickenpox, but other children may have blisters that become infected. Others may develop pneumonia. There is no way to tell in advance how severe your child's symptoms will be.

Before vaccines were available, about 50 children died every year from chickenpox, and about 1 in 500 children who got chickenpox was hospitalized.

Natural immunity occurs when your child is exposed to a disease and becomes infected. It is true that natural immunity usually results in better immunity than vaccination, but the risks are much greater. A natural chickenpox infection may result in pneumonia, whereas the vaccine might only cause a sore arm for a couple of days.

I Got the Whooping Cough and Other Recommended Vaccines While Pregnant. Why Does My Baby Need These Too?

The protection (antibodies) you passed to your baby before birth will give her or him some early protection against whooping cough and flu. However, these antibodies will only give her or him short-term protection. It is very important for your baby to get vaccines on time so she or he can start building her or his own protection against these serious diseases.

Chapter 5

Promoting Wellness

Chapter Contents

Section 5.1

Promoting Healthy Habits

This section includes text excerpted from "Helping Your Child: Tips for Parents," National Institute of Diabetes and Digestive and Kidney Diseases (NIDDK), January 2012. Reviewed September 2019.

How Can You Help Your Child Form Healthy Habits?

Parents play a big part in shaping children's habits on eating and physical activity. When parents eat foods that are lower in fat and added sugars and high in fiber, children learn to like these foods as well. If your child does not like a new food right away, do not be upset. Children often need to see a new food many times before they will try it. Parents have an effect on children's physical activity habits as well.

Be a Role Model

A powerful example for your child is to be active yourself. You can set a good example by going for a walk or bike ride instead of watching television (TV), playing a video game, or surfing the Internet. Playing ball or jumping rope with your children shows them that being active is fun.

Talk about Being Healthy

Take the time to talk to your children about how a certain food or physical activity may help them. For example, when going for your daily walk, bring your children with you and let them pick the route. Discuss how walking helps you feel better and is a fun way to spend time together. It also offsets calories eaten and inactive time spent in front of TV screens or computers. Use your children's food choices as teaching moments. Speak up when you see unhealthy eating habits. Direct children to healthier options or say, "You can have a little of that, but not too much." Talk to them about why an overly salty or heavily sugared snack is not the best choice. You can also praise your children when they choose a healthy item, such as fruit or yogurt. Use comments like these:

- "Great choice!"

- "You are giving your body what it needs with that snack!"

- "I like those too."

With physical activity, try upbeat phrases, such as these to keep your child excited:

- "You run so fast, I can hardly keep up!"
- "You are building a strong, healthy heart!"
- "Let's walk 10 more minutes to make ourselves stronger."

Believe in the Power to Change

Know that eating healthy and moving more are the basics of being fit. Work together as a family to form healthy habits.

Promote Good Health beyond Your Family

Other adults may play a role in your child's life, too. You can share ideas about healthy habits with them. For instance, many parents work outside the home and need other adults to help with child care. Caregivers like other family members, daycare providers, babysitters, or friends may shape your child's eating and activity habits. Talk to your child's caregivers to make sure they offer healthy snacks and meals. Check that caregivers are also providing plenty of active playtime and limiting time with TV or inactive video games.

If your child is in school, you can help promote healthy eating and physical activity in several other ways:

- Find out more about the school's breakfast and lunch programs. Ask for input on menu choices.

- Support physical education and after-school sports at your child's school.

- Take turns with other parents watching your children play outside.

Consider Other Influences

Your children's friends and the media can also affect eating and activity choices. Children may choose to go to fast-food places or play video games with their friends instead of playing tag or other active games. TV ads try to persuade children to eat high-fat foods and sugary drinks. You can teach your children to be aware of these pressures. To do so, speak with your children about choices while you watch TV and surf the Internet with them. Talk about how media outlets sell products or values through famous football or basketball players, cartoon figures, and made-up images. Use programs and ads to spark chats about your values. These talks may help your child make healthy choices outside the home.

Section 5.2

Nutrition for Children

This section includes text excerpted from "Helping Your Child: Tips for Parents," National Institute of Diabetes and Digestive and Kidney Diseases (NIDDK), January 2012. Reviewed September 2019.

What Should Your Child Eat?

Just like adults, children need to eat a wide variety of foods. Every five years, the U.S. government releases a set of guidelines on healthy eating. The guidelines suggest balancing calories with physical activity. The guidelines also recommend improving eating habits to promote health, reduce the risk of disease, and reduce overweight and obesity. The guidelines encourage Americans ages two years and older to eat a variety of healthy foods. Suggested items include the following:

- Fruits, vegetables, unsalted nuts and seeds, and whole grains

- Fat-free or low-fat milk and milk products

- Lean meats, poultry, seafood, beans and peas, soy products, and eggs

The guidelines also suggest reducing salt (sodium), refined grains, added sugars, and solid fats (such as lard, butter, and margarine). Added sugars and solid fats often occur in pizzas, sodas, sugar-sweetened drinks, desserts, such as cookies or cake, and fast foods. These foods are the main sources of high fat and sugar among children and teens. Another important guideline is to make sure your children eat breakfast to spark the energy they need to focus in school. Not eating breakfast is often linked to overweight and obesity, especially in children and teens.

How Can You Help Your Child Eat More Healthily?

Some tips to consider are these:

Use Less Fat, Salt, and Sugar

- Cook with fewer solid fats. Use olive or canola oil instead of butter or margarine. Bake or roast instead of frying. You can get a crunchy texture with "oven-frying" recipes that involve little or no oil.

- Choose and prepare foods with less salt. Keep the salt shaker off the table. Have fruits and vegetables on hand for snacks instead of salty snacks, such as chips.

- Limit the amount of sugar your child eats. Choose cereals with low sugar or with dried fruits as the source of sugar.

- Reshape the plate.
  - Make half of what is on your child's plate fruits and vegetables.
  - Avoid over-sized portions.

Four for Fitness

Experts note that most Americans do not get enough potassium, calcium, vitamin D, and dietary fiber. Calcium builds strong bones and teeth. Potassium helps lower blood pressure and reduces bone loss. Vitamin D supports bone health. Dietary fiber promotes normal digestion and may help reduce the risk of heart disease, obesity, and type 2 diabetes.

Here are some ways you can boost your children's intake of these nutrients.

- **Dish up more fruit for breakfast, snacks, and desserts.** Add dark green, red, and orange vegetables to stews and soups. Add beans (black, kidney, pinto), peas, and lentils to casseroles and salads.

- **Serve more low-fat milk and milk products.** If your child cannot digest much lactose, serve lactose-free products or fat-free milk and yogurt. (Lactose is the sugar in milk that may cause some people stomach pain and bloating when they drink milk or eat milk products.) Your child can also try soy or rice drinks enriched with calcium or vitamin D.

- **Stay active during daylight hours.** Be active with your child outside in the sunlight to improve vitamin D levels naturally.

- **Include fish.** Serve fresh, frozen, or canned salmon, shrimp, and light tuna (not albacore). For young children, you may serve fish in small portions totaling up to 12 ounces each week.

- **Intake dietary fiber.** Replace at least half of the refined grains (breads, pasta, and rice) your child eats with whole-grain foods. Eat more bran. Check "Nutrition Facts" labels to find products high in dietary fiber. Look at the ingredients list to be sure that whole grains are one of the first items.

Think about the Drink

- Serve water or low-fat or fat-free milk more often as the drink of the first choice.

- Reduce the amount of sugar-sweetened sodas and fruit-flavored drinks that your child drinks.

- Offer fresh fruit, which has more fiber than juice, more often than 100 percent fruit juice.

Offer Healthy Snacks

- Try to keep healthy food in the house for snacks and meals for the whole family.

- Offer such snacks as sliced apples, oranges, pears, and celery sticks. Or try whole-grain bread served with low-fat cheese, peanut butter, or soy-nut butter.

- Give your children a healthy snack or two in addition to their three daily meals to keep them energized.

- Read nutrition labels. Some foods, such as snack bars, are not as healthy as they seem.

Limit Fast Food

- Order a side fruit bowl or salad instead of fries.

- Ask for sandwiches to be prepared without sauce.

- Order "small." Avoid super-sizing.

Share Food Time as Family Time

- Eat sit-down, family meals together and serve everyone the same thing.

- Involve your children in planning and preparing meals. Children may be more willing to eat the dishes they help prepare.

- Try to limit how much you eat out to control the calories, salt, and fat your children eat. To serve more homemade meals, cook large batches of soup, stew, or casseroles and freeze them as a time saver.

- Limit eating at home to specific areas, such as the kitchen or dining room.

Section 5.3

Physical Fitness and Health

This section includes text excerpted from "Physical Activity Facts," Centers for Disease Control and Prevention (CDC), April 9, 2018.

Physical Activity Behaviors of Young People

- Less than one-quarter (24%) of children 6 to 17 years of age participate in 60 minutes of physical activity every day.

- In 2017, only 26.1 percent of high-school students participated in at least 60 minutes per day of physical activity on all 7 days of the previous week.

- In 2017, 51.1 percent of high-school students participated in muscle-strengthening exercises (e.g., push-ups, sit-ups, weight lifting) on 3 or more days during the previous week.

- In 2017, 51.7 percent of high-school students attended physical-education classes in an average week, and only 29.9

percent of high-school students attended physical-education classes daily.

Consequences of Physical Inactivity

Physical inactivity can:

- Lead to energy imbalance (e.g., expend less energy through physical activity than consumed through diet) and can increase the risk of becoming overweight or obese

- Increase the risk of factors for cardiovascular disease, including hyperlipidemia (e.g., high cholesterol and triglyceride levels), high blood pressure, obesity, and insulin resistance and glucose intolerance

- Increase the risk for developing type 2 diabetes

- Increase the risk of developing breast, colon, endometrial, and lung cancers

- Lead to low-bone density, which in turn, leads to osteoporosis

The *Physical Activity Guidelines for Americans*, second edition, recommend that children and adolescents 6 to 17 years of age do 60 minutes or more of moderate-to-vigorous physical activity daily.

Recommendations for Physical Activity

- **Aerobic.** Most of the 60 minutes or more per day should be either moderate- or vigorous-intensity aerobic physical activity and should include vigorous-intensity physical activity on at least 3 days a week.

- **Muscle-strengthening.** As part of their 60 minutes or more of daily physical activity, children and adolescents should include muscle-strengthening physical activity on at least 3 days a week.

- **Bone-strengthening.** As part of their 60 minutes or more of daily physical activity, children and adolescents should include bone-strengthening physical activity on at least 3 days a week.

These guidelines state that children and adolescents be provided opportunities and encouragement to participate in physical activities that are appropriate for their age, that is enjoyable and that offer variety.

The national recommendation for schools is to have a comprehensive approach for addressing physical education and physical activity in schools. This approach is called "Comprehensive School Physical Activity Programs (CSPAP)."

Benefits of Physical Activity

Regular physical activity can help children and adolescents improve cardio-respiratory fitness, build strong bones and muscles, control weight, reduce symptoms of anxiety and depression, and reduce the risk of developing health conditions, such as:

- Heart disease
- Cancer
- Type 2 diabetes
- High blood pressure
- Osteoporosis
- Obesity

Physical Activity and Academic Achievement

- Students who are physically active tend to have better grades, school attendance, cognitive performance (e.g., memory), and classroom behaviors (e.g., on-task behavior).
- Higher physical activity and physical fitness levels are associated with improved cognitive performance (e.g., concentration, memory) among students.

Section 5.4

Obesity in Children

This section contains text excerpted from the following sources:
Text in this section begins with excerpts from "Obesity in Children,"
MedlinePlus, National Institutes of Health (NIH), November 29,
2016. Reviewed September 2019; Text under the heading "Childhood
Obesity Facts" is excerpted from "Childhood Obesity Facts," Centers
for Disease Control and Prevention (CDC), April 29, 2019; Text under
the heading "Helping Your Child Who Is Overweight" is excerpted
from "Helping Your Child Who Is Overweight," National Institute of
Diabetes and Digestive and Kidney Diseases (NIDDK), September
2016. Reviewed September 2019.

"Obesity" means having too much body fat. It is different from being
"overweight," which means weighing too much. Both terms mean that
a person's weight is greater than what is considered healthy for her or
his height. Children grow at different rates, so it is not always easy to
know when a child has obesity or is overweight. Ask your healthcare
provider to check whether your child's weight and height are in a
healthy range.

Childhood Obesity Facts

In the United States, the percentage of children and adolescents
affected by obesity has more than tripled since the 1970s. Data from
2015 to 2016 show that nearly 1 in 5 school-age children and young
people (6 to 19 years) in the United States have obesity.

Many factors contribute to childhood obesity, including:

- Genetics
- Metabolism—how your body changes food and oxygen into
  energy it can use
- Eating and physical activity behaviors.
- Community and neighborhood design and safety
- Short sleep duration
- Negative childhood events

Genetic factors are difficult to change. However, people and places
can play a role in helping children achieve and maintain a healthy
weight. Changes in the environments where young people spend their

time—such as homes, schools, and community settings—can make it easier for youth to access nutritious foods and be physically active. Schools can adopt policies and practices that help young people eat more fruits and vegetables, eat fewer foods and beverages that are high in added sugars or solid fats, and increase daily minutes of physical activity. These kinds of school-based and after-school programs and policies can be cost-effective and even cost-saving.

Helping Your Child Who Is Overweight
How Can I Tell If My Child Is Overweight?

Being able to tell whether a child is overweight is not always easy. Children grow at different rates and at different times. Also, the amount of a child's body fat changes with age and differs between girls and boys.

One way to tell if your child is overweight is to calculate her or his body mass index (BMI). BMI is a measure of body weight relative to height. The BMI calculator uses a formula that produces a score often used to tell whether a person is underweight, a normal weight, overweight, or obese. The BMI of children is age- and sex-specific and known as the "BMI-for-age."

Body mass index-for-age uses growth charts created by the Centers for Disease Control and Prevention (CDC). Doctors use these charts to track a child's growth. The charts use a number called a "percentile" to show how your child's BMI compares with the BMI of other children.

The main BMI categories for children and teens are:

- **Healthy weight:** 5th to 84th percentile

- **Overweight:** 85th to 94th percentile

- **Obese:** 95th percentile or higher

Why Should I Be Concerned If My Child Is Overweight?

You should be concerned if your child has extra weight because weighing too much may increase the chances that your child will develop health problems now or later in life.

In the short run, for example, she or he may have breathing problems or joint pain, making it hard to keep up with friends. Some children may develop health problems, such as type 2 diabetes, high blood pressure, and high cholesterol. Some children also may experience teasing, bullying, depression, or low self-esteem.

Children who are overweight are at higher risk of entering adulthood with too much weight. The chances of developing health problems such as heart disease and certain types of cancer are higher among adults with too much weight.

Body mass index is a screening tool and does not directly measure body fat or an individual child's risk of health problems. If you are concerned about your child's weight, talk with your child's doctor or other healthcare professional. She or he can check your child's overall health and growth over time and tell you if weight management may be helpful. Many children who are still growing in length do not need to lose weight; they may need to decrease the amount of weight they gain while they grow taller. Do not put your child on a weight-loss diet unless your child's doctor tells you to.

How Can I Help My Child Be More Active?

Try to make physical activity fun for your child. Children need about 60 minutes of physical activity a day, although the activity does not have to be all at once. Several short 10- or even 5-minute spurts of activity throughout the day are just as good. If your child is not used to being active, encourage her or him to start out slowly and buildup to 60 minutes a day.

To encourage daily physical activity:

- Let your child choose a favorite activity to do regularly, such as climbing a jungle gym at the playground or joining a sports team or dance class

- Help your child find simple, fun activities to do at home or on her or his own, such as playing tag, jumping rope, playing catch, shooting baskets, or riding a bike (wear a helmet)

- Limit time with the computer, television, cell phone, and other devices to two hours a day

- Let your child and other family members plan active outings, such as a walk or hike to a favorite spot

Where Can I Go for Help?

If you have tried to change your family's eating, drinking, physical activity, and sleep habits and your child has not reached a healthy weight, ask your child's healthcare professional about other options. She or he may be able to recommend a plan for healthy eating and physical activity or refer you to a weight-management specialist, registered dietitian, or program. Your local hospital, a community-health clinic, or health department also may offer weight-management programs for children and teens or information about where you can enroll in one.

What Should I Look for in a Weight-Management Program?

When choosing a weight-management program for your child, look for a program that:

- Includes a variety of healthcare providers on staff, such as doctors, psychologists, and registered dietitians
- Evaluates your child's weight, growth, and health before enrollment and throughout the program
- Adapts to your child's specific age and abilities. Programs for elementary school-aged children should be different from those for teens.
- Helps your family keep healthy eating, drinking, and physical-activity habits after the program ends

How Else Can I Help My Child?

You can help your child by being positive and supportive throughout any process or program you choose to help her or him achieve a healthy weight. Help your child set specific goals and track progress. Reward successes with praise and hugs.

Tell your child that she or he is loved, special, and important. Children's feelings about themselves are often based on how they think their parents and other caregivers feel about them.

Listen to your child's concerns about her or his weight. She or he needs support, understanding, and encouragement from caring adults.

Section 5.5

Healthy Sleep Habits

This section includes text excerpted from "Sleep and Health," Centers for Disease Control and Prevention (CDC), September 18, 2018.

Adequate sleep contributes to a student's overall health and well-being. Students should get the proper amount of sleep at night to help stay focused, improve concentration, and improve academic performance.

Children and adolescents who do not get enough sleep have a higher risk for many health problems, including obesity, diabetes, poor mental health, and injuries. They are also more likely to have attention and behavior problems, which can contribute to poor academic performance in school.

How Much Sleep Do Students Need?

How much sleep someone needs depends on their age. The American Academy of Sleep Medicine (AASM) has made the following recommendations for children and adolescents:

Table 5.1. Recommended Sleep for Students

Age Group	Recommended Hours of Sleep per Day
6 to 12 years	9 to 12 hours per 24 hours
13 to 18 years	8 to 10 hours per 24 hours

Insufficient Sleep among Students

The data from the 2015 national and state Youth Risk Behavior Surveys (YRBS), a Centers for Disease Control and Prevention (CDC) study, shows that a majority of middle-school and high-school students reported getting less than the recommended amount of sleep for their age.

Middle-School Students (Grades 6 to 8)

- Students in 9 states were included in the study.

- About 6 out of 10 students (57.8%) did not get enough sleep on school nights.

High-School Students (Grades 9 to 12)

- National sample.

- About 7 out of 10 students (72.7%) did not get enough sleep on school nights.

What Parents Can Do

- **Model and encourage habits that help promote good sleep.** Setting a regular bedtime and rise time, including on weekends, is recommended for everyone—children, adolescents, and adults alike. Adolescents with parent-set bedtimes usually get more sleep than those whose parents do not set bedtimes.

- **Dim lighting.** Adolescents who are exposed to more light (such as room lighting or from electronics) in the evening are less likely to get enough sleep.

- **Implement a media curfew.** Technology use (computers, video gaming, or mobile phones) may also contribute to late bedtimes. Parents should consider banning technology use after a certain time or removing these technologies from the bedroom.

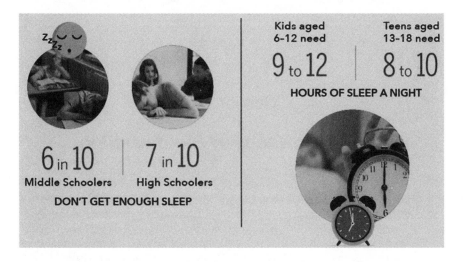

Figure 5.1. *Sleep Recommendations for Children* (Source: "Do Your Children Get Enough Sleep?" Centers for Disease Control and Prevention (CDC).)

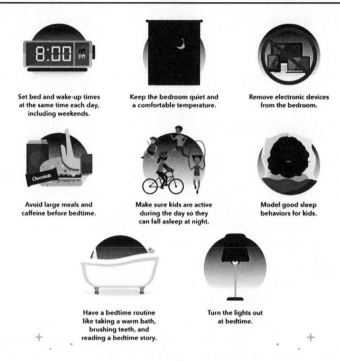

Figure 5.2. *Tips for Good Sleep* (Source: "Do Your Children Get Enough Sleep?" Centers for Disease Control and Prevention (CDC).)

Section 5.6

The Importance of Handwashing

This section contains text excerpted from the following sources: Text in this section begins with excerpts from "Handwashing: A Family Activity," Centers for Disease Control and Prevention (CDC), July 25, 2016. Reviewed September 2019; Text beginning with the heading "When Should You Wash Your Hands?" is excerpted from "When and How to Wash Your Hands," Centers for Disease Control and Prevention (CDC), March 7, 2016. Reviewed September 2019.

For kids, washing hands can be a fun and entertaining activity. It is simple enough for even very young children to understand.

Handwashing gives children and adults a chance to take an active role in their own health. Once kids learn how to properly wash their hands, they can—and often do—show their parents and siblings and encourage them to wash hands, too.

Parents can help keep their families healthy by:

- Teaching them good hand-washing technique
- Reminding their kids to wash their hands
- Washing their own hands with their kids

Improving Health

Hand-washing education in the community:

- Reduces the number of people who get sick with diarrhea by 31 percent
- Reduces diarrheal illness in people with weakened immune systems by 58 percent
- Reduces respiratory illnesses, such as colds, in the general population by 21 percent

Saving Time and Money

Handwashing is one of the best ways to avoid getting sick and spreading illness to others.

- Reduces illness increases productivity due to:
- Less time spent at the doctor's office
- More time spent at work or school

Helping Families Thrive

Children who have been taught handwashing at school bring that knowledge home to parents and siblings. This can help family members get sick less often and miss less work and school.

Despite widespread knowledge of the importance of handwashing, there is still room for improvement. A study showed that only 31 percent of men and 65 percent of women washed their hands after using a public restroom.

When Should You Wash Your Hands?

- Before, during, and after preparing food

- Before eating food

- Before and after caring for someone who is sick

- Before and after treating a cut or wound

- After using the toilet

- After changing diapers or cleaning up a child who has used the toilet

- After blowing your nose, coughing, or sneezing

- After touching an animal, animal feed, or animal waste

- After handling pet food or pet treats

- After touching garbage

How Should You Wash Your Hands?

- **Wet** your hands with clean, running water (warm or cold), turn off the tap, and apply soap.

- **Lather** your hands by rubbing them together with the soap. Be sure to lather the backs of your hands, between your fingers, and under your nails.

- **Scrub** your hands for at least 20 seconds. Need a timer? Hum the "Happy Birthday" song from beginning to end twice.

- **Rinse** your hands well under clean, running water.

- **Dry** your hands using a clean towel or air dry them.

What Should You Do If You Do Not Have Soap and Clean, Running Water?

Washing hands with soap and water is the best way to reduce the number of germs on them in most situations. If soap and water are not available, use an alcohol-based hand sanitizer that contains at least 60 percent alcohol. Alcohol-based hand sanitizers can quickly reduce the number of germs on hands in some situations, but sanitizers do not eliminate all types of germs and might not remove harmful chemicals.

Hand sanitizers are not as effective when hands are visibly dirty or greasy.

How Do You Use Hand Sanitizers?

- Apply the product to the palm of one hand (read the label to learn the correct amount).
- Rub your hands together.
- Rub the product over all surfaces of your hands and fingers until your hands are dry.

Caution! Swallowing alcohol-based hand sanitizers can cause alcohol poisoning. Keep it out of reach of young children.

Section 5.7

The Effects of Secondhand Smoke on Children

This section includes text excerpted from "How We Can Protect Our Children from Secondhand Smoke: A Parent's Guide," Centers for Disease Control and Prevention (CDC), January 14, 2019.

Secondhand smoke comes from lit cigarettes and cigars. It also comes from smoke breathed out by smokers. When children breathe secondhand smoke, it is like they are smoking, too. Secondhand smoke is made of thousands of chemicals. Many are poisons that stay in your body.

Secondhand Smoke Threatens Children

Scientists reporting to the U.S. Surgeon General found that secondhand smoke harms everyone, especially children. They also learned that:

- An estimated 58 million nonsmoking Americans, including 14 million children aged 3 to 11 years, are exposed to secondhand smoke.

- They breathe it at home, daycare, and in cars.

- Children are almost twice as likely as nonsmoking adults to be exposed to secondhand smoke.

Here are just a few of the chemicals and poisons in tobacco smoke.

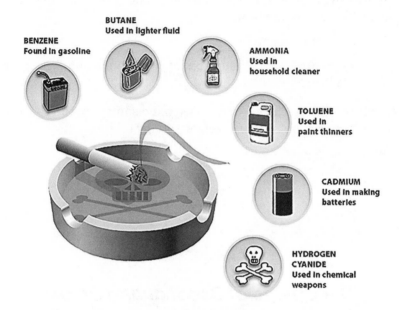

Figure 5.3. *Secondhand Smoke Exposure-Sources*

14 million children aged 3 to 11 years are exposed to secondhand smoke.

How Does Secondhand Smoke Hurt Your Children?

Tobacco smoke harms babies, even before they are born. It harms children, too, because their lungs and bodies are still growing.

- Babies who breathe secondhand smoke are more likely to die unexpectedly from sudden infant death syndrome (SIDS), also called "crib death."

- Babies and children who breathe secondhand smoke are sick more often with bronchitis, pneumonia, and ear infections.

- For children with asthma, breathing secondhand smoke can trigger an attack. The attack can be severe enough to send a child to the hospital. Sometimes an asthma attack is so severe that a child dies.

No One Can Hide from Secondhand Smoke at Home

Smoking in another room (for eg., a bathroom or bedroom) pollutes all the air in your home. In an apartment, smoke in one room can go through the whole building.

- Smoking outside in a hall or stairwell does not protect children inside. Smoke goes under doors, windows, and through cracks.

- To protect the children inside, homes and apartment buildings must be smoke-free.

No Amount of Secondhand Smoke Is Safe

- Even when you cannot smell it, cigarette smoke can still harm your child.

- Opening a window or using a fan does not protect children.

- Air purifiers and air fresheners do not remove smoke's poisons.

- Smoke from one cigarette can stay in a room for hours. Do not smoke at home, even when children are not there.

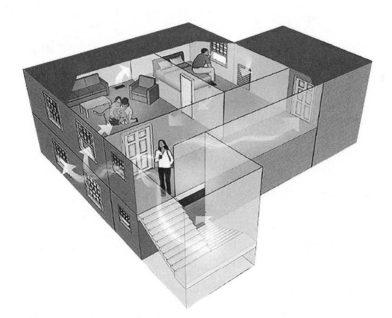

Figure 5.4. *How Secondhand Smoke Spreads in a House*

Children Must Be Protected from Secondhand Smoke Everywhere

At Home

If you take care of children in your home, do not allow anyone to smoke there. Do not let babysitters or family and friends smoke around your children.

In Day Care

Make sure smoking is not allowed in your child's daycare.

At School

Make sure your child's school is smoke-free inside and out. All school events should be "No Smoking."

In Public

Choose restaurants and businesses that are smoke-free. "No Smoking" sections in restaurants do not protect children from secondhand smoke.

In Your Car

Do not allow anyone to smoke if children are riding in your car. Rolling down a window does not protect them.

Take Simple Steps to Protect Your Children from Secondhand Smoke

Children respect and learn from your actions and words. As caregivers, you teach your children by the choices you make.

- Ask people not to smoke around your children.

- Support family and friends who also want to stop smoking.

- Decide to have a smoke-free home and car, and ask family and friends to respect your decision.

- Get rid of all the ashtrays in your home.

- Teach your children to stay away from secondhand smoke. Encourage your teens not to smoke.

- Make the decision to quit smoking. Get help from your doctor, family, and friends. Call this free quitline: 800-784-8669.

Section 5.8

Protecting Children from the Sun

This section includes text excerpted from "How Can I Protect My Children from the Sun?" Centers for Disease Control and Prevention (CDC), June 24, 2019.

Just a few serious sunburns can increase your child's risk of skin cancer later in life. Kids do not have to be at the pool, beach, or on vacation to get too much sun. Their skin needs protection from the sun's harmful ultraviolet (UV) rays whenever they are outdoors.

- **Seek shade.** UV rays are strongest and most harmful during midday, so it is best to plan indoor activities then. If this is not possible, seek shade under a tree, an umbrella, or a pop-up tent. Use these options to prevent sunburn, not to seek relief after it has happened.

- **Cover up.** When possible, long-sleeved shirts and long pants and skirts can provide protection from UV rays. Clothes made from tightly woven fabric offer the best protection. A wet T-shirt offers much less UV protection than a dry one, and darker colors may offer more protection than lighter colors. Some clothing certified under international standards comes with information on its ultraviolet protection factor.

- **Get a hat.** Hats that shade the face, scalp, ears, and neck are easy to use and give great protection. Baseball caps are popular among kids, but they do not protect their ears and neck. If your child chooses a cap, be sure to protect exposed areas with sunscreen.

- **Wear sunglasses.** They protect your child's eyes from UV rays, which can lead to cataracts later in life. Look for sunglasses that wrap around and block as close to 100 percent of both UVA and UVB rays as possible.

- **Apply sunscreen.** Use sunscreen with at least SPF 15 and UVA and UVB (broad spectrum) protection every time your child goes outside. For the best protection, apply sunscreen generously 30 minutes before going outdoors. Do not forget to protect ears, noses, lips, and the tops of feet. Reapply every 2 hours and after swimming, sweating, or toweling off.

Take sunscreen with you to reapply during the day, especially after your child swims or exercises. This applies to waterproof and water-resistant products as well.

Follow the directions on the package for using a sunscreen product on babies less than six months old. All products do not have the same ingredients; if you or your child's skin reacts badly to one product, try another one or call a doctor. Your baby's best defense against sunburn is avoiding the sun or staying in the shade.

Keep in mind, sunscreen is not meant to allow kids to spend more time in the sun than they would otherwise. Try combining sunscreen with other options to prevent UV damage.

Too Much Sun Hurts

- **Turning pink?** Unprotected skin can be damaged by the sun's UV rays in as little as 15 minutes. Yet it can take up to 12 hours for skin to show the full effect of sun exposure. So, if your child's skin looks "a little pink" today, it may be burned tomorrow morning. To prevent further burning, get your child out of the sun.

- **Tan?** There is no other way to say it—tanning your skin is damaging your skin. Any change in the color of your child's skin after time outside—whether sunburn or suntan—indicates damage from UV rays.

- **Cool and cloudy?** Children still need protection. UV rays, not the temperature, do the damage. Clouds do not block UV rays; they filter them—and sometimes only slightly.

- **Oops!** Kids often get sunburned when they are outdoors unprotected for longer than expected. Remember to plan ahead, and keep sun protection handy—in your car, bag, or child's backpack.

Chapter 6

Preventing Childhood Injuries

Chapter Contents

Section 6.1

Preventing Burns

This section includes text excerpted from "Burn Prevention," Centers
for Disease Control and Prevention (CDC), February 6, 2019.

We all want to keep our children safe and secure and help them
live to their full potential. Knowing how to prevent leading causes of
child injury, such as burns, is a step toward this goal.

Every day, over 300 children ages 0 to 19 are treated in emergency
rooms for burn-related injuries and 2 children die as a result of being
burned.

Younger children are more likely to sustain injuries from scald
burns that are caused by hot liquids or steam, while older children
are more likely to sustain injuries from flame burns that are caused
by direct contact with fire.

Thankfully, there are ways you can help protect the children you
love from burns.

Prevention Tips
To Prevent Burns from Fires and Scalding

- **Be "alarmed."** Install and maintain smoke alarms in your
  home—on every floor and near all rooms family members sleep
  in. Test your smoke alarms once a month to make sure they are
  working properly. Use long-life batteries when possible.

- **Have an escape plan.** Create and practice a family fire-escape
  plan, and involve kids in the planning. Make sure everyone
  knows at least two ways out of every room and identify a central
  meeting place outside.

- **Cook with care,** Use safe cooking practices, such as never
  leaving food unattended on the stove. Also, supervise or restrict
  children's use of stoves, ovens, and microwaves.

- **Check the water heater temperature.** Set your water
  heater's thermostat to 120°F or lower. Infants and small
  children may not be able to get away from water that may be
  too hot, and maintaining a constant thermostat setting can
  help control the water temperature throughout your home—
  preventing it from getting too high. Test the water at the tap if
  possible.

Section 6.2

Preventing Drowning

This section includes text excerpted from "Drowning Prevention,"
Centers for Disease Control and Prevention (CDC), February 6, 2019.

We all want to keep our children safe and secure and help them live to their full potential. Knowing how to prevent leading causes of child injury, such as drowning, is a step toward this goal.

When most of us are enjoying time at the pool or beach, injuries are not the first thing on our minds. Yet, drowning is a leading cause of injury death for young children ages 1 to 14, and 3 children die every day as a result of drowning. In fact, drowning kills more children 1 to 4 than anything else except birth defects.

Thankfully, parents can play a key role in protecting the children they love from drowning.

Prevention Tips
Learn Life-Saving Skills

Everyone should know the basics of swimming (floating, moving through the water) and cardiopulmonary resuscitation (CPR).

Fence It Off

Install a four-sided isolation fence, with self-closing and self-latching gates, around backyard swimming pools. This can help keep children away from the area when they are not supposed to be swimming. Pool fences should completely separate the house and play area from the pool.

Make Life Jackets a Must

Make sure kids wear life jackets in and around natural bodies of water, such as lakes or the ocean, even if they know how to swim. Life jackets can be used in and around pools for weaker swimmers too.

Be on the Lookout

When kids are in or near water (including bathtubs), closely supervise them at all times. Because drowning happens quickly and quietly, adults watching kids in or near water should avoid distracting activities, such as playing cards, reading books, talking on the phone, and using alcohol or drugs.

75

Section 6.3

Preventing Falls

This section includes text excerpted from "Fall Prevention," Centers
for Disease Control and Prevention (CDC), February 6, 2019.

We all want to keep our children safe and secure and help them
live to their full potential. Knowing how to prevent leading causes of
child injury, such as falls, is a step toward this goal.

Falls are the leading cause of nonfatal injuries for all children ages
0 to 19. Every day, approximately 8,000 children are treated in the
U.S. emergency rooms for fall-related injuries. This adds up to almost
2.8 million children each year.

Thankfully, many falls can be prevented, and parents and caregivers can play a key role in protecting children.

Prevention Tips
Play Safely

Falls on the playground are a common cause of injury. Check to
make sure that the surfaces under playground equipment are safe,
soft, and consist of appropriate materials (such as wood chips or sand,
not dirt or grass). The surface materials should be an appropriate
depth and well-maintained.

Make Your Home Safer

Use home safety devices, such as guards on windows that are above
ground level, stair gates, and guard rails. These devices can help keep
a busy, active child from taking a dangerous tumble.

Keep Sports Safe

Make sure your child wears protective gear during sports and recreation. For example, when in-line skating, use wrist guards, knee
and elbow pads, and a helmet.

Supervision Is Key

Supervise young children at all times around fall hazards, such as
stairs and playground equipment, whether you are at home or out to
play.

Section 6.4

Playground Safety

This section includes text excerpted from "Playground Safety,"
Centers for Disease Control and Prevention (CDC), February 6, 2019.

Each year in the United States, emergency departments (EDs) treat more than 200,000 children ages 14 and younger for playground-related injuries. More than 20,000 of these children are treated for a traumatic brain injury (TBI), including concussion. Overall, more research is needed to better understand what specific activities are putting kids at risk of injury and what changes in playground equipment and surfaces might help prevent injuries.

Occurrence and Consequences of Playground-Related Injuries
All Emergency Department-Treated, Playground-Related Injuries

- About 56 percent of playground-related injuries that are treated in EDs are fractures and contusions/abrasions.

- About 75 percent of injuries related to playground equipment occur on public playgrounds. Most occur at a place of recreation or school.

Playground-Related Traumatic Brain Injuries

- The overall rate of ED visits for playground-related TBI has significantly increased during 2005 to 2013.

- About two-thirds of playground-related TBIs occurred at school and places or recreation or sports and often involved monkey bars, climbing equipment, or swings.

- Most ED visits for playground-related TBIs occur during weekdays, Monday through Friday.

- Playground-related TBI ED visits occurred frequently during the months of April, May, and September.

Deaths

Between 2001 and 2008, the Consumer Product Safety Commission (CPSC) investigated 40 deaths associated with playground equipment.

The average age of children who died was 6 years old. Of these, 27 (68%) died from strangulation and 6 (15%) died from falls to the playground surface. Most strangulation involved the combination of slides or swings and jump ropes, other ropes, dog leashes, or clothes drawstrings.

What Can Be Done?

Take steps to keep kids safe by:

- Checking that playgrounds have soft material under them such as wood chips, sand, or mulch

- Reading playground signs and using playground equipment that is right for your child's age

- Making sure there are guardrails in good condition to help prevent falls

- Looking out for things in the play area that can trip your child, such as tree stumps or rocks

Section 6.5

Sports Safety

This section includes text excerpted from "Sports Safety," Centers for Disease Control and Prevention (CDC), February 6, 2019.

Taking part in sports and recreation activities is an important part of a healthy, physically active lifestyle for kids. But, injuries can, and do, occur. More than 2.6 million children 0 to 19 years old are treated in the emergency department (ED) each year for sports and recreation-related injuries.

Thankfully, there are steps that parents can take to help make sure kids stay safe on the field, the court, or wherever they play or participate in sports and recreation activities.

Prevention Tips
Gear Up

When children are active in sports and recreation, make sure they use the right protective gear for their activity, such as helmets, wrist guards, knee or elbow pads.

Use the Right Stuff

Be sure that sports protective equipment is in good condition, fits appropriately and is worn correctly all the time—for example, avoid missing or broken buckles or compressed or worn padding. Poorly fitting equipment may be uncomfortable and may not offer the best protection.

Get an Action Plan in Place

Be sure your child's sports program or school has an action plan that includes information on how to teach athletes ways to lower their chances of getting a concussion and other injuries.

Pay Attention to Temperature

Allow time for child athletes to gradually adjust to hot or humid environments to prevent heat-related injuries or illness. Parents and coaches should pay close attention to make sure that players are hydrated and appropriately dressed.

Be a Good Model

Communicate positive safety messages and serve as a model of safe behavior, including wearing a helmet and following the rules.

Section 6.6

Preventing Poisoning

This section includes text excerpted from "Poisoning Prevention,"
Centers for Disease Control and Prevention (CDC), February 6, 2019.

Every day, over 300 children in the United States ages 0 to 19 are treated in an emergency department (ED), and two children die, as a result of being poisoned. It is not just chemicals in your home marked with clear warning labels that can be dangerous to children.

Everyday items in your home, such as household cleaners and medicines, can be poisonous to children as well. Medication dosing mistakes and unsupervised ingestions are common ways that children are poisoned. Active, curious children will often investigate—and sometimes try to eat or drink—anything that they can get into.

Thankfully, there are ways you can help poison-proof your home and protect the children you love.

Prevention Tips
Lock Them Up and Away

Keep medicines and toxic products such as cleaning solutions and detergent pods in their original packaging where children cannot see or get them.

Know the Number

Put the nationwide poison control center (PCC) phone number, 800-222-1222, on or near every telephone in your home and program it into your cell phone. Call the PCC if you think a child has been poisoned but they are awake and alert; they can be reached 24 hours a day, 7 days a week. Call 911 if you have a poison emergency and your child has collapsed or is not breathing.

Read the Label

Follow label directions carefully and read all warnings when giving medicines to children.

Do Not Keep It If You Do Not Need It

Safely dispose of unused, unneeded, or expired prescription drugs and over-the-counter (OTC) drugs, vitamins, and supplements. To dispose of medicines, mix them with coffee grounds or kitty litter and throw them away. You can also turn them in at a local take-back program or during National Drug Take-Back events.

Section 6.7

Road Traffic Safety

This section includes text excerpted from "Road Traffic Safety,"
Centers for Disease Control and Prevention (CDC), August 12, 2019.

We all want to keep our children safe and secure and help them live to their full potential. Knowing how to prevent leading causes of child injury, such as road-traffic injuries, is a step toward this goal.

Every hour, nearly 150 children between 0 and 19 years of age are treated in emergency departments (EDs) for injuries sustained in motor vehicle crashes. More children ages 5 to 19 die from crash-related injuries than from any other type of injury.

Thankfully, parents can play a key role in protecting the children they love from road traffic injuries.

Prevention Tips
Know the Stages

Make sure children are properly buckled up in a car seat, booster seat, or seat belt, whichever is appropriate for their age, height, and weight.

Birth up to Age 2: Rear-Facing Car Seat

For the best possible protection, infants and children should be buckled in a rear-facing car seat, in the back seat, until age 2 or when they reach the upper weight or height limits of their particular seat. Check the seat's owner's manual and/or labels on the seat for weight and height limits.

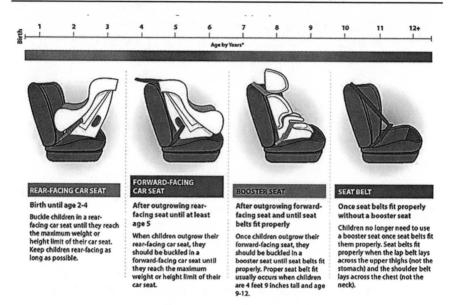

Figure 6.1. *Age- and Size-Appropriate Car Seat or Booster Seat*

Using the correct car seat or booster seat can be a lifesaver. Make sure your child is always buckled in an age- and size-appropriate car seat or booster seat. Keep children ages 12 and under properly buckled in the back seat. Never place a rear-facing car seat in front of an active airbag.

*Recommended age ranges for each seat type vary to account for differences in child growth and height/weight limits of car seats and booster seats.

Age 2 up to at Least Age 5: Forward-Facing Car Seat

When children outgrow their rear-facing seats they should be buckled in a forward-facing car seat, in the back seat, until at least age 5 or when they reach the upper weight or height limit of their particular seat. Check the seat's owner's manual and/or labels on the seat for weight and height limits.

Age 5 up until Seat Belts Fit Properly: Booster Seat

Once children outgrow their forward-facing seat, (by reaching the upper height or weight limit of their seat), they should be buckled in a belt-positioning booster seat until seat belts fit properly. Seat belts fit properly when the lap belt lays across the upper thighs (not the stomach) and the shoulder belt lays across the chest (not the neck). Remember to keep children properly buckled in the back seat for the best possible protection.

Once Seat Belts Fit Properly without a Booster Seat: Seat Belt

Children no longer need to use a booster seat once seat belts fit them properly. Seat belts fit properly when the lap belt lays across the upper thighs (not the stomach) and the shoulder belt lays across the chest (not the neck). For the best possible protection keep children properly buckled in the back seat.

Install and Use Car and Booster Seats Properly

Install and use car seats and booster seats according to the seat's owner's manual or get help installing them from a certified Child Passenger Safety Technician.

Seat Children in the Back Seat

Buckle all children aged 12 and under in the back seat.

Do Not Seat Children in Front of an Airbag

Airbags can kill young children riding in the front seat. Never place a rear-facing car seat in front of an airbag.

Seat Children in the Middle of the Back Seat

Buckle children in the middle of the back seat when possible, because it is the safest spot in the vehicle.

Use Proper Restraints Every Trip

Buckle children in car seats, booster seats, or seat belts on every trip, no matter how short.

Parents and Caregivers: Always Wear a Seat Belt

Set a good example by always using a seat belt themselves.

Chapter 7

Fevers and Febrile Seizures in Children

Chapter Contents

Section 7.1

Fevers

This section contains text excerpted from the following sources:
Text in this section begins with excerpts from "Fever," MedlinePlus,
National Institutes of Health (NIH), December 15, 2016. Reviewed
September 2019; Text beginning with the heading "Acetaminophen
to Reduce Fever in Children" is excerpted from "Reducing Fever
in Children: Safe Use of Acetaminophen," U.S. Food and Drug
Administration (FDA), July 21, 2011. Reviewed September 2019.

A fever is a body temperature that is higher than normal. A normal temperature can vary from person to person, but it is usually around 98.6°F. A fever is not a disease. It is usually a sign that your body is trying to fight an illness or infection.

Infections cause most fevers. You get a fever because your body is trying to kill the virus or bacteria that caused the infection. Most of those bacteria and viruses do well when your body is at your normal temperature. But if you have a fever, it is harder for them to survive. Fever also activates your body's immune system.

Other causes of fevers include:

- Medicines, including some antibiotics, blood pressure medicines, and antiseizure medicines

- Heat illness

- Cancers

- Autoimmune diseases

- Some childhood immunizations

Treatment depends on the cause of your fever. If the fever is very high, your healthcare provider may recommend taking an over-the-counter (OTC) medicine, such as acetaminophen or ibuprofen. Adults can also take aspirin, but children with fevers should not take aspirin. It is also important to drink enough liquids, to prevent dehydration.

Acetaminophen to Reduce Fever in Children

You are in the drug store, looking for a fever-reducing medicine for your children. They range in age from six months to seven years, and you want to buy one product you can use for all of them. So you buy liquid acetaminophen in concentrated drops for infants, figuring you can use the dropper for the baby and a teaspoon for the oldest.

This could be a dangerous mistake.

This use of concentrated drops in much larger amounts—as would be given with a teaspoon—can cause fatal overdoses, says Sandra Kweder, M.D., Deputy Director of the U.S. Food and Drug Administration's (FDA) Office of New Drugs (OND).

You cannot just give an older child more of an infant's medicine, adds Kweder. "Improper dosing is one of the biggest problems in giving acetaminophen to children."

Confusion about dosing is partly caused by the availability of different formulas, strengths, and dosage instructions for different ages of children.

Sold as a single active ingredient under such brand names as Tylenol, acetaminophen is commonly used to reduce fever and relieve pain. It is also used in combination with other ingredients in products to relieve multiple symptoms, such as cough and cold medicines. Acetaminophen can be found in more than 600 (OTC, or nonprescription) and prescription medicines.

Acetaminophen is generally safe and effective if you follow the directions on the package, but if you give a child even a little more than directed or give more than one medicine that contains acetaminophen, it can cause nausea and vomiting, says Kweder.

In some cases—in both adults and children—it can cause liver failure and death. In fact, acetaminophen poisoning is a leading cause of liver failure in the United States.

Advice from Outside Experts

The FDA's Advisory Panel of outside experts met to discuss how to minimize medication errors and make children's OTC medicines that contain acetaminophen safer to use.

The Panel recommended:

• That liquid, chewable, and tablet forms be made in just one strength. There are seven strengths available for these forms combined.

• That dosing instructions to reduce fever be developed for children as young as 6 months. The instructions apply to children 2 to 12 years of age and for those under 2, only state "consult a doctor."

- That dosing instructions be based on weight, not just age

- Setting standards for dosing devices, such as spoons and cups, for children's medicines. Some use milliliters (mL) while others use cubic centimeters (cc) or teaspoons (tsp).

"The FDA is considering these recommendations," says Kweder, and for those that the agency adopts, "we will work with manufacturers to try to get them in place on a voluntary basis." The process of getting a regulation finalized could take several years, she adds, so having the drug industry act voluntarily would help make acetaminophen safer sooner.

Drugmakers have already agreed to phase out the concentrated infant drops to reduce confusion for parents who try to use them for older children. The Consumer Healthcare Products Association (CHPA), a trade group representing the makers of OTC medicines, announced plans to convert liquid acetaminophen products for children to just one strength (160 mg/5 mL). In addition, the industry is voluntarily standardizing the unit of measurement "mL" on dosing devices for these products.

Tips for Giving Acetaminophen to Children

- Never give your child more than one medicine containing acetaminophen at a time. To find out if an OTC medicine contains acetaminophen, look for "acetaminophen" on the Drug Facts label under the section called "Active Ingredients." For prescription pain relievers, ask the pharmacist if the medicine contains acetaminophen.

- Choose the right OTC medicine based on your child's weight and age. The "Directions" section of the Drug Facts label tells you if the medicine is right for your child and how much to give. If a dose for your child's weight or age is not listed on the label or you cannot tell how much to give, ask your pharmacist or doctor what to do.

- Never give more of an acetaminophen-containing medicine than directed. If the medicine does not help your child feel better, talk to your doctor, nurse, or pharmacist.

- If the medicine is a liquid, use the measuring tool that comes with the medicine—not a kitchen spoon.

- Keep a daily record of the medicines you give to your child. Share this information with anyone who is helping care for your child.

- If your child swallows too much acetaminophen, get medical help right away, even if your child does not feel sick. For immediate help, call the 24-hour Poison Control Center (PCC) at 800-222-1222, or call 911.

Section 7.2

Febrile Seizures

This section includes text excerpted from "Febrile Seizures Fact Sheet," National Institute of Neurological Disorders and Stroke (NINDS), May 13, 2019.

What Are Febrile Seizures?

Febrile seizures are seizures or convulsions that occur in young children and are triggered by fever. Young children between the ages of about six months and five years old are the most likely to experience febrile seizures; this risk peaks during the second year of life. The fever may accompany common childhood illnesses, such as a cold, the flu, or an ear infection. In some cases, a child may not have a fever at the time of the seizure but will develop one a few hours later.

The vast majority of febrile seizures are convulsions. Most often during a febrile seizure, a child will lose consciousness and both arms and legs will shake uncontrollably. Less common symptoms include eye-rolling, rigid (stiff) limbs, or twitching on only one side or a portion of the body, such as an arm or a leg. Sometimes during a febrile seizure, a child may lose consciousness but will not noticeably shake or move.

Most febrile seizures last only a few minutes and are accompanied by a fever above 101°F (38.3°C). Although they can be frightening for parents, brief febrile seizures (less than 15 minutes) do not cause any long-term health problems. Having a febrile seizure does not mean a child has epilepsy since that disorder is characterized by reoccurring seizures that are not triggered by fever. Even prolonged seizures (lasting more than 15 minutes) generally have a good outcome but carry an increased risk of developing epilepsy.

How Common Are Febrile Seizures?

Febrile seizures are the most common type of convulsions in infants and young children and occur in two to five percent of American children before age five. Approximately 40 percent of children who experience one febrile seizure will have a recurrence. Children at highest risk for recurrence are those who have:

- Their first febrile seizure at a young age (younger than 18 months)

- A family history of febrile seizures

- A febrile seizure as the first sign of an illness

- A relatively low-temperature increase with their first febrile seizure

A prolonged initial febrile seizure does not substantially boost the risk of reoccurring febrile seizures. However, if another does occur, it is more likely to be prolonged.

What Should Be Done for a Child Having a Febrile Seizure?

It is important that parents and caretakers remain calm, take first-aid measures, and carefully observe the child. If a child is having a febrile seizure, parents and caregivers should do the following:

- **Note the start time of the seizure.** If the seizure lasts longer than five minutes, call an ambulance. The child should be taken immediately to the nearest medical facility for diagnosis and treatment.

- **Call an ambulance** if the seizure is less than five minutes but the child does not seem to be recovering quickly.

- **Gradually place the child on a protected surface,** such as the floor or ground, to prevent accidental injury. Do not restrain or hold a child during a convulsion.

- **Position the child on her or his side or stomach to prevent choking.** When possible, gently remove any objects from the child's mouth. Nothing should ever be placed in the child's mouth during a convulsion. These objects can obstruct the child's airway and make breathing difficult.

- **Seek immediate medical attention** if this is the child's first febrile seizure and take the child to the doctor once the seizure has ended to check for the cause of the fever. This is especially urgent if the child shows symptoms of a stiff neck, extreme lethargy, or abundant vomiting, which may be signs of meningitis, an infection over the brain surface.

Are Febrile Seizures Harmful?

The vast majority of febrile seizures are short and do not cause any long-term damage. During a seizure, there is a small chance that the child may be injured by falling or may choke on food or saliva in the mouth. Using proper first aid for seizures can help avoid these hazards.

There is no evidence that short febrile seizures cause brain damage. Large studies have found that even children with prolonged febrile seizures have normal school achievement and perform as well on intellectual tests as their siblings who do not have seizures. Even when the seizures last a long time, most children recover completely.

Multiple or prolonged seizures are a risk factor for epilepsy but most children who experience febrile seizures do not go on to develop the reoccurring seizures that are characteristic of epilepsy. Some children, including those with cerebral palsy, delayed development, or other neurological abnormalities as well as those with a family history of epilepsy are at increased risk of developing epilepsy whether or not they have febrile seizures. Febrile seizures may be more common in these children but do not contribute much to the overall risk of developing epilepsy.

Children who experience a brief, full-body febrile seizure are slightly more likely to develop epilepsy than the general population. Children who have a febrile seizure that lasts longer than 10 minutes; a focal seizure (a seizure that starts on one side of the brain); or seizures that reoccur within 24 hours, have a moderately increased risk (about 10%) of developing epilepsy as compared to children who do not have febrile seizures.

Of greatest concern is the small group of children with very prolonged febrile seizures lasting longer than 30 minutes. In these children, the risk of epilepsy is as high as 30 to 40 percent, though the condition may not occur for many years. Studies suggest that prolonged febrile seizures can injure the hippocampus, a brain structure involved with temporal lobe epilepsy (TLE).

How Are Febrile Seizures Evaluated?

Before diagnosing febrile seizures in infants and children, doctors sometimes perform tests to be sure that the seizures are not caused by an underlying or more serious health condition. For example, meningitis, an infection of the membranes surrounding the brain, can cause both fever and seizures that can look like febrile seizures but are much more serious. If a doctor suspects a child has meningitis a spinal tap may be needed to check for signs of the infection in the cerebrospinal fluid (fluid surrounding the brain and spinal cord). If there has been severe diarrhea or vomiting, dehydration could be responsible for seizures. Also, doctors often perform other tests, such as examining the blood and urine, to pinpoint the cause of the child's fever.

If the seizure is either very prolonged or is accompanied by a serious infection, or if the child is younger than six months of age, the clinician may recommend hospitalization. In most cases, however, a child who has a febrile seizure usually will not need to be hospitalized.

Can Subsequent Febrile Seizures Be Prevented?

Experts recommend that children who have experienced a febrile seizure not take any antiseizure medication to prevent future seizures, as the side effects of these daily medications outweigh any benefits. This is especially true since most febrile seizures are brief and harmless.

If a child has a fever, most parents will use fever-lowering drugs, such as acetaminophen or ibuprofen to make the child more comfortable. However, available studies show this does not reduce the risk of having another febrile seizure.

Although the majority of children with febrile seizures do not need medication, children especially prone to febrile seizures may be treated with medication, such as Diazepam, when they have a fever. This medication may lower the risk of having another febrile seizure. It is usually well-tolerated, although it occasionally can cause drowsiness, a lack of coordination, or hyperactivity. Children vary widely in their susceptibility to such side effects.

A child whose first febrile seizure is a prolonged one does not necessarily have a higher risk of having reoccurring prolonged seizures. But if the child has another seizure, it is likely to be prolonged. Because very long febrile seizures are associated with the potential for injury and an increased risk of developing epilepsy, some doctors may prescribe medication to these children to prevent prolonged seizures. The parents of children who have experienced a long febrile may wish to talk to their doctor about this treatment option.

What Research Is Being Done on Febrile Seizures?

Researchers are exploring the biological, environmental, and genetic risk factors that might make children susceptible to febrile seizures. They are also working to pinpoint factors that can help predict which children are likely to have reoccurring or prolonged febrile seizures.

Investigators continue to monitor the long-term impact that febrile seizures might have on intelligence, behavior, school achievement, and the development of epilepsy. For example, the National Institute of Neurological Disorders and Stroke (NINDS)-funded scientists are assessing the effects of febrile seizures, especially very prolonged febrile seizures, on brain structures, such as the hippocampus, an area of the brain that plays a role in memory and learning. They are also working to determine the impact of these seizures on the development of epilepsy and memory.

Children who have experienced prolonged febrile seizures are more likely to develop a particular type of epilepsy called "TLE," which is often difficult to treat. TLE is associated with scarring of the hippocampus and usually presents in adolescents or young adults, some of whom have a history of long febrile seizures as young children. Scientists are trying to identify which children will go on to develop TLE in order to develop better treatments to prevent this condition. Investigators are also trying to develop drugs to prevent the occurrence of brain injury, epilepsy, and memory problems following prolonged febrile seizures.

Chapter 8

Caring for Children in an Emergency

Regardless of your child's age, she or he may feel upset or have other strong emotions after an emergency. Some children react right away, while others may show signs of difficulty much later. How children react or common signs of distress can vary according to age. Knowing how to help children cope after an emergency can help them stay healthy in future emergencies.

An emergency can happen anywhere and at any time. It is important for parents to know what steps they can take before, during, and after an emergency to protect their family. Parents ensure that family members are ready and know what to do when emergencies happen.

Before an Emergency
A Little Preparation Now Can Make a Big Difference Later

Here are some steps you can take to help keep your family safe and healthy when an emergency happens:

- **Prepare an emergency kit** that includes a three-day supply of necessities for each person in your family, and include such

This chapter includes text excerpted from "Before, during and after an Emergency," Centers for Disease Control and Prevention (CDC), July 18, 2019.

necessities as food, medicine, water, games, flashlight, and special toys to help keep your children calm during an emergency.

- **Make a plan to contact family members**, especially if you are not together when an emergency strikes. If your children are old enough, teach them how to call 911 and memorize important phone numbers. Create a reunification plan as part of the family communication plan to reunite you with your loved ones as soon as it is safe to do so.

- **Review with your children the different types of emergencies that can happen in your area and the warning signs for those emergencies.** For example, if tornadoes are common, your children should know what to do during a tornado. This includes knowing the signs of an approaching storm and instructions on how to take shelter during a tornado.

- **Be informed, stay informed, and get vital information**, such as emergency warnings and alerts, from reliable news sources and your local emergency-management agency.

Help Protect Your Child during the School Day

In the United States, about 69 million children are separated from their parents or caregivers every workday to attend school or child care. You can help protect your children, even when you are not with them, through the following steps:

- **Find out the school or childcare center's emergency plans.** Every school and childcare center should have a written emergency plan with information, such as how to contact parents in an emergency and where children will go if evacuated. Also, ask how you can contact the school or childcare center during an emergency and how parents and caregivers will reunite with their children.

- **Update your emergency contact information.** Make sure that the school has up-to-date emergency contact information for your child. Notify the school every time your address or phone number changes. Keeping a backpack emergency card (Figure 8.1) with your child is one way to make sure that emergency contact information—as well as other important information such as medications and allergies—is handy.

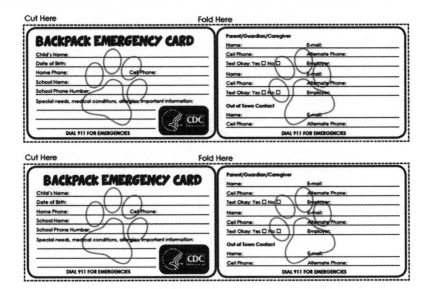

Figure 8.1. *Backpack Emergency Card Template*

It is important to have your emergency contact information with you in case of an emergency. Complete the cards and keep one in your wallet and one in your child's backpack.

During an Emergency

Each emergency is different and may require different actions to keep you and your family safe. Local authorities will share safety instructions and updates on television, radio, the Internet, or social media pages, such as Twitter and Facebook. Depending on the emergency, authorities may ask you to stay where you are ("shelter in place"), or they may recommend that you go somewhere else ("evacuate").

If you have children in a school in the exposed area, school authorities may evacuate your children to a safer place or emergency shelter. In these cases, do not go to your children during the emergency. This can put you and your children at greater risk. Wait until emergency or school authorities say it is safe for you to pick up your children.

After an Emergency
Reuniting after an Emergency

Children may be away from their parents—or accidentally separated—during an emergency. Having a reunification plan and knowing reunification resources can help you reunite with your loved ones as soon as it is safe to do so.

Helping Children Cope

Regardless of your child's age, she or he may feel upset or have other strong emotions after an emergency. Some children react right away, while others may show signs of difficulty much later. How children react or common signs of distress can vary according to age. Knowing how to help children cope after an emergency can help them stay healthy in future emergencies.

Part Two

Childhood Infections and Related Concerns

Chapter 9

Foodborne Illness

What Is Foodborne Illness?

Foodborne illness is a preventable public-health challenge that causes an estimated 48 million illnesses and 3,000 deaths each year in the United States. It is an illness that comes from eating contaminated food. The onset of symptoms may occur within minutes to weeks and often presents itself as flu-like symptoms, as the ill person may experience symptoms, such as nausea, vomiting, diarrhea, or fever. Because the symptoms are often flu-like, many people may not recognize that the illness is caused by harmful bacteria or other pathogens in food.

Everyone is at risk of getting a foodborne illness. However, some people are at greater risk for experiencing a more serious illness or even death should they get a foodborne illness. Those at greater risk are infants, young children, pregnant women, and their unborn babies, older adults, and people with weakened immune systems (such as those with human immunodeficiency virus (HIV), acquired immunodeficiency syndrome (AIDS), cancer, diabetes, kidney disease, and transplant patients). Some people may become ill after ingesting only

This chapter contains text excerpted from the following sources: Text beginning with the heading "What Is Foodborne Illness?" is excerpted from "Foodborne Illness: What Consumers Need to Know," Food Safety and Inspection Service (FSIS), U.S. Department of Agriculture (USDA), August 7, 2013. Reviewed September 2019; Text under the heading "How Children Are Affected by Foodborne Illness" is excerpted from "People at Risk: Children under Five," Foodsafety.gov, U.S. Department of Health and Human Services (HHS), April 26, 2019.

a few harmful bacteria; others may remain symptom-free after ingesting thousands.

How Do Bacteria Get in Food?

Microorganisms may be present on food products when you purchase them. For example, plastic-wrapped boneless chicken breasts and ground meat were once part of live chickens or cattle. Raw meat, poultry, seafood, and eggs are not sterile. Neither is fresh produce, such as lettuce, tomatoes, sprouts, and melons.

Thousands of types of bacteria are naturally present in our environment. Microorganisms that cause disease are called "pathogens." When certain pathogens enter the food supply, they can cause foodborne illness. Not all bacteria cause disease in humans. For example, some bacteria are used beneficially in making cheese and yogurt.

Foods, including safely cooked and ready-to-eat foods, can become cross-contaminated with pathogens transferred from raw egg products and raw meat, poultry, and seafood products and their juices, other contaminated products, or from food handlers with poor personal hygiene. Most cases of foodborne illness can be prevented with proper cooking or processing of food to destroy pathogens.

How Children Are Affected by Foodborne Illness

Children younger than five years are at an increased risk for foodborne illness and related health complications because their immune systems are still developing. Young children with developing immune systems cannot fight off infections as well as adults can. In addition, young children produce less stomach acid that kills harmful bacteria, making it easier for them to get sick.

Food poisoning can be particularly dangerous for young children because food poisoning often causes vomiting or diarrhea or both. Since children's bodies are small, they can quickly lose a lot of body fluid, causing dehydration.

Food safety for young children depends on the food-safety behaviors of their parents and caregivers. Handwashing is especially important, by children and those caring for them.

In children under five-years-old, *E. coli* infections are more likely to lead to hemolytic uremic syndrome (HUS), a severe complication that can cause chronic kidney disease (CKD), kidney failure, and death. Symptoms of HUS are urinating less often, feeling very tired, and losing pink color in cheeks and inside the lower eyelids. These new

Table 9.1. Foodborne Bacteria

Bacteria	Associated Foods	Symptoms and Potential Impact	Prevention
Campylobacter jejuni	Contaminated water, raw or unpasteurized milk, and raw or undercooked meat, poultry, or shellfish.	Diarrhea (sometimes bloody), cramping, abdominal pain, and fever that appear 2 to 5 days after eating; may last 7 days. May spread to the bloodstream and cause a life-threatening infection.	Cook meat and poultry to a safe minimum internal temperature; do not drink or consume unpasteurized milk or milk products; wash your hands after coming in contact with feces.
Clostridium botulinum	Improperly canned foods, garlic in oil, vacuum-packed and tightly wrapped food.	Bacteria produce a nerve toxin that causes illness, affecting the nervous system. Toxin affects the nervous system. Symptoms usually appear 18 to 36 hours, but can sometimes appear as few as 6 hours or as many as 10 days after eating; double vision, blurred vision, drooping eyelids, slurred speech, difficulty swallowing, dry mouth, and muscle weakness. If untreated, these symptoms may progress causing muscle paralysis and even death.	Do not use damaged canned foods or canned foods showing signs of swelling, leakage, punctures, holes, fractures, extensive deep rusting, or crushing/denting severe enough to prevent normal stacking. Follow safety guidelines when home canning food. Boil home-canned foods for 10 minutes before eating to ensure safety. (Note: Safe home canning guidelines may be obtained from State University or County Extension Office).
Clostridium perfringens	Meats, meat products, and gravy Called "the cafeteria germ" because many outbreaks result from food left for long periods in steam tables or at room temperature.	Intense abdominal cramps nausea and diarrhea may appear 6 to 24 hours after eating; usually last about 1 day, but for immune comprised individuals, symptoms may last 1 to 2 weeks. Complications and/or death can occur only very rarely.	Keep hot foods hot and cold foods cold! Once the food is cooked, it should be held hot, at an internal temperature of 140°F or above. Use a food thermometer to make sure. Discard all perishable foods left at room temperature longer than 2 hours; 1 hour in temperatures above 90°F.

Table 9.1. Continued

Bacteria	Associated Foods	Symptoms and Potential Impact	Prevention
Cryptosporidium	Soil, food, water, contaminated surfaces. Swallowing contaminated water, including that from recreational sources, (e.g., a swimming pool or lake); eating uncooked or contaminated food; placing a contaminated object in the mouth.	Dehydration, weight loss, stomach cramps or pain, fever, nausea, and vomiting; respiratory symptoms may also be present. Symptoms begin 2 to 10 days after becoming infected, and may last 1 to 2 weeks. Immune-comprised individuals may experience a more serious illness.	Wash your hands before and after handling raw meat products, and after changing diapers, going to the bathroom, or touching animals. Avoid water that might be contaminated. (Do not drink untreated water from shallow wells, lakes, rivers, springs, ponds, and streams.)
Escherichia coli O157:H7	Uncooked beef (especially ground beef), unpasteurized milk and juices (e.g., "fresh" apple cider); contaminated raw fruits and vegetables, or water. Person to person contamination can also occur.	Severe diarrhea (often bloody diarrhea), abdominal cramps, and vomiting. Usually little or no fever. Can begin 2 to 8 days, but usually 3 to 4 days after consumption of contaminated food or water and lasts about 5 to 7 days depending on severity. Children under 5 are at greater risk of developing hemolytic uremic syndrome (HUS), which causes acute kidney failure.	Cook hamburgers and ground beef to a safe minimum internal temperature of 160°F. Drink only pasteurized milk, juice, or cider. Rinse fruits and vegetables under running tap water, especially those that will not be cooked. Wash your hands with warm water and soap after changing diapers, using the bathroom, handling pets or having any contact with feces.

Table 9.1. Continued

Bacteria	Associated Foods	Symptoms and Potential Impact	Prevention
	Ready-to-eat foods such as hot dogs, luncheon meats, cold cuts, fermented or dry sausage, and other deli-style meat and poultry. Also, soft cheeses made with unpasteurized milk. Smoked seafood and salads made in the store such as ham salad, chicken salad, or seafood salad.	Fever, muscle aches, and sometimes gastrointestinal symptoms such as nausea or diarrhea. If the infection spreads to the nervous system, symptoms such as headache, stiff neck, confusion, loss of balance, or convulsions can occur. Those at risk (including pregnant women and newborns, older adults, and people with weakened immune systems) may later develop more serious illness; death can result from Listeria. Can cause severe problems with pregnancy, including miscarriage or death in newborns.	Cook raw meat, poultry, and seafood to a safe minimum internal temperature; prevent cross-contamination, separating ready to eat foods from raw eggs, and raw meat, poultry, seafood, and their juices; wash your hands before and after handling raw meat, poultry, seafood, and egg products. Those with a weakened immune system should avoid eating hot dogs, and deli meats, unless they are reheated to 165 ºF or steaming hot. Do not drink raw (unpasteurized) milk or foods that have unpasteurized milk in them, e.g., soft cheeses). Do not eat deli salads made in-store, such as ham, egg, tuna or seafood salad.
Listeria monocytogenes			
Salmonella (over 2300 types)	Raw or undercooked eggs, poultry, and meat; unpasteurized milk and juice; cheese and seafood; and contaminated fresh fruits and vegetables.	Diarrhea, fever, and abdominal cramps usually appear 12 to 72 hours after eating; may last 4 to 7 days. In people with a weakened immune system, the infection may be more severe and lead to serious complications, including death.	Cook raw meat, poultry, and egg products to a safe temperature. Do not eat raw or undercooked eggs. Avoid consuming raw or unpasteurized milk or other dairy products. Produce should be thoroughly washed before consuming.

Table 9.1. Continued

Bacteria	Associated Foods	Symptoms and Potential Impact	Prevention
Shigella (over 30 types)	Person-to-person by fecal–oral route; fecal contamination of food and water. Most outbreaks result from food, especially salads, prepared and handled by workers using poor personal hygiene.	The disease referred to as "shigellosis" or bacillary dysentery. Diarrhea (watery or bloody), fever, abdominal cramps; 1 to 2 days from ingestion of bacteria and usually resolves in 5 to 7 days	Hand washing is a very important step to prevent shigellosis. Always wash your hands with warm water and soap before handling food and after using the bathroom, changing diapers or having contact with an infected person.
Staphylococcus aureus	Commonly found on the skin and in the noses of up to 25% of healthy people and animals. Person-to-person through food from improper food handling. Multiply rapidly at room temperature to produce a toxin that causes illness. Contaminated milk and cheeses.	Severe nausea, abdominal cramps, vomiting, and diarrhea occur 30 minutes to 6 hours after eating; recovery from 1 to 3 days—longer if severe dehydration occurs.	Because the toxins produced by this bacterium are resistant to heat and cannot be destroyed by cooking, preventing the contamination of food before the toxin can be produced is important. Keep hot foods hot (over 140°F) and cold foods cold (40°F or under); wash your hands with warm water and soap and wash kitchen counters with hot water and soap before and after preparing food.
Vibrio vulnificus	Uncooked or raw seafood (fish or shellfish); oysters	In a healthy person, symptom includes diarrhea, stomach pain, and vomiting may result in a blood infection and death for those with a weakened immune system particularly with underlying liver disease.	Do not eat raw oysters or other raw shellfish; cook shellfish (oysters, clams, mussels) thoroughly. Prevent cross-contamination by separating cooked seafood and other foods from raw seafood and its juices. Refrigerate cooked shellfish within two hours after cooking.

symptoms usually develop after about a week of *E. coli* illness, when the diarrhea is improving.

Choose and Prepare Safe Food

Learn about safer food choices for people with a higher risk for foodborne illness, including young children. If you prepare food for children under the age of five you should always follow the four steps:

Clean: Wash hands, utensils, and surfaces often. Germs can spread and survive in many places.

Separate: Raw meat, poultry, seafood, and eggs can spread illness-causing bacteria to ready-to-eat foods, so keep them separate.

Cook: Food is safely cooked only when the internal temperature is high enough to kill germs that can make you sick.

Chill: Refrigerate promptly. Bacteria that cause food poisoning to multiply quickest is between 40°F and 140°F.

Safe Storage and Microwaving of Puréed and Solid Baby Foods

Follow these precautions when microwaving baby's food:

- Do not microwave baby foods in the jar. Instead, transfer the food to a dish before microwaving it. This way the food can be stirred and taste-tested for temperature.

- Microwave four ounces of solid food in a dish for about 15 seconds on high power. Always stir, let stand 30 seconds, and taste-test before feeding. Food that is "baby-ready" should taste or feel lukewarm.

- Do not heat baby-food meats, meat sticks, or eggs in the microwave. Use the stovetop instead. These foods have a high-fat content, and since microwaves heat fats faster than other substances, these foods can cause splattering and overheating.

Safety Tips for Preparing and Storing Infant Formula
Preparing Formula

- Carefully read and follow the instructions on the infant formula container.

- Wash your hands well before preparing bottles or feeding your baby.

- Clean and sanitize the workspace where you will prepare the infant formula.

- Use clean, sanitized bottles.

- If you use powdered infant formula, use water from a safe source to mix it. If you are not sure if your tap water is safe to use for preparing infant formula, contact your local health department.

- Use the amount of water listed on the instructions of the infant formula container. Always measure the water first and then add the powder.

- If your baby is very young (younger than 3 months old), was born prematurely, or has a weakened immune system, you may want to take extra precautions in preparing your infant's formula to protect against *Cronobacter*, a rare but serious infection that can be caused by germs in powdered infant formula.

- Use prepared infant formula within 2 hours of preparation and within 1 hour from when feeding begins.

- If you do not start to use it within 2 hours, immediately store the bottle in the fridge and use it within 24 hours.

- Throw away formula left in the bottle after feeding your baby.

Table 9.2. Safe Storage of Puréed and Solid Baby Food

Purees and Solids (Opened or Freshly Made)	Refrigerator	Freezer
Strained fruits and vegetables	2 to 3 days	6 to 8 months
Strained meats and eggs	1 day	1 to 2 months
Meat/vegetable combinations	1 to 2 days	1 to 2 months
Homemade baby foods	1 to 2 days	1 to 2 months

Heating Breast Milk or Formula

Baby's milk or infant formula does not need to be warmed before feeding, but some people like to warm their baby's bottle. If you do decide to warm the bottle, here is advice on how to warm it safely:

In hot tap water: Place the bottle under hot, running tap water until the desired temperature is reached. This should take one to two minutes.

On the stove: Heat water in a pan. Remove the pan from the heat and set the bottle in it until it is warm.

When heating baby's milk, always shake the liquid to even out the temperature and test on top of your hand—not the wrist (this is one of the areas least sensitive to heat)—before feeding. Milk that is "baby-ready" should feel lukewarm.

Never heat breast milk or infant formula in the microwave. Microwaves heat baby's milk and food unevenly, which results in hot spots that can burn a baby's mouth and throat.

Chapter 10

Streptococcal Bacterial Infections

Chapter Contents

Section 10.1

Impetigo

This section includes text excerpted from "How to Treat Impetigo
and Control This Common Skin Infection," U.S. Food and Drug
Administration (FDA), November 1, 2016. Reviewed September 2019.

It is a scary sight when your child comes home from day care or
elementary school with red sores and oozing fluid-filled blisters. Do
not be alarmed if it is impetigo. Impetigo—one of the most common
childhood diseases—can be treated with medications approved by the
U.S. Food and Drug Administration (FDA).

Impetigo is a common bacterial skin infection that can produce
blisters or sores anywhere on the body, but usually on the face (around
the nose and mouth), neck, hands, and diaper area. It is contagious,
preventable, and manageable with antibiotics, says pediatrician
Thomas D. Smith, MD, of the FDA.

What Causes Impetigo

Two types of bacteria found on our skin cause impetigo: *Staphylococcus aureus* and *Streptococcus pyogenes* (which also causes strep
throat). Most of us go about our lives carrying around these bacteria
without a problem, Smith says. But then a minor cut, scrape, or insect
bite allows the bacteria to cause an infection, resulting in impetigo.

Anyone can get impetigo—and more than once, Smith says.
Although impetigo is a year-round disease, it occurs most often during
the warm-weather months. There are more than three million cases
of impetigo in the United States every year.

"We typically see impetigo with kids two to six years old, probably
because they get more cuts and scrapes and scratch more. And that
spreads the bacteria," Smith says.

Treating Impetigo

Look for these signs of impetigo:

- Itchy red sores that fill with fluid and then burst open, forming a
  yellow crust

- Itchy rash

- Fluid-filled blisters

If you see these symptoms, visit your healthcare provider. Impetigo is usually treated with topical or oral antibiotics. If your child has multiple lesions or if there is an outbreak, your doctor might prescribe an oral antibiotic. There is no over-the-counter (OTC) treatment for impetigo.

Controlling and Preventing Impetigo

Untreated, impetigo often clears up on its own after a few days or weeks, Smith says. The key is to keep the infected area clean with soap and water and not to scratch it. The downside of not treating impetigo is that some people might develop more lesions that spread to other areas of their bodies.

And you can infect others. "To spread impetigo, you need fairly close contact—not casual contact—with the infected person or the objects they touched," he says. Avoid spreading impetigo to other people or other parts of your body by:

• Cleaning the infected areas with soap and water

• Loosely covering scabs and sores until they heal

• Gently removing crusty scabs

• Washing your hands with soap and water after touching infected areas or infected persons

Because impetigo spreads by skin-to-skin contact, there often are small outbreaks within a family or a classroom, Smith says. Avoid touching objects that someone with impetigo has used, such as utensils, towels, sheets, clothing, and toys. If you have impetigo, keep your fingernails short so the bacteria cannot live under your nails and spread. Also, do not scratch the sores.

Call your healthcare provider if the symptoms do not go away or if there are signs the infection has worsened, such as fever, pain, or increased swelling.

Section 10.2

Pneumococcal Disease

This section includes text excerpted from "Pneumococcal
Disease," Centers for Disease Control and
Prevention (CDC), September 6, 2017.

What Is Pneumococcal Disease?

Pneumococcal disease is an infection caused by *Streptococcus pneumoniae* bacteria, sometimes referred to as "pneumococcus." Pneumococcus can cause many types of illnesses, including ear infections and meningitis. There are vaccines to prevent pneumococcal disease in children.

Types of Infection

Streptococcus pneumoniae bacteria, or pneumococcus, can cause many types of illnesses. Some of these illnesses can be life-threatening.

Pneumococcus is the most common cause of bloodstream infections, pneumonia, meningitis, and middle ear infections in young children.

You have probably heard of pneumonia, which is an infection of the lungs. Many different bacteria, viruses, and even fungi, can cause pneumonia. Pneumococcus is one of the most common causes of severe pneumonia.

Besides pneumonia, pneumococcus can cause other types of infections too, such as:

- Ear infections

- Sinus infections

- Meningitis (infection of the tissue covering the brain and spinal cord)

- Bacteremia (bloodstream infection)

Doctors consider some of these infections "invasive." Invasive disease means that germs invade parts of the body that are normally free from germs. For example, pneumococcal bacteria can invade the bloodstream, causing bacteremia, and the tissues and fluids covering the brain and spinal cord, causing meningitis. When this happens, the disease is usually very severe, requiring treatment in a hospital and even causing death in some cases.

Risk Factors and Transmission of Pneumococcal Disease

Anyone can get pneumococcal disease, but some people are at greater risk for disease than others. Being a certain age or having some medical conditions can put you at increased risk for pneumococcal disease.

Children at Risk for Pneumococcal Disease

Children at increased risk for pneumococcal disease include those:

- Younger than two years old
- Who have certain illnesses (sickle cell disease (SCD), human immunodeficiency virus (HIV) infection, diabetes, immune-compromising conditions, nephrotic syndrome, or chronic heart, lung, kidney, or liver disease)
- With cochlear implants or cerebrospinal fluid (CSF) leaks (escape of the fluid that surrounds the brain and spinal cord)

Transmission of Pneumococcal Disease

Pneumococcal bacteria spread from person-to-person by direct contact with respiratory secretions, such as saliva or mucus. Children have the bacteria in their nose or throat at one time or another without being ill. Doctors call this "carriage" and do not know why it only rarely leads to sickness.

Symptoms and Complications of Pneumococcal Disease

There are many types of pneumococcal disease. Symptoms and complications depend on the part of the body that is infected.

Symptoms

Pneumococcal pneumonia (lung infection) is the most common serious form of pneumococcal disease. Symptoms include:

- Fever and chills
- Cough
- Rapid breathing or difficulty breathing
- Chest pain

Pneumococcal meningitis is an infection of the tissue covering the brain and spinal cord. Symptoms include:

- Stiff neck

- Fever

- Headache

- Photophobia (eyes being more sensitive to light)

- Confusion

In babies, meningitis may cause poor eating and drinking, low alertness, and vomiting.

Pneumococcal bacteremia is a blood infection. Symptoms include:

- Fever

- Chills

- Low alertness

Sepsis is a complication caused by the body's overwhelming and life-threatening response to an infection, which can lead to tissue damage, organ failure, and death. Symptoms include:

- Confusion or disorientation

- Shortness of breath

- High heart rate

- Fever, shivering, or feeling very cold

- Extreme pain or discomfort

- Clammy or sweaty skin

Pneumococcus bacteria cause up to half of the middle ear infections (otitis media). Symptoms include:

- Ear pain

- A red, swollen eardrum

- Fever

- Sleepiness

Complications

Most pneumococcal infections are mild. However, some can be deadly or result in long-term problems, such as brain damage or hearing loss.

Meningitis is the most severe type of invasive pneumococcal disease. Of children younger than 5 years old who get pneumococcal meningitis, about 1 out of 15 dies of the infection. The chance of death from pneumococcal meningitis is higher among elderly patients. Others may have long-term problems, such as hearing loss or developmental delay.

Bacteremia is a type of invasive pneumococcal disease that infects the blood. About 1 out of 100 children younger than 5 years old with this bloodstream infection dies of it. The chance of death from pneumococcal bacteremia is higher among elderly patients.

Pneumonia is an infection of the lungs that can cause mild to severe illness in people of all ages. Complications of pneumococcal pneumonia include:

- Infection of the space between the membranes that surround the lungs and chest cavity (empyema)

- Inflammation of the sac surrounding the heart (pericarditis)

- Blockage of the airway that allows air into the lungs (endobronchial obstruction), with collapse within the lungs (atelectasis) and collection of pus (abscess) in the lungs

About 5 out of 100 people with noninvasive pneumococcal pneumonia will die from it. Doctors consider pneumococcal pneumonia noninvasive if there is not bacteremia or empyema occurring at the same time.

Sinus and **ear infections** are usually mild and are more common than the more severe forms of pneumococcal disease. However, some children develop repeated ear infections and may need ear tubes.

Diagnosis and Treatment of Pneumococcal Disease

Early diagnosis and treatment are very important for invasive pneumococcal disease. It is important to know if it is pneumococcal disease because the treatment will change depending on the cause. In the case of pneumococcal disease, antibiotics can help prevent severe illness.

Diagnosis of Pneumococcal Disease

If doctors suspect invasive pneumococcal diseases such as meningitis or bloodstream infections, they collect samples of cerebrospinal fluid or blood and send them to a laboratory for testing.

Identifying pneumococcus bacteria from the sample collected helps doctors confirm that pneumococcus is the cause of the illness. Additionally, growing the bacteria in a laboratory is important for identifying the specific type of bacteria that is causing the infection. It is also important for deciding which antibiotic will work best.

For other pneumococcal infections such as ear and sinus infections, healthcare professionals usually diagnose them based on history and physical exam findings that support pneumococcal infection.

Treatment of Pneumococcal Disease

Antibiotics can treat pneumococcal disease. However, many types of pneumococcal bacteria have become resistant to some of the antibiotics used to treat these infections.

Antibiotic treatment for invasive pneumococcal infections typically includes "broad-spectrum" antibiotics until results of antibiotic sensitivity testing are available. Broad-spectrum antibiotics work against a wide range of bacteria. Once the sensitivity of the bacteria is known, a more targeted (or "narrow-spectrum") antibiotic may be selected.

With the success of the pneumococcal conjugate vaccine, there is much less antibiotic-resistant pneumococcal infections. In addition to the vaccine, the appropriate use of antibiotics may also slow or reverse drug-resistant pneumococcal infections.

Prevention of Pneumococcal Disease

The best way to prevent pneumococcal disease is to get the vaccine(s). Pneumococcal vaccines help protect against some of the more than 90 types of pneumococcal bacteria.

Vaccination

The pneumococcal conjugate vaccine (PCV13 or Prevnar 13®) protects against the 13 types of pneumococcal bacteria that cause most of the severe illness in children and adults. The vaccine can also help prevent some ear infections. The CDC recommends PCV13 for all children at 2, 4, 6, and 12 to 15 months old.

The pneumococcal polysaccharide vaccine (PPSV23 or Pneumovax 23®) protects against 23 types of pneumococcal bacteria. The CDC recommends this vaccine for children and adults 2 through 64 years old who are at increased risk for pneumococcal disease.

It is also important to get an influenza vaccine every year because having the flu increases your chances of getting pneumococcal disease.

Antibiotics

It is not common for people to develop pneumococcal disease after being exposed to someone with pneumococcal infection. Therefore, the CDC does not recommend prophylactic (preventative) antibiotics for contacts of patients with such infections.

Previous Infection

Because there are more than 90 known pneumococcal serotypes (strains or types) that cause disease, a previous pneumococcal infection will not protect you from future infection. Therefore, the CDC still recommends pneumococcal vaccines for children who have had the pneumococcal disease in the past.

Section 10.3

Rheumatic Fever

This section includes text excerpted from "Rheumatic Fever: All You Need to Know," Centers for Disease Control and Prevention (CDC), November 1, 2018.

Rheumatic fever (acute rheumatic fever) is a disease that can affect the heart, joints, brain, and skin. Rheumatic fever can develop if strep throat and scarlet-fever infections are not treated properly. Early diagnosis of these infections and treatment with antibiotics are key to preventing rheumatic fever.

How You Get Rheumatic Fever

Rheumatic fever may develop after strep throat or scarlet-fever infections that are not treated properly. Bacteria called "group A *Streptococcus*" or "group A strep" cause strep throat and scarlet fever. It usually takes about one to five weeks after strep throat or scarlet fever for rheumatic fever to develop. Rheumatic fever is thought to be caused by a response of the body's defense system—the immune system. The immune system responds to the earlier strep throat or scarlet-fever infection and causes a generalized inflammatory response.

Rheumatic Fever Is Not Contagious

Children cannot catch rheumatic fever from someone else because it is an immune response and not an infection. However, people with strep throat or scarlet fever can spread group A strep to others, primarily through respiratory droplets.

Common Signs and Symptoms

Symptoms of rheumatic fever can include:

- Fever
- Painful, tender joints (arthritis), most commonly in the knees, ankles, elbows, and wrists
- Symptoms of congestive heart failure, including chest pain, shortness of breath, fast heartbeat
- Fatigue
- Jerky, uncontrollable body movements (called "chorea")
- Painless lumps (nodules) under the skin near joints (this is a rare symptom)
- Rash that appears as pink rings with a clear center (this is a rare symptom)

In addition, someone with rheumatic fever can have:

- A new heart murmur
- An enlarged heart
- Fluid around the heart

Children Most Often Affected

Although anyone can get rheumatic fever, it is more common in school-age children (5 through 15 years old). Rheumatic fever is very rare in children younger than three years old and adults.

Infectious illnesses, including group A strep, tend to spread wherever large groups of people gather together. Crowded conditions can increase the risk of getting strep throat or scarlet fever, and thus rheumatic fever. These settings include:

- Schools

- Day-care centers

- Military training facilities

Someone who had rheumatic fever in the past is more likely to get rheumatic fever again if they get strep throat or scarlet fever again.

Many Tests, Considerations Help Doctors Diagnose Rheumatic Fever

There is no single test used to diagnose rheumatic fever. Instead, doctors can look for signs of illness, check the patient's medical history, and use many tests, including:

- A throat swab to look for a group A strep infection

- A blood test to look for antibodies that would show if the patient recently had a group A strep infection

- A test of how well the heart is working (electrocardiogram or EKG)

- A test that creates a movie of the heart muscle working (echocardiography or echo)

Treatment Focuses on Managing Inflammation Symptoms

Doctors treat symptoms of rheumatic fever with medicines such as aspirin to reduce fever, pain, and general inflammation. In addition, all patients with rheumatic fever should get antibiotics that treat group A strep infections. Children who develop rheumatic heart disease with symptoms of heart failure may require medicines to help manage this as well.

Serious Complications Include Long-Term Heart Damage

If rheumatic fever is not treated promptly, long-term heart damage (called "rheumatic heart disease") may occur. Rheumatic heart disease weakens the valves between the chambers of the heart. Severe rheumatic heart disease can require heart surgery and result in death.

Protect Yourself and Others

Having a group A strep infection does not protect someone from getting infected again in the future. People can also get rheumatic fever more than once. However, there are things people can do to protect themselves and others.

Good Hygiene Helps Prevent Group A Strep Infections

The best way to keep from getting or spreading group A strep infections such as strep throat or scarlet fever is to wash your hands often, especially after coughing or sneezing and before preparing foods or eating.

Antibiotics Are Key to Treatment and Prevention

The main ways to prevent rheumatic fever are to:

- Treat group A strep infections such as strep throat and scarlet fever with antibiotics
- Prevent group A strep infections in the first place
- Use preventive antibiotics for people who had rheumatic fever in the past

Preventive antibiotics help protect people who had rheumatic fever from getting it again. Doctors also call this prophylaxis or "secondary prevention." People may need antibiotic prophylaxis over a period of many years (often until 21 years old). Prophylaxis can include daily antibiotics by mouth or a shot into the muscle every few weeks.

Section 10.4

Scarlet Fever

This section includes text excerpted from "Scarlet Fever:
All You Need to Know," Centers for Disease Control
and Prevention (CDC), November 1, 2018.

If your child has a sore throat and a rash, it may be scarlet fever (also called "scarlatina"). Your child's doctor can do a quick strep test to find out. If your child has scarlet fever, antibiotics can help your child feel better faster and prevent long-term health problems. Antibiotics can also help protect others from getting sick.

Bacteria Cause Scarlet Fever

Bacteria called "group A *Streptococcus* or group A strep" cause scarlet fever. The bacteria sometimes make a poison (toxin), which causes a rash—the "scarlet" of scarlet fever.

How You Get Scarlet Fever

Group A strep live in the nose and throat and can easily spread to other people. It is important to know that all infected people do not have symptoms or seem sick. People who are infected spread the bacteria by coughing or sneezing, which creates small respiratory droplets that contain the bacteria.

Children can get sick if they:

- Breathe in those droplets

- Touch something with droplets on it and then touch their mouth or nose

- Drink from the same glass or eat from the same plate as a sick person

- Touch sores on the skin caused by group A strep (impetigo)

Rarely, people can spread group A strep through food that is not handled properly. Experts do not believe pets or household items, such as toys, spread these bacteria.

Common Signs and Symptoms of Scarlet Fever

- Very red, sore throat

- Fever (101°F or higher)
- Whitish coating on the tongue early in the illness
- "Strawberry" (red and bumpy) tongue
- Red skin rash that has a sandpaper feel
- Bright red skin in the creases of the underarm, elbow, and groin (the area where your stomach meets your thighs)
- Swollen glands in the neck

Other general symptoms:

- Headache or body aches
- Nausea, vomiting, or abdominal pain

Children and Certain Adults Are at Increased Risk

Anyone can get scarlet fever, but there are some factors that can increase the risk of getting this infection.

Scarlet fever such as strep throat is more common in children than adults. It is most common in children 5 through 15 years old. It is rare in children younger than 3 years old.

Close contact with another person with scarlet fever is the most common risk factor for illness. For example, if someone has scarlet fever, it often spreads to other people in their household.

Infectious illnesses tend to spread wherever large groups of people gather together. Crowded conditions can increase the risk of getting a group A strep infection. These settings include:

- Schools
- Day-care centers
- Military training facilities

Doctors Can Test for and Treat Scarlet Fever

Many viruses and bacteria can cause an illness that includes a red rash and a sore throat. Only a rapid strep test or a throat culture can determine if group A strep is the cause.

A rapid strep test involves swabbing the throat and testing the swab. The test quickly shows if group A strep is causing the illness. If the test is positive, doctors can prescribe antibiotics. If the test is negative, but a doctor still suspects scarlet fever, then the doctor can take a throat culture swab. A throat culture takes time to see if group A strep bacteria grow from the swab. While it takes more time, a throat culture sometimes finds infections that the rapid strep test misses. Culture is important to use in children and teens since they can get a rheumatic fever from an untreated scarlet fever infection.

Antibiotics Get You Well Fast

Doctors treat scarlet fever with antibiotics. Either penicillin or amoxicillin is recommended as the first choice for those who are not allergic to penicillin. Doctors can use other antibiotics to treat scarlet fever in those who are allergic to penicillin.

Benefits of antibiotics include:

- Decreasing how long someone is sick

- Decreasing symptoms (feeling better)

- Preventing the bacteria from spreading to others

- Preventing serious complications such as rheumatic fever

Long-Term Health Problems Are Not Common But Can Happen

Complications are rare but can occur after having scarlet fever. This can happen if the bacteria spread to other parts of the body. Complications can include:

- Abscesses (pockets of pus) around the tonsils

- Swollen lymph nodes in the neck

- Ear, sinus, and skin infections

- Pneumonia (lung infection)

- Rheumatic fever (a heart disease)

- Poststreptococcal glomerulonephritis (a kidney disease)

- Arthritis (joint inflammation)

Treatment with antibiotics can prevent most of these health problems.

Protect Yourself and Others

A person can get scarlet fever more than once. Having scarlet fever does not protect someone from getting it again in the future. While there is no vaccine to prevent scarlet fever, there are things people can do to protect themselves and others.

Good Hygiene Helps Prevent Group A Strep Infections

The best way to keep from getting or spreading group A strep is to wash your hands often. This is especially important after coughing or sneezing and before preparing foods or eating. To practice good hygiene you should:

- Cover your mouth and nose with a tissue when you cough or sneeze

- Put your used tissue in the wastebasket

- Cough or sneeze into your upper sleeve or elbow, not your hands, if you do not have a tissue

- Wash your hands often with soap and water for at least 20 seconds

- Use an alcohol-based hand rub if soap and water are not available

You should also wash glasses, utensils, and plates after someone who is sick uses them. These items are safe for others to use once washed.

Antibiotics Help Prevent Spreading the Infection to Others

A person with scarlet fever should stay home from work, school, or day care until they:

- No longer have a fever

- Have taken antibiotics for at least 24 hours

Take the prescription exactly as the doctor says to. Do not stop taking the medicine, even if you or your child feel better, unless the doctor says to stop.

Section 10.5

Strep Throat

This section includes text excerpted from "Strep Throat:
All You Need to Know," Centers for Disease Control
and Prevention (CDC), November 1, 2018.

Bacteria Cause Strep Throat

Viruses are the most common cause of a sore throat. However, strep throat is an infection in the throat and tonsils caused by bacteria called "group A *Streptococcus* (group A strep)."

How You Get Strep Throat

Group A strep live in the nose and throat and can easily spread to other people. It is important to know that all infected people do not have symptoms or seem sick. People who are infected spread the bacteria by coughing or sneezing, which creates small respiratory droplets that contain the bacteria.

Children can get sick if they:

- Breathe in those droplets

- Touch something with droplets on it and then touch their mouth or nose

- Drink from the same glass or eat from the same plate as a sick person

- Touch sores on the skin caused by group A strep (impetigo)

Rarely, people can spread group A strep through food that is not handled properly. Experts do not believe pets or household items, such as toys, spread these bacteria.

Pain and Fever without a Cough Are Common Signs and Symptoms

In general, strep throat is a mild infection, but it can be very painful. The most common symptoms of strep throat include:

- Sore throat that can start very quickly

- Pain when swallowing

- Fever

- Red and swollen tonsils, sometimes with white patches or streaks of pus

- Tiny, red spots (petechiae) on the roof of the mouth (the soft or hard palate)

- Swollen lymph nodes in the front of the neck

Other symptoms in children may include headache, stomach pain, nausea, or vomiting. Someone with strep throat may also have a rash known as "scarlet fever" (also called "scarlatina").

The following symptoms suggest a virus is the cause of the illness instead of strep throat:

- Cough

- Runny nose

- Hoarseness (changes in your voice that make it sound breathy, raspy, or strained)

- Conjunctivitis (also called "pink eye")

It usually takes two to five days for someone exposed to group A strep to become ill.

Children and Certain Adults Are at Increased Risk

Anyone can get strep throat, but there are some factors that can increase the risk of getting this common infection.

Strep throat is more common in children than adults. It is most common in children 5 through 15 years old. It is rare in children younger than 3 years old.

Close contact with another person with strep throat is the most common risk factor for illness. For example, if someone has strep throat, it often spreads to other people in their household.

Infectious illnesses tend to spread wherever large groups of people gather together. Crowded conditions can increase the risk of getting a group A strep infection. These settings include:

- Schools

- Day-care centers

- Military training facilities

A Simple Test Gives Fast Results

Only a rapid strep test or throat culture can determine if group A strep is the cause. A doctor cannot tell if someone has strep throat just by looking at her or his throat.

A rapid strep test involves swabbing the throat and running a test on the swab. The test quickly shows if group A strep is causing the illness. If the test is positive, doctors can prescribe antibiotics. If the test is negative, but the doctor still suspects strep throat, then the doctor can take a throat culture swab. A throat culture takes time to see if group A strep bacteria grow from the swab. While it takes more time, a throat culture sometimes finds infections that the rapid strep test misses. Culture is important to use in children and teens since they can get a rheumatic fever from an untreated strep throat infection.

Antibiotics Get You Well Fast

Doctors treat strep throat with antibiotics. Either penicillin or amoxicillin is recommended as the first choice for children who are not allergic to penicillin. Doctors can use other antibiotics to treat strep throat in children who are allergic to penicillin.

Benefits of antibiotics include:

- Decreasing how long someone is sick

- Decreasing symptoms (feeling better)

- Preventing the bacteria from spreading to others

- Preventing serious complications such as rheumatic fever

Someone who tests positive for strep throat but has no symptoms (called a "carrier") usually does not need antibiotics. They are less likely to spread the bacteria to others and very unlikely to get complications. If a carrier gets a sore throat illness caused by a virus, the rapid strep test can be positive. In these cases, it can be hard to know what is causing the sore throat. If someone keeps getting a sore throat after taking the right antibiotics, they may be a strep carrier and have a viral throat infection. Talk to a doctor if you think your child may be a strep carrier.

Serious Complications Are Not Common But Can Happen

Complications can occur after a strep throat infection. This can happen if the bacteria spread to other parts of the body.

Complications can include:

- Abscesses (pockets of pus) around the tonsils
- Swollen lymph nodes in the neck
- Sinus infections
- Ear infections
- Rheumatic fever (a heart disease)
- Poststreptococcal glomerulonephritis (a kidney disease)

Protect Yourself and Others

Children can get strep throat more than once. Having strep throat does not protect someone from getting it again in the future. While there is no vaccine to prevent strep throat, there are things children can do to protect themselves and others.

Good Hygiene Helps Prevent Group A Strep Infections

The best way to keep from getting or spreading group A strep is to wash your hands often. This is especially important after coughing or sneezing and before preparing foods or eating. To practice good hygiene you should:

- Cover your mouth and nose with a tissue when you cough or sneeze
- Put your used tissue in the wastebasket
- Cough or sneeze into your upper sleeve or elbow, not your hands, if you do not have a tissue
- Wash your hands often with soap and water for at least 20 seconds
- Use an alcohol-based hand rub if soap and water are not available

You should also wash glasses, utensils, and plates after someone who is sick uses them. These items are safe for others to use once washed.

Antibiotics Help Prevent Spreading the Infection to Others

Children with strep throat should stay home from work, school, or day care until they:

- No longer have a fever

- Have taken antibiotics for at least 24 hours

Take the prescription exactly as the doctor says to. Do not stop taking the medicine, even if you or your child feel better unless the doctor says to stop.

Wash your hands often to help prevent germs from spreading.

Chapter 11

Other Bacterial Infections

Chapter Contents

Section 11.1

Cat Scratch Disease

This section includes text excerpted from "Cat Scratch Disease FAQs," Centers for Disease Control and Prevention (CDC), January 11, 2016. Reviewed September 2019.

What Is Cat Scratch Disease?

Cat scratch disease (CSD) is a bacterial infection caused by *Bartonella henselae* bacteria. Most infections usually occur after scratches from domestic or feral cats, especially kittens. CSD occurs wherever cats and fleas are found. The most common symptoms include fever; enlarged, tender lymph nodes that develop one to three weeks after exposure; and a scab or pustule at the scratch site. In the United States, most cases occur in the fall and winter and illness is most common in children less than 15 years old.

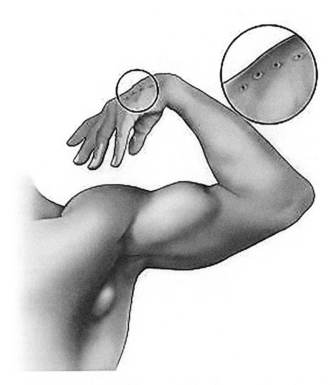

Figure 11.1. *Swollen Lymph Node in Armpit and Cat Scratch on Hand*

Symptoms of Cat Scratch Disease

- Low-grade fever
- Enlarged, tender lymph nodes that develop one to three weeks after exposure
- A papule or pustule at the site of the scratch

Rarely, eye infections, severe muscle pain, or encephalitis (swelling of the brain) may occur.

Transmission of Cat Scratch Disease

Children can get CSD from the scratches of domestic or feral cats, particularly kittens. The disease occurs most frequently in children under 15. Cats can be infested with infected fleas that carry *Bartonella* bacteria. These bacteria can be transmitted from a cat to a person during a scratch. Some evidence suggests that CSD may be spread directly to people by the bite of infected cat fleas, although this has not been proven.

Cat scratch disease occurs worldwide, wherever cats live. Stray cats may be more likely than pets to carry *Bartonella*. In the United States, most cases of CSD occur in the fall and winter.

Ticks may carry some species of *Bartonella* bacteria, but there is currently no causal evidence that ticks can transmit *Bartonella* infection to people through their bites.

Prevention of Cat Scratch Disease

- Avoid rough play with cats, particularly strays and kittens, to prevent scratches. This is especially important for people who have weakened immune systems. Wash hands promptly after handling cats.
- Treat cats for fleas using fipronil and other spot-on treatments. Check with your veterinarian. Products that contain permethrin should not be used on cats.
- Use a flea collar or similar topical preventive on dogs (fipronil, methoprene, imidacloprid, or permethrin), especially if you have both cats and dogs in your household.
- Keep cats indoors and away from stray cats.
- People who have weakened immune systems should avoid owning cats less than one-year-old.

Treatment of Catscratch Disease

The use of antibiotics to shorten the course of disease is debated. Most cases of CSD resolve without treatment, although some patients may develop complications from disseminated disease. Azithromycin has been shown to decrease lymph node volume more rapidly compared to no treatment. The recommended dose of azithromycin for CSD for children is ≤ 45.5 kg: 10 mg/kg on day 1, followed by 5 mg/kg for 4 days.

A number of other antibiotics are effective against *Bartonella* infections, including penicillins, tetracyclines, cephalosporins, and aminoglycosides. Since aminoglycosides are bactericidal, they are typically used as first-line treatment for *Bartonella* infections other than CSD. Often, with serious infections, more than one antibiotic is used.

Trench fever, Carrión's disease, and endocarditis due to *Bartonella* spp. are serious infections that require antibiotic treatment.

Section 11.2

Diphtheria

This section includes text excerpted from "Diphtheria," Centers for Disease Control and Prevention (CDC), December 17, 2018.

Diphtheria is an infection caused by the bacterium *Corynebacterium diphtheriae*. Diphtheria causes a thick covering in the back of the throat. It can lead to difficulty breathing, heart failure, paralysis, and even death. The Centers for Disease Control and Prevention (CDC) recommends vaccines for infants, children, and teens to prevent diphtheria.

Starting in the 1920s, diphtheria rates dropped quickly in the United States and other countries with the widespread use of vaccines. In the past decade, there were less than 5 cases of diphtheria in the United States reported to CDC. However, the disease continues to cause illness globally. In 2016, countries reported about 7,100 cases of diphtheria to the World Health Organization (WHO), but there are likely many more cases.

Causes and Transmission of Diphtheria

Diphtheria spreads (transmits) from person to person, usually through respiratory droplets, such as from coughing or sneezing. Rarely, people can get sick from touching open sores (skin lesions) or clothes that touched open sores of someone sick with diphtheria. A person also can get diphtheria by coming in contact with an object, such as a toy, that has the bacteria that cause diphtheria on it.

Symptoms of Diphtheria

Bacteria that cause diphtheria can get into and attach to the lining of the respiratory system, which includes parts of the body that help you breathe. When this happens, the bacteria can produce a poison (toxin) that can cause:

- Weakness
- Sore throat
- Fever
- Swollen glands in the neck

The poison destroys healthy tissues in the respiratory system. Within two to three days, the dead tissue forms a thick, gray coating that can build up in the throat or nose. Medical experts call this thick gray coating a "pseudomembrane." It can cover tissues in the nose, tonsils, voice box, and throat, making it very hard to breathe and swallow.

The poison may also get into the bloodstream and cause damage to the heart, nerves, and kidneys.

Complications of Diphtheria

Complications from diphtheria may include:

- Blocking of the airway
- Damage to the heart muscle (myocarditis)
- Nerve damage (polyneuropathy)
- Loss of the ability to move (paralysis)
- Lung infection (respiratory failure or pneumonia)

For some people, diphtheria can lead to death. Even with treatment, about 1 in 10 diphtheria patients die. Without treatment, up to half of the patients can die from the disease.

Diagnosis and Treatment of Diphtheria

Doctors usually decide if a person has diphtheria by looking for common signs and symptoms. They can use a swab from the back of the throat and test it for the bacteria that cause diphtheria. A doctor can also take a sample from a skin lesion (such as a sore) and try and grow the bacteria. If the bacteria grow, the doctor can be sure a patient has diphtheria.

It is important to start treatment right away if a doctor suspects diphtheria and not to wait for laboratory confirmation. In the United States, before there was a treatment for diphtheria, up to half of the people who got the disease died from it.

Diphtheria treatment today involves:

- Using diphtheria antitoxin to stop the poison (toxin) produced by the bacteria from damaging the body

- Using antibiotics to kill and get rid of the bacteria

People with diphtheria are usually no longer able to infect others 48 hours after they begin taking antibiotics. However, it is important to finish taking the full course of antibiotics to make sure the bacteria are completely removed from the body. After the patient finishes the full treatment, the doctor will run tests to make sure the bacteria are not in the patient's body anymore.

Prevention of Diphtheria

Getting vaccinated is the best way to prevent diphtheria. In the United States, there are four vaccines used to prevent diphtheria: Diphtheria-tetanus-pertussis (DTaP), Tetanus, diphtheria, and pertussis (Tdap), diphtheria and tetanus (DT), and tetanus and diphtheria (TD). Each of these vaccines prevents diphtheria and tetanus; DTaP and Tdap also help prevent pertussis (whooping cough). Healthcare professionals give DTaP and DT to children younger than seven years old, while older children and teens get Tdap.

Babies and Children

The current childhood immunization schedule by the CDC for diphtheria includes five doses of DTaP for children younger than seven years old.

Preteens and Teens

The adolescent immunization schedule by the CDC recommends that preteens get a booster dose of Tdap at 11 or 12 years old. Teens who did not get Tdap when they were 11 or 12 years old should get a dose the next time they see their doctor.

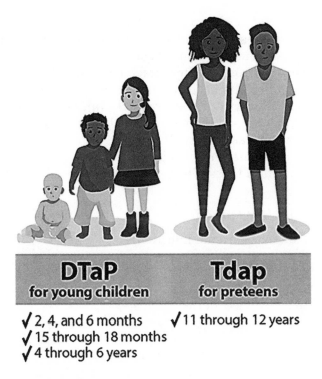

DTaP
for young children

Tdap
for preteens

✓ 2, 4, and 6 months   ✓ 11 through 12 years
✓ 15 through 18 months
✓ 4 through 6 years

Figure 11.2. *Diptheria Vaccines for Children* (Source: "People of All Ages Need Diphtheria Vaccines," Centers for Disease Control and Prevention (CDC).)

Section 11.3

Haemophilus influenza Type B

This section includes text excerpted from "*Haemophilus influenzae* Disease (Including Hib)," Centers for Disease Control and Prevention (CDC), February 13, 2018.

Haemophilus influenzae, a type of bacteria, can cause many different kinds of infections. These infections range from mild ear infections to severe diseases, such as bloodstream infections.

Doctors consider some of these infections "invasive." Invasive disease happens when the bacteria invade parts of the body that are normally free from germs. For example, *H. influenzae* can invade the spinal fluid, causing meningitis, or the bloodstream, causing bacteremia. Invasive disease is usually severe, requiring treatment in a hospital, and can sometimes result in death.

The most common types of invasive disease caused by *H. influenzae* are:

- Pneumonia* (lung infection)

- Bacteremia (bloodstream infection)

- Meningitis (infection of the tissue covering of the brain and spinal cord)

- Epiglottitis (swelling in the throat)

- Cellulitis (skin infection)

- Infectious arthritis (inflammation of the joint)

H. influenzae can also be a common cause of ear infections in children.

*Doctors consider pneumonia an invasive infection when H. influenzae *also infects the blood or pleural fluid (fluid surrounding the lungs).*

Causes of Haemophilus influenzae *Infections*

Haemophilus influenzae disease refers to any infection caused by *H. influenzae* bacteria. There are six identifiable types of *H. influenzae* (named a through f) and other nonidentifiable types (called "nontypeable"). The one that people are most familiar with is *H. influenzae* type b or Hib.

These bacteria live in people's nose and throat and usually cause no harm. However, the bacteria can sometimes move to other parts of the body and cause infection.

Experts do not know how long it takes after *H. influenzae* enters a person's body for someone to get sick. However, it could take as little as a few days before symptoms appear.

How It Spreads

People spread *H. influenzae*, including Hib, to others through respiratory droplets. This happens when someone who has the bacteria in their nose or throat coughs or sneezes. People who are not sick but have the bacteria in their noses and throats can still spread the bacteria. That is how *H. influenzae* spreads most of the time.

The bacteria can also spread to people who have close or lengthy contact with a person with *H. influenzae* disease.

People at Increased Risk

H. influenzae, including Hib, disease occurs mostly in babies and children younger than five years old.

Signs and Symptoms of Haemophilus influenzae Infections

Haemophilus influenzae, including *H. influenzae* type b or Hib, can cause many different kinds of infections. Symptoms depend on the part of the body that is infected.

Pneumonia

Symptoms of pneumonia (lung infection) usually include:

- Fever and chills
- Cough
- Shortness of breath or difficulty breathing
- Sweating
- Chest pain
- Headache
- Muscle pain or aches
- Excessive tiredness

Bacteremia

Bacteremia is an infection of the bloodstream. Symptoms of bacteremia include:

- Fever and chills
- Excessive tiredness
- Pain in the belly
- Nausea with or without vomiting
- Diarrhea
- Anxiety
- Shortness of breath or difficulty breathing
- Altered mental status (confusion)

Bacteremia from *H. influenzae* can occur with or without pneumonia.

Meningitis

Meningitis is an infection of the tissue covering the brain and spinal cord. Symptoms of meningitis typically include sudden onset of:

- Fever
- Headache
- Stiff neck
- Nausea with or without vomiting
- Photophobia (eyes being more sensitive to light)
- Altered-mental status (confusion)

Babies with meningitis may be irritable, vomit, feed poorly, or appear to be slow or inactive. In young babies, doctors may also test the child's reflexes, which can be abnormal with meningitis.

Diagnosis of Haemophilus influenzae *Infections*

Doctors usually diagnose *Haemophilus influenzae*, including *H. influenzae type b* or Hib, infection with one or more laboratory tests. The most common testing methods use a sample of body fluids, such as blood or spinal fluid.

Treatment of Haemophilus influenzae *Infections*

People diagnosed with *H. influenzae*, including Hib, disease take antibiotics, usually for 10 days, to treat the infection. Depending on how serious the infection is, people with *H. influenzae* infection may need care in a hospital. Other treatments may include:

- Breathing support

- Medication to treat low blood pressure

- Wound care for parts of the body with damaged skin

When *H. influenzae* cause milder infections, such as bronchitis or ear infections, doctors may give antibiotics to prevent complications.

Complications of Haemophilus influenzae *Infections*

Even with appropriate treatment, some *H. influenzae* infections can result in long-term problems or death. For example, blood infections (bacteremia) can result in loss of limbs. Meningitis (infection of the tissue covering the brain and spinal cord) can cause brain damage or hearing loss. A small number (3 to 6 in 100) of children with meningitis caused by Hib die from the disease.

Complications are rare and typically not severe for bronchitis and ear infections caused by *H. influenzae*.

Prevention of Haemophilus influenzae *Infections*
Vaccine

A vaccine can prevent *Haemophilus influenzae type b* (Hib) disease. Before the vaccine, Hib was the most common cause of serious *H. influenzae* disease. However, the Hib vaccine does not prevent disease caused by the other types of *H. influenzae*.

The CDC recommends Hib vaccine for all children younger than two years old in the United States. Babies start getting the Hib vaccine at two months old (they need multiple doses for best protection).

Older children and adults usually do not need a Hib vaccine. However, the CDC recommends Hib vaccination for people with certain medical conditions. Talk to your or your child's healthcare professional about what is best for your specific situation.

Reinfection

People can get *H. influenzae* more than once. Therefore, the CDC recommends Hib vaccination for all children younger than two years old who had Hib disease. Vaccinating young children gives them the best protection when they are at increased risk for Hib disease.

Preventive Antibiotics

H. influenzae can spread to people who have close or lengthy contact with a person with *H. influenzae* disease. In certain cases, close contacts of someone with *H. influenzae* disease should receive antibiotics to prevent them from getting sick. A doctor or local health department will make recommendations for who should receive antibiotics.

Vaccine

A vaccine can prevent *H. influenzae* type b (Hib) disease. Before the vaccine, Hib was the most common cause of serious *H. influenzae* disease. However, the Hib vaccine does not prevent disease caused by the other types of H. influenzae.

The CDC recommends Hib vaccine for all children younger than two years old in the United States. Babies start getting the Hib vaccine at two months old (they need multiple doses for best protection).

Older children and adults usually do not need a Hib vaccine. However, the CDC recommends Hib vaccination for people with certain medical conditions. Talk to your or your child's healthcare professional about what is best for your specific situation.

Reinfection

People can get H. influenzae more than once. Therefore, the CDC recommends Hib vaccination for all children younger than two years old who had Hib disease. Vaccinating young children gives them the best protection when they are at increased risk for Hib disease.

Preventive Antibiotics

H. influenzae can spread to people who have close or lengthy contact with a person with *H. influenzae* disease. In certain cases, close contacts of someone with *H. influenzae* disease should receive antibiotics to prevent them from getting sick. A doctor or local health department will make recommendations for who should receive antibiotics.

Section 11.4

Lyme Disease

This section includes text excerpted from "Lyme Disease," Centers for Disease Control and Prevention (CDC), June 3, 2019.

Lyme disease is caused by the bacterium *Borrelia burgdorferi* and is transmitted to humans through the bite of infected black-legged ticks. Typical symptoms include fever, headache, fatigue, and a characteristic skin rash called "erythema migrans." If left untreated, infection can spread to joints, the heart, and the nervous system.

Lyme disease is diagnosed based on symptoms, physical findings (e.g., rash), and the possibility of exposure to infected ticks. Laboratory testing is helpful if used correctly and performed with validated methods. Most cases of Lyme disease can be treated successfully with a few weeks of antibiotics. Steps to prevent Lyme disease include using insect repellent, removing ticks promptly, applying pesticides, and reducing tick habitat. The ticks that transmit Lyme disease can occasionally transmit other tick-borne diseases as well.

Signs and Symptoms of Untreated Lyme Disease

Untreated Lyme disease can produce a wide range of symptoms, depending on the stage of infection. These include fever, rash, facial paralysis, and arthritis. Seek medical attention if you observe any of these symptoms and have had a tick bite, live in an area known for Lyme disease, or have recently traveled to an area where Lyme disease occurs.

Early Signs and Symptoms (3 to 30 Days after Tick Bite)

- Fever, chills, headache, fatigue, muscle and joint aches, and swollen lymph nodes

- Erythema migrans (EM) rash:

  - Occurs in approximately 70 to 80 percent of infected persons

  - Begins at the site of a tick bite after a delay of 3 to 30 days (average is about 7 days)

  - Expands gradually over a period of days reaching up to 12 inches or more (30 cm) across

- May feel warm to the touch but is rarely itchy or painful
- Sometimes clears as it enlarges, resulting in a target or "bull's-eye" appearance
- May appear on any area of the body

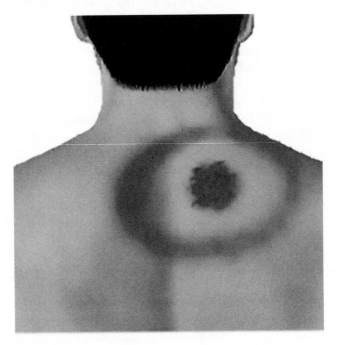

Figure 11.3. *"Classic" Erythema Migrans Rash*

Later Signs and Symptoms (Days to Months after Tick Bite)

- Severe headaches and neck stiffness
- Additional EM rashes on other areas of the body
- Arthritis with severe joint pain and swelling, particularly the knees and other large joints.
- Facial palsy (loss of muscle tone or droop on one or both sides of the face)
- Intermittent pain in tendons, muscles, joints, and bones
- Heart palpitations or an irregular heartbeat (Lyme carditis)

- Episodes of dizziness or shortness of breath
- Inflammation of the brain and spinal cord
- Nerve pain
- Shooting pains, numbness, or tingling in the hands or feet
- Problems with short-term memory

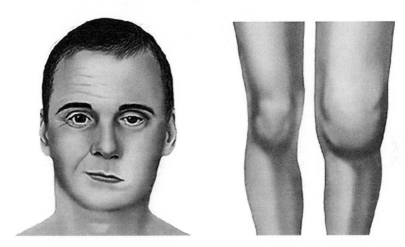

Figure 11.4. *Facial Palsy and Swollen Knee*

Causes of Lyme Disease

The Lyme disease bacterium, *Borrelia burgdorferi*, is spread through the bite of infected ticks. The black-legged tick (or deer tick, *Ixodes scapularis*) spreads the disease in the northeastern, mid-Atlantic, and north-central United States. The western black-legged tick (*Ixodes pacificus*) spreads the disease on the Pacific Coast.

Ticks can attach to any part of the human body but are often found in hard-to-see areas such as the groin, armpits, and scalp. In most cases, the tick must be attached for 36 to 48 hours or more before the Lyme disease bacterium can be transmitted.

Most humans are infected through the bites of immature ticks called "nymphs." Nymphs are tiny (less than 2 mm) and difficult to see; they feed during the spring and summer months. Adult ticks can also transmit Lyme disease bacteria, but they are much larger and are more likely to be discovered and removed before they have had time to transmit the bacteria. Adult *Ixodes* ticks are most active during the cooler months of the year.

Diagnosis and Testing of Lyme Disease

When assessing a patient for Lyme disease, healthcare providers should consider:

- The signs and symptoms of Lyme disease
- The likelihood that the patient has been exposed to infected black-legged ticks
- The possibility that other illnesses may cause similar symptoms
- Results of laboratory tests, when indicated

Laboratory Testing

The Centers for Disease Control and Prevention (CDC) currently recommends a two-step testing process for Lyme disease. Both steps are required and can be done using the same blood sample. If this first step is negative, no further testing is recommended. If the first step is positive or indeterminate (sometimes called "equivocal"), the second step should be performed. The overall result is positive only when the first test is positive (or equivocal) and the second test is positive (or equivocal).

Key Points to Remember

- Most Lyme disease tests are designed to detect antibodies made by the body in response to infection.
- Antibodies can take several weeks to develop, so patients may test negative if infected only recently.
- Antibodies normally persist in the blood for months or even years after the infection is gone; therefore, the test cannot be used to determine a cure.
- Infection with other diseases, including some tickborne diseases, or some viral, bacterial, or autoimmune diseases, can result in false-positive test results.

Treatment of Lyme Disease

People treated with appropriate antibiotics in the early stages of Lyme disease usually recover rapidly and completely. Antibiotics commonly used for oral treatment include doxycycline, amoxicillin, or cefuroxime axetil. People with certain neurological or cardiac forms of illness may require intravenous treatment with antibiotics, such as ceftriaxone or penicillin.

Treatment regimens listed in the following table are for localized (early) Lyme disease.

These regimens are guidelines only and may need to be adjusted depending on a person's age, medical history, underlying health conditions, or allergies.

Table 11.1. Treatment for Early Lyme Disease

Age Category	Drug	Dosage	Maximum	Duration, Days
	Amoxicillin	50 mg/kg per day orally, divided into 3 doses	500 mg per dose	14 to 21
	Doxycycline	4 mg/kg per day orally, divided into 2 doses	100 mg per dose	10 to 21*
Children	Cefuroxime axetil	30 mg/kg per day orally, divided into 2 doses	500 mg per dose	14 to 21

Note: *For people intolerant of amoxicillin, doxycycline, and cefuroxime axetil, the macrolides azithromycin, clarithromycin, or erythromycin may be used, although they have a lower efficacy. People treated with macrolides should be closely monitored to ensure that symptoms resolve*
*Recent publications suggest the efficacy of shorter courses of treatment for early Lyme disease.

The National Institutes of Health (NIH) has funded several studies on the treatment of Lyme disease that show most people recover when treated within a few weeks of antibiotics taken by mouth. In a small percentage of cases, symptoms such as fatigue (being tired) and muscle aches can last for more than six months. This condition is known as "post-treatment Lyme disease syndrome" (PTLDS), although it is often called "chronic Lyme disease."

Section 11.5

Methicillin-Resistant Staphylococcus aureus

This section includes text excerpted from "Methicillin-Resistant
Staphylococcus aureus (MRSA)," National Institute of
Allergy and Infectious Diseases (NIAID), June 22, 2015.
Reviewed September 2019.

During the past four decades, a type of bacteria has evolved from
a controllable nuisance into a serious public health concern. This bacterium is known as "methicillin-resistant *Staphylococcus aureus*," or
MRSA. About one-third of people in the world have *S. aureus* bacteria
on their bodies at any given time, primarily in the nose and on the
skin. The bacteria can be present without causing an active infection.
Of the people with *S. aureus* present, about one percent has MRSA,
according to the Centers for Disease Control and Prevention (CDC).

Methicillin-resistant *Staphylococcus aureus* can be categorized
according to where the infection was acquired: hospital-acquired
MRSA (HA-MRSA) or community-associated MRSA (CA-MRSA).

Hospital-Acquired MRSA

Hospital-acquired MRSA is acquired in the hospital setting and
is one of many hospital-acquired infections exhibiting increased
antimicrobial resistance. HA-MRSA has increased during the past
decade due to a number of factors including an increased number of
immunocompromised and elderly patients; an increase in the number of invasive procedures, e.g., advanced surgical operations and
life-support treatments; and failures in infection control measures,
such as hand washing prior to patient contact and removal of nones-
sential catheters.

Community-Associated MRSA

Community-associated MRSA is caused by newly emerging strains
unlike those responsible for HA-MRSA and can cause infections in otherwise healthy persons with no links to healthcare systems. CA-MRSA
infections typically occur as skin or soft tissue infections, but can
develop into more invasive, life-threatening infections. CA-MRSA is
occurring with increasing frequency in the United States and around
the world and tends to occur in conditions where people are in close
physical contact, such as athletes involved in football and wrestling,

soldiers kept in close quarters, inmates, childcare workers, and residents of long-term care facilities.

Methicillin-resistant *Staphylococcus aureus* has attracted the attention of the medical research community, illustrating the urgent need to develop better ways to diagnose and treat bacterial infections.

Transmission of MRSA

Over the years *S. aureus* has evolved to the point where experts refer to MRSA in terms ranging from a considerable public-health burden to a crisis. The bacteria have been classified into two categories based on where the infection is first acquired.

Hospital-Acquired MRSA (HA-MRSA)

Hospital-acquired MRSA has been recognized for decades and primarily affects people in healthcare settings, such as those who have had surgery or medical devices surgically implanted. This source of MRSA is typically problematic for the elderly, for people with weakened immune systems, and for patients undergoing kidney dialysis or using venous catheters or prosthetics.

A study published in 2005 found that nearly one percent of all hospital in-patient stays, or 292,045 per year, were associated with *S. aureus* infection. The study reviewed nearly 14 million patient discharge diagnoses from 2000 and 2001. Patients with diagnoses of *S. aureus* infection, when compared with those without the infection, had about three times the length of stay, three times the total cost, and five times the risk of in-hospital death. Notably, the S. aureus infections in this hospital study resulted in 14,000 deaths.

Community-Associated MRSA (CA-MRSA)

Community-associated MRSA has only been known since the 1990s. CA-MRSA is of great concern to public health professionals because of who it can affect. Unlike the hospital sources, which usually can be traced to a specific exposure, the origin of CA-MRSA infection can be elusive. CA-MRSA skin infections are known to spread in crowded settings; in situations where there is close skin-to-skin contact; when personal items, such as towels, razors, and sporting equipment is shared; when personal hygiene is compromised; and when healthcare is limited.

Outbreaks of CA-MRSA have involved bacterial strains with specific microbiologic and genetic differences from traditional HA-MRSA

151

strains, and these differences suggest that community strains might spread more easily from person to person than HA-MRSA. While CA-MRSA is resistant to penicillin and methicillin, they can still be treated with other common-use antibiotics.

Community-associated MRSA most often enters the body through a cut or scrape and appears in the form of a skin or soft tissue infection, such as a boil or abscess. The involved site is red, swollen, and painful and is often mistaken for a spider bite. Though rare, CA-MRSA can develop into more serious invasive infections, such as bloodstream infections or pneumonia, leading to a variety of other symptoms including shortness of breath, fever, chills, and death. CA-MRSA can be particularly dangerous in children because their immune systems are not fully developed.

You should pay attention to minor skin problems, such as pimples, insect bites, cuts, and scrapes, in children. If the wound appears to be infected, see a healthcare provider.

Researchers continue to study information about these cases in an attempt to determine why certain groups of people become ill when exposed to these strains. Researchers also continue to try to understand why high-incidence areas may appear. For example, for unknown reasons, severe outbreaks have occurred in Alaska, Georgia, and Louisiana.

Diagnosis of MRSA

To diagnose *S. aureus*, a sample is obtained from the infection site and sent to a microbiology laboratory for testing. If *S. aureus* is found, the organism should be further tested to determine which antibiotic would be effective for treatment.

Doctors often diagnose MRSA by checking a tissue sample or nasal secretions for signs of drug-resistant bacteria. Current diagnostic procedures involve sending a sample to a lab where it is placed in a dish of nutrients that encourage bacterial growth (a culture). It takes about 48 hours for the bacteria to grow. However, newer tests that can detect staph deoxyribonucleic acid (DNA) in a matter of hours are now becoming more widely available. This will help healthcare providers decide on the proper treatment regimen for a patient more quickly, after an official diagnosis has been made.

In the hospital, you might be tested for MRSA if you show signs of infection, or if you are transferred to a hospital from another healthcare setting where MRSA is known to be present. You also might be tested if you have had a previous history of MRSA.

Treatment of MRSA

Healthcare providers can treat many *S. aureus* skin infections by draining the abscess or boil and may not need to use antibiotics. Draining of skin boils or abscesses should only be done by a healthcare provider.

For mild to moderate skin infections, incision and drainage by a healthcare provider is the first-line treatment. Before prescribing antibiotics, your provider will consider the potential for antibiotic resistance. Thus, if MRSA is suspected, your provider will avoid treating you with beta-lactam antibiotics, a class of antibiotic observed not to be effective in killing the staph bacteria.

For severe infection, doctors will typically use vancomycin intravenously.

Prevention of MRSA

The best defense against spreading MRSA is to practice good hygiene, as follows:

- Keep your hands clean by washing thoroughly with soap and water. Scrub them briskly for at least 15 seconds, then dry them with a disposable towel and use another towel to turn off the faucet. When you do not have access to soap and water, carry a small bottle of hand sanitizer containing at least 62 percent alcohol.

- Always shower promptly after exercising.

- Keep cuts and scrapes clean and covered with a bandage until healed. Keep wounds that are draining or have pus covered with clean, dry bandages. Follow your healthcare provider's instructions on proper care of the wound. Pus from infected wounds can contain *S. aureus* and MRSA, so keeping the infection covered will help prevent the spread to others. Bandages or tape can be discarded with the regular trash.

- Avoid contact with other people's wounds or bandages.

- Avoid sharing personal items, such as towels, washcloths, razors, clothes, or uniforms.

- Wash sheets, towels, and clothes that become soiled with water and laundry detergent; use bleach and hot water if possible. Drying clothes in a hot dryer, rather than air-drying, also helps kill bacteria in clothes.

Tell any healthcare providers who treat you if you have or had an *S. aureus* or MRSA skin infection. If you have a skin infection that requires treatment, ask your healthcare provider if you should be tested for MRSA. Many healthcare providers prescribe drugs that are not effective against antibiotic-resistant staph, which delays treatment and creates more resistant germs.

Healthcare providers are fighting back against MRSA infection by tracking bacterial outbreaks and by investing in products, such as antibiotic-coated catheters and gloves that release disinfectants.

Section 11.6

Mycoplasma *Infection*

This section includes text excerpted from "*Mycoplasma pneumoniae* Infection," Centers for Disease Control and Prevention (CDC), January 2017.

Mycoplasma pneumoniae (*M. pneumoniae*) is a type of bacteria that can cause several different types of infection including chest colds and pneumonia (lung infection). To best protect yourself and others from this bacteria, practice good hygiene by washing your hands often and covering your mouth when you cough or sneeze.

Signs and Symptoms of Mycoplasma *Infection*

Mycoplasma pneumoniae causes illness by damaging the lining of the respiratory system (nose, throat, windpipe, and lungs). *M. pneumoniae* infections have long incubation periods (the time between first catching the bacteria and developing symptoms). Symptoms appear and worsen after a period of one to four weeks. The most common type of illness is tracheobronchitis, commonly known as a "chest cold." Symptoms of a chest cold often include:

- Sore throat

- Being tired (fatigue)

- Fever

- Headache

- Slowly worsening cough that can last for weeks or months

Children younger than five years old often do not have a fever, but may wheeze, vomit, or have diarrhea.

Mycoplasma pneumoniae can sometimes cause mild pneumonia, often referred to as "walking pneumonia" since the illness usually does not require treatment in a hospital. Less often *M. pneumoniae* causes more serious pneumonia, which does need treatment in a hospital. Symptoms of pneumonia caused by *M. pneumoniae* include fatigue, fever, pain when breathing, and a dry cough that produces little mucus.

Mycoplasma pneumoniae can rarely cause swelling in the brain (encephalitis). Symptoms of encephalitis typically include fever and severe headache, but can also include confusion, seizures (jerking or twitching of the muscles or staring), or problems with movement.

Certain People Are at Increased Risk

People of all ages are at risk for getting *M. pneumoniae* infection, but it is most common among young adults and school-aged children. *M. pneumoniae* infections most often spread among families who live in the same household as well as people who work or live in crowded settings, such as schools, nursing homes, and hospitals. People with weakened immune systems, those who have asthma, or those who are recovering from a respiratory illness are at increased risk for getting a more serious illness from this infection.

Spreads from Person to Person

Mycoplasma pneumoniae is spread when a person who is sick coughs or sneezes while in close contact with others who then breathe in the bacteria. Most people who are exposed for a short amount of time do not get sick. However, it is common for this illness to spread between family members who live together. If you are sick, be sure to cover your mouth when you cough or sneeze to help prevent spreading the bacteria to others.

Treatment of Mycoplasma Infection

Most cases of *M. pneumoniae* infection are mild and get better on their own without treatment. Antibiotics (medicines that kill bacteria in the body) are used to treat more serious infections, such as pneumonia.

Section 11.7

Pertussis

This section contains text excerpted from the following sources: Text in this section begins with excerpts from "Pertussis (Whooping Cough)," Centers for Disease Control and Prevention (CDC), August 7, 2017; Text beginning with the heading "Why Should My Child Get the DTaP Shot?" is excerpted from "For Parents: Vaccines for Your Children," Centers for Disease Control and Prevention (CDC), August 14, 2015. Reviewed September 2019.

Pertussis also known as "whooping cough," is a highly contagious respiratory disease. It is caused by the bacterium *Bordetella pertussis*.

Pertussis is known for uncontrollable, violent coughing which often makes it hard to breathe. After coughing fits, someone with pertussis often needs to take deep breaths, which result in a "whooping" sound. Pertussis can affect people of all ages, but can be very serious, even deadly, for babies less than a year old.

The best way to protect against pertussis is by getting vaccinated.

Causes of Pertussis

Pertussis is a very contagious disease caused by a type of bacteria called *"Bordetella pertussis."* These bacteria attach to the cilia (tiny, hair-like extensions) that line part of the upper respiratory system. The bacteria release toxins (poisons), which damage the cilia and cause the airways to swell.

Transmission of Pertussis

Pertussis is a very contagious disease only found in humans. Pertussis spreads from person to person. People with pertussis usually spread the disease to another person by coughing or sneezing or when spending a lot of time near one another where you share breathing space. Many babies who get pertussis are infected by older siblings, parents, or caregivers who might not even know they have the disease.

Infected people are most contagious up to about two weeks after the cough begins. Antibiotics may shorten the amount of time someone is contagious.

While pertussis vaccines are the most effective tool to prevent this disease, no vaccine is 100 percent effective. When pertussis circulates in the community, there is a chance that a fully vaccinated person, of any age, can catch this disease. If you have gotten the pertussis vaccine but still get sick, the infection is usually not as bad.

Signs and Symptoms of Pertussis

Pertussis (whooping cough) can cause serious illness in babies, children, teens, and adults. Symptoms of pertussis usually develop within 5 to 10 days after you are exposed. Sometimes pertussis symptoms do not develop for as long as three weeks.

Early Symptoms

The disease usually starts with cold-like symptoms and maybe a mild cough or fever. In babies, the cough can be minimal or not even there. Babies may have a symptom known as "apnea." Apnea is a pause in the child's breathing pattern. Pertussis is most dangerous for babies. About half of babies younger than one year who get the disease need care in the hospital.

Early symptoms can last for one to two weeks and usually include:

- Runny nose

- Low-grade fever (generally minimal throughout the course of the disease)

- Mild, occasional cough

- Apnea—a pause in breathing (in babies)

Pertussis in its early stages appears to be nothing more than the common cold. Therefore, healthcare professionals often do not suspect or diagnose it until more severe symptoms appear.

Later-Stage Symptoms

After one to two weeks and as the disease progresses, the traditional symptoms of pertussis may appear and include:

- Paroxysms (fits) of many, rapid coughs followed by a high-pitched "whoop" sound

- Vomiting (throwing up) during or after coughing fits

- Exhaustion (very tired) after coughing fits

Pertussis can cause violent and rapid coughing, over and over, until the air is gone from your lungs. When there is no more air in the lungs, you are forced to inhale with a loud "whooping" sound. This extreme coughing can cause you to throw up and be very tired. Although you are often exhausted after a coughing fit, you usually appear fairly well in-between. Coughing fits generally become more common and bad as the illness continues, and can occur more often at night. The coughing fits can go on for up to 10 weeks or more. In China, pertussis is known as the "100 day cough."

The "whoop" is often not there if you have a milder (less serious) disease. The infection is generally milder in teens and adults, especially those who have gotten the pertussis vaccine.

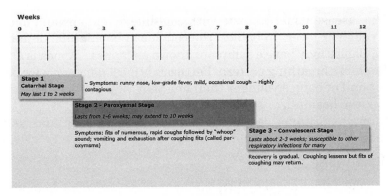

Figure 11.5. *Disease Progression: Pertussis*

Recovery

Recovery from pertussis can happen slowly. The cough becomes milder and less common. However, coughing fits can return with other respiratory infections for many months after the pertussis infection started.

Complications in Babies and Children

Pertussis (whooping cough) can cause serious and sometimes deadly complications in babies and young children, especially those who have not received all recommended pertussis vaccines.

About half of babies younger than one-year-old who get pertussis need care in the hospital. The younger the baby, the more likely they will need treatment in the hospital. Of those babies who are treated in the hospital with pertussis about:

- 1 out of 4 (23%) get pneumonia (lung infection)

- 1 out of 100 (1.1%) will have convulsions (violent, uncontrolled shaking)

- 3 out of 5 (61%) will have apnea (slowed or stopped breathing)

- 1 out of 300 (0.3%) will have encephalopathy (disease of the brain)

- 1 out of 100 (1%) will die

Diagnosis of Pertussis

Healthcare providers diagnose pertussis (whooping cough) by considering if you have been exposed to pertussis and by doing a:

- History of typical signs and symptoms

- Physical examination

- Laboratory test which involves taking a sample of mucus (with a swab or syringe filled with saline) from the back of the throat through the nose

- Blood test

Treatment of Pertussis

Healthcare providers generally treat pertussis with antibiotics and early treatment is very important. Treatment may make your infection less serious if you start it early before coughing fits begin. Treatment can also help prevent spreading the disease to close contacts (people who have spent a lot of time around the infected person). Treatment after three weeks of illness is unlikely to help. The bacteria are gone from your body by then, even though you usually will still have symptoms. This is because the bacteria have already done damage to your body.

There are several antibiotics (medications that can help treat diseases caused by bacteria) available to treat pertussis. If a healthcare professional diagnoses you or your child with pertussis, they will explain how to treat the infection.

Pertussis can sometimes be very serious, requiring treatment in the hospital. Babies are at greatest risk for serious complications from pertussis.

Prevention of Pertussis

The best way to protect babies and children from pertussis (whooping cough) is to make sure everyone gets vaccinated. Diphtheria-tetanus-pertussis shot (DTaP) is the recommended pertussis vaccine for babies and children. This is a combination vaccine that protects children against three diseases: diphtheria, tetanus, and pertussis. For maximum protection against pertussis, children need five DTaP shots, which begin at two months old.

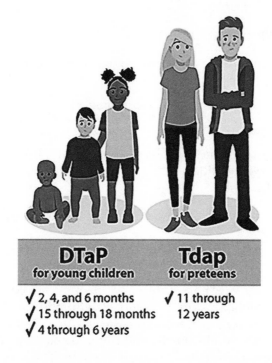

Figure 11.6. *Pertussis Vaccines for Children* (Source: "People of All Ages Need Whooping Caugh Vaccines," Centers for Disease Control and Prevention (CDC).)

Parents can also help protect their children by keeping them away, as much as possible, from anyone who has cold symptoms or a cough. Pregnant women should get the Tdap shot to help protect babies until they are old enough to receive DTaP vaccines.

Why Should My Child Get the Diphtheria-Tetanus-Pertussis Shot?

The DTaP shot:

- Helps protect your child from whooping cough, a potentially serious and even deadly disease, as well as diphtheria and tetanus

- Helps to prevent your child from having violent coughing fits from whooping cough

- Helps keep your child from missing school or childcare (and keeps you from missing work to care for your sick child)

Is the Diphtheria-Tetanus-Pertussis Shot Shot Safe?

Yes. The DTaP shot is very safe. Vaccines, like any medicine, can have side effects. Most children who get the DTaP shot have no side effects.

What Are the Side Effects?

Most children do not have any side effects from the shot. The side effects that do occur are usually mild and may include:

- Redness, swelling, or pain where the shot was given

- Fever

- Vomiting

These types of side effects happen in about one out of every four children who get the shot.

More serious side effects are very rare but can include:

- A fever over 105 degrees

- Nonstop crying for three hours or more

- Seizures (jerking, twitching of the muscles, or staring)

Section 11.8

Tetanus

This section includes text excerpted from "Tetanus," Centers for
Disease Control and Prevention (CDC), February 28, 2019.

Tetanus is an infection caused by bacteria called *"Clostridium tetani."* When the bacteria invade the body, they produce a poison (toxin) that causes painful muscle contractions. Another name for tetanus is "lockjaw." It often causes a person's neck and jaw muscles to lock, making it hard to open the mouth or swallow. The Centers for Disease Control and Prevention (CDC) recommends vaccines for infants, children, teens, and adults to prevent tetanus.

Tetanus is different from other vaccine-preventable diseases because it does not spread from person to person. The bacteria are usually found in soil, dust, and manure and enter the body through breaks in the skin—usually cuts or puncture wounds caused by contaminated objects.

Today, tetanus is uncommon in the United States, with an average of about 30 reported cases each year. Nearly all cases of tetanus are among people who did not get all the recommended tetanus vaccinations. This includes people who have never received a tetanus vaccine and adults who do not stay up to date on their 10-year booster shots.

Causes and Transmission of Tetanus

Tetanus is an infection caused by a bacterium called *"Clostridium tetani."* Spores of tetanus bacteria are everywhere in the environment, including soil, dust, and manure. The spores develop into bacteria when they enter the body.

Common Ways Tetanus Gets into Your Body

The spores can get into the body through broken skin, usually through injuries from contaminated objects. Tetanus bacteria are more likely to infect certain breaks in the skin. These include:

- Wounds contaminated with dirt, poop (feces), or spit (saliva)

- Wounds caused by an object puncturing the skin (puncture wounds), such as a nail or needle

- Burns
- Crush injuries
- Injuries with dead tissue

Other Ways Tetanus Gets into Your Body

Tetanus bacteria can also infect the body through breaks in the skin caused by:

- Clean superficial wounds (when only the topmost layer of skin is scraped off)
- Surgical procedures
- Insect bites
- Dental infections
- Compound fractures (a break in the bone where it is exposed)
- Chronic sores and infections
- Intravenous (IV) drug use
- Intramuscular injections (shots given in a muscle)

Time from Exposure to Illness

The incubation period—time from exposure to illness—is usually between 3 and 21 days (average 10 days). However, it may range from 1 day to several months, depending on the kind of wound. Most cases occur within 14 days. In general, doctors see shorter incubation periods with:

- More heavily contaminated wounds
- More serious disease
- A worse outcome (prognosis)

Symptoms and Complications of Tetanus

People often call tetanus "lockjaw" because one of the most common signs of this infection is the tightening of the jaw muscles. Tetanus infection can lead to serious health problems, including being unable to open the mouth and having trouble swallowing and breathing.

163

Symptoms

Symptoms of tetanus include:

- Jaw cramping
- Sudden, involuntary muscle tightening (muscle spasms)— often in the stomach
- Painful muscle stiffness all over the body
- Trouble swallowing
- Jerking or staring (seizures)
- Headache
- Fever and sweating
- Changes in blood pressure and heart rate

Complications

Serious health problems that can happen because of tetanus include:

- Uncontrolled/involuntary tightening of the vocal cords (laryngospasm)
- Broken bones (fractures)
- Infections are gotten by a patient during a hospital visit (hospital-acquired infections)
- Blockage of the main artery of the lung or one of its branches by a blood clot that has traveled from elsewhere in the body through the bloodstream (pulmonary embolism)
- Pneumonia, a lung infection that develops by breathing in foreign materials (aspiration pneumonia)
- Breathing difficulty, possibly leading to death (1 to 2 in 10 cases are fatal)

Diagnosis and Treatment of Tetanus

Diagnosis

Doctors can diagnose tetanus by examining the patient and looking for certain signs and symptoms. There are no hospital lab tests that can confirm tetanus.

Treatment

Tetanus is a medical emergency requiring:

- Care in the hospital
- Immediate treatment with a medicine called human "tetanus immune globulin" (TIG)
- Aggressive wound care
- Drugs to control muscle spasms
- Antibiotics
- Tetanus vaccination

Depending on how serious the infection is, a machine to help you breathe may be required.

Prevention of Tetanus

Vaccination and good wound care are important to help prevent tetanus infection. Doctors can also use a medicine to help prevent tetanus in cases where someone is seriously hurt and does not have protection from tetanus vaccines.

Vaccination

Being up to date with your tetanus vaccine is the best tool to prevent tetanus. Protection from vaccines, as well as a prior infection, do not last a lifetime. This means that if you had tetanus or got the vaccine before, you still need to get the vaccine regularly to keep a high level of protection against this serious disease. The CDC recommends tetanus vaccines for people of all ages, with booster shots throughout life.

Good Wound Care

Immediate and good wound care can also help prevent infection.

- Do not delay first aid of even minor, noninfected wounds, such as blisters, scrapes, or any break in the skin.
- Wash hands often with soap and water or use an alcohol-based hand rub if washing is not possible.
- Consult your doctor if you have concerns and need further advice.

165

Section 11.9

Tuberculosis

This section includes text excerpted from "Tuberculosis (TB),"
Centers for Disease Control and Prevention (CDC), October 10, 2014.
Reviewed September 2019.

Tuberculosis (TB) disease in children under 15 years of age (also called "pediatric tuberculosis") is a public-health problem of special significance because it is a marker for recent transmission of TB. Also of special significance, infants and young children are more likely than older children and adults to develop life-threatening forms of TB disease (e.g., disseminated TB, TB meningitis). Among children, the greatest numbers of TB cases are seen in children less than five years of age, and in adolescents older than 10 years of age.

Basic Tuberculosis Facts

Tuberculosis is caused by a bacterium called *"Mycobacterium tuberculosis."* TB bacteria are spread from person to person through the air. The TB bacteria are put into the air when a person with TB disease of the lungs or throat coughs, sneezes, speaks, or sings. People nearby may breathe in these bacteria and become infected.

People with TB disease of the lungs or throat can spread bacteria to others with whom they spend time every day. However, children are less likely to spread TB bacteria to others. This is because the forms of TB disease most commonly seen in children are usually less infectious than the forms seen in adults.

Not everyone infected with TB bacteria becomes sick. As a result, two TB-related conditions exist:

Latent Tuberculosis Infection

Persons with latent TB infection:

- Usually have a skin test or blood test indicating TB infection

- Have TB bacteria in their bodies, but the bacteria are not active

- Are not sick and do not have symptoms

- Cannot spread bacteria to others

- Are often given medicine to prevent them from developing TB disease

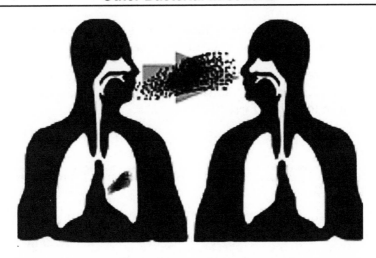

Figure 11.7. *How Tuberculosis Spreads* (Source: "Questions and Answers about TB," Centers for Disease Control and Prevention (CDC).)

Tuberculosis Disease

If TB bacteria become active in the body and multiply, the person will get sick with TB disease.

Persons with TB disease:

- Usually, have a skin test or blood test indicating TB infection

- Are sick from TB bacteria that are active (meaning that they are multiplying and destroying tissue in their body)

- Usually, have symptoms of TB disease

- Must be given medicine to treat TB disease

Once infected with TB bacteria, children are more likely to get sick with TB disease and to get sick more quickly than adults. In comparison to children, TB disease in adults is usually due to past TB infection that becomes active years later, when a person's immune system becomes weak for some reason (e.g., HIV infection, diabetes).

Confirming the diagnosis of TB disease in children with a laboratory test can be challenging. This is because:

- It is difficult to collect sputum specimens from infants and young children

- The laboratory tests used to find TB in sputum are less likely to have a positive result in children; this is due to the fact that children are more likely to have TB disease caused by a smaller number of bacteria (paucibacillary disease)

For these reasons, the diagnosis of TB disease in children is often made without laboratory confirmation and instead based on a combination of the following factors:

- Clinical signs and symptoms typically associated with TB disease

- Positive tuberculin skin test (TST) or positive TB blood test (IGRA)

- Chest x-ray that has patterns typically associated with TB disease

- History of contact with a person with infectious TB disease

Testing for Tuberculosis in Children

In the absence of symptoms, usually, the only sign of TB infection is a positive reaction to the TB skin test or TB blood test. TB skin testing is considered safe in children, and is preferred over TB blood tests for children less than five years of age.

All children with a positive test for TB infection, symptoms of TB, or a history of contact with a person with infectious TB disease should undergo a medical evaluation. Medical evaluations for TB disease include a chest x-ray and physical examination to exclude TB disease, and must be done before beginning treatment for latent TB infection.

Signs and Symptoms of Tuberculosis Disease in Children

Signs and symptoms of TB disease in children include:

- Cough
- Feelings of sickness or weakness, lethargy, and/or reduced playfulness
- Weight loss or failure to thrive
- Fever
- Night sweats

The most common form of TB disease occurs in the lungs, but TB disease can affect other parts of the body as well. Symptoms of TB disease in other parts of the body depend on the area affected. Infants, young children, and immunocompromised children (e.g., children with HIV) are at the highest risk of developing the most severe forms of TB, such as TB meningitis or disseminated TB disease.

Treatment of Tuberculosis Disease in Children

A pediatric TB expert should be involved in the treatment of TB in children and in the management of infants, young children, and immunocompromised children who have been exposed to someone with infectious TB disease. It is very important that children or anyone being treated for latent TB infection or TB disease finish the medicine and take the drugs exactly as instructed.

Latent Tuberculosis Infection

Treatment is recommended for children with latent TB infection to prevent them from developing TB disease. Infants, young children, and immunocompromised children with latent TB infection or children in close contact with someone with infectious TB disease, require special consideration because they are at increased risk for getting TB disease. Consultation with a pediatric TB expert is recommended before treatment begins.

Children over two years of age can be treated for latent TB infection with once-weekly isoniazid-rifapentine for 12 weeks. Alternative treatments for latent TB infection in children include four months of daily rifampin or nine months of daily isoniazid. The regimens are equally acceptable; however, healthcare providers should prescribe the more convenient shorter regimens, when possible. Patients are more likely to complete shorter treatment regimens.

Tuberculosis Disease

Tuberculosis disease is treated by taking several anti-TB medicines for six to nine months. It is important to note that if a child stops taking the drugs before completion, the child can become sick again. If drugs are not taken correctly, the bacteria that are still alive may become resistant to those drugs. TB that is resistant to drugs is harder and more expensive to treat, and treatment lasts much longer (up to 18 to 24 months).

Vaccines

Bacille Calmette-Guerin (BCG) is a vaccine to prevent TB disease. BCG is used in many countries to prevent childhood TB disease. However, the BCG vaccine is not generally used in the United States, because of the low risk of infection with TB bacteria and the variable effectiveness of the vaccine. The BCG vaccine should only be considered for very select persons who meet specific criteria and in consultation with a TB doctor.

Statistics

In the United States, a total of 9,582 cases of TB were reported in 2013, of which 485 (5%) cases were among children less than 15 years of age. Worldwide, it is estimated that there are at least 1 million cases of TB among children less than 15 years of age each year. In high TB burden settings outside of the United States, children account for an estimated 15 to 20 percent of TB cases.

Chapter 12

Viral Infections

Chapter Contents

Section 12.1

Adenovirus Infections

This section includes text excerpted from "Adenoviruses," Centers for Disease Control and Prevention (CDC), April 26, 2018.

What Is an Adenoviruses Infection?

Adenoviruses are common viruses that cause a range of illnesses. They can cause cold-like symptoms, sore throat, bronchitis, pneumonia, diarrhea, and pink eye (conjunctivitis).

You can get an adenovirus infection at any age. People with weakened immune systems or existing respiratory or cardiac disease are more likely than others to get very sick from an adenovirus infection.

Symptoms of Adenovirus Infections

Adenoviruses can cause a wide range of illnesses such as:

- Common cold

- Sore throat

- Bronchitis

- Pneumonia

- Diarrhea

- Pink eye

- Fever

- Bladder inflammation or infection

- Inflammation of stomach and intestines

- Neurologic disease or conditions that affect the brain and spinal cord

Adenoviruses can cause mild to severe illness, though serious illness is less common. People with weakened immune systems, or existing respiratory or cardiac disease, are at higher risk of developing severe illness from an adenovirus infection.

Transmission of Adenovirus Infections

Adenoviruses are usually spread from an infected person to others through:

- Close personal contact, such as touching or shaking hands

- The air by coughing and sneezing

- Touching an object or surface with adenoviruses on it, then touching your mouth, nose, or eyes before washing your hands

Some adenoviruses can spread through an infected person's stool, for example, during diaper changing. Adenovirus can also spread through the water, such as swimming pools, but this is less common.

Sometimes the virus can be shed (released from the body) for a long time after a person recovers from an adenovirus infection, especially among people who have weakened immune systems. This "virus shedding" usually occurs without any symptoms, even though the person can still spread adenovirus to other people.

Prevention of Adenovirus Infections

Follow simple steps to protect yourself and others
You can protect yourself and others from adenoviruses and other respiratory illnesses by following a few simple steps:

- Wash your hands often with soap and water

- Avoid touching your eyes, nose, or mouth with unwashed hands

- Avoid close contact with people who are sick

If you are sick you can help protect others:

- Stay home when you are sick

- Cover your mouth and nose when coughing or sneezing

- Avoid sharing cups and eating utensils with others

- Refrain from kissing others

- Wash your hands often with soap and water, especially after using the bathroom

Frequent handwashing is especially important in childcare settings and healthcare facilities.

Maintain proper chlorine levels to prevent outbreaks. Adenoviruses are resistant to many common disinfectant products and can remain infectious for long periods on surfaces and objects. It is important to keep adequate levels of chlorine in swimming pools to prevent outbreaks of conjunctivitis caused by adenoviruses.

Treatment of Adenovirus Infections

There is no specific treatment for people with adenovirus infection. Most adenovirus infections are mild and may require only care to help relieve symptoms.

Section 12.2

Chickenpox

This section contains text excerpted from the following sources:
Text in this section begins with excerpts from "About Chickenpox,"
Centers for Disease Control and Prevention (CDC), December 31,
2018; Text under the heading "Vaccines Used to Reduce Chickenpox"
is excerpted from "Chickenpox (Varicella)," Vaccines.gov, U.S.
Department of Health and Human Services (HHS), January 2018.

Chickenpox is a highly contagious disease caused by the varicella-zoster virus (VZV). It can cause an itchy, blister-like rash. The rash first appears on the chest, back, and face, and then spreads over the entire body, causing between 250 and 500 itchy blisters. Chickenpox can be serious, especially in babies, adolescents, adults, pregnant women, and people with a weakened immune system. The best way to prevent chickenpox is to get the chickenpox vaccine.

Chickenpox used to be very common in the United States. In the early 1990s, an average of 4 million people got chickenpox, 10,500 to 13,000 were hospitalized, and 100 to 150 died each year.

Chickenpox vaccine became available in the United States in 1995. Each year, more than 3.5 million cases of chickenpox, 9,000 hospitalizations, and 100 deaths are prevented by chickenpox vaccination in the United States.

Signs and Symptoms of Chickenpox

Anyone who has not had chickenpox or gotten the chickenpox vaccine can get the disease. Chickenpox illness usually lasts about four to seven days.

The classic symptom of chickenpox is a rash that turns into itchy, fluid-filled blisters that eventually turn into scabs. The rash may first show up on the chest, back, and face, and then spread over the entire body, including inside the mouth, eyelids, or genital area. It usually takes about one week for all of the blisters to become scabs.

Other typical symptoms that may begin to appear one to two days before rash include:

- Fever

- Tiredness

- Loss of appetite

- Headache

Children usually miss five to six days of school or childcare due to chickenpox.

Chickenpox in Vaccinated People

Some people who have been vaccinated against chickenpox can still get the disease. However, the symptoms are usually milder, with fewer or no blisters (or just red spots), mild or no fever, and shorter duration of illness. But some vaccinated people who get chickenpox may have a disease similar to unvaccinated people.

People at Risk for Severe Chickenpox

Some people who get chickenpox may have more severe symptoms and may be at higher risk for complications.

Complications of Chickenpox

Complications from chickenpox can occur, but they are not common in healthy people who get the disease.

People who may get a serious case of chickenpox and may be at high risk for complications include:

- Infants

- Adolescents

- Adults

- Pregnant women

- People with weakened immune systems because of illness or medications, for example,

  - People with human immunodeficiency virus (HIV)/acquired immunodeficiency syndrome (AIDS) or cancer

  - Patients who have had transplants

  - People on chemotherapy, immunosuppressive medications, or long-term use of steroids

Serious complications from chickenpox include:

- Bacterial infections of the skin and soft tissues in children, including group A *Streptococcal* infections

- Infection of the lungs (pneumonia)

- Infection or inflammation of the brain (encephalitis, cerebellar ataxia)

- Bleeding problems (hemorrhagic complications)

- Bloodstream infections (sepsis)

- Dehydration

Some people with serious complications from chickenpox can become so sick that they need to be hospitalized. Chickenpox can also cause death.

Deaths are very rare now due to the vaccine program. However, some deaths from chickenpox continue to occur in healthy, unvaccinated children and adults. In the past, many of the healthy adults who died from chickenpox contracted the disease from their unvaccinated children.

Transmission of Chickenpox

Chickenpox is a highly contagious disease caused by the VZV. The virus spreads easily from people with chickenpox to others who have never had the disease or never been vaccinated. The virus spreads mainly through close contact with someone who has chickenpox.

The VZV also causes shingles. Chickenpox can be spread from people with shingles to others who have never had chickenpox or received the chickenpox vaccine. This can happen through close contact with someone who has shingles.

A person with chickenpox is contagious beginning 1 to 2 days before rash onset until all the chickenpox lesions have crusted (scabbed). Vaccinated people who get chickenpox may develop lesions that do not crust. These people are considered contagious until no new lesions have appeared for 24 hours.

It takes about 2 weeks (from 10 to 21 days) after exposure to a person with chickenpox or shingles for someone to develop chickenpox. If a vaccinated person gets the disease, they can still spread it to others. For most people, getting chickenpox once provides immunity for life. However, for a few people, it is possible to get chickenpox more than once; although, this is not common.

Prevention and Treatment of Chickenpox

The best way to prevent chickenpox is to get the chickenpox vaccine. Everyone—including children, adolescents, and adults—should get two doses of chickenpox vaccine if they have never had chickenpox or were never vaccinated.

Chickenpox vaccine is very safe and effective at preventing the disease. Most people who get the vaccine will not get chickenpox. If a vaccinated person does get chickenpox, the symptoms are usually milder with fewer or no blisters (they may have just red spots) and mild or no fever.

The chickenpox vaccine prevents almost all cases of severe illness. Since the varicella vaccination program began in the United States, there has been an over 90 percent decrease in chickenpox cases, hospitalizations, and deaths.

Treatments at Home for People with Chickenpox

There are several things that you can do at home to help relieve chickenpox symptoms and prevent skin infections. Calamine lotion and a cool bath with added baking soda, uncooked oatmeal, or colloidal oatmeal may help relieve some of the itching. Try to minimize scratching to prevent the virus from spreading to others and potential bacterial infection from occurring. Keeping fingernails trimmed short may help prevent skin infections caused by scratching blisters.

Over-the-Counter Medications

Do not use aspirin or aspirin-containing products to relieve fever from chickenpox. The use of aspirin in children with chickenpox has been associated with Reye syndrome, a severe disease that affects the liver and brain and can cause death. Instead, use nonaspirin medications, such as acetaminophen, to relieve fever from chickenpox. The American Academy of Pediatrics (AAP) recommends avoiding treatment with ibuprofen if possible because it has been associated with life-threatening bacterial skin infections.

Vaccines Used to Reduce Chickenpox

Chickenpox used to be very common in the United States. But the good news is that the vaccine has greatly reduced the number of people who get it. Two doses of the chickenpox vaccine are about 94 percent effective at preventing it. Most people who get the vaccine do not get chickenpox—and those who do usually get a much milder version of the disease.

There are two vaccines that protect against chickenpox:

- The chickenpox vaccine protects children and adults from chickenpox

- The measles, mumps, and rubella vaccine (MMRV) protects children from measles, mumps, rubella, and chickenpox

Importance of the Chickenpox Vaccine

Chickenpox is very contagious—it spreads easily from person to person. And while it is usually mild, it can cause serious complications, such as pneumonia (lung infection). Certain people—such as infants, people with weakened immune systems, and pregnant women—are at increased risk for complications.

The chickenpox virus can also cause shingles later in life. Shingles is a disease that causes a painful skin rash and can affect the nervous system. Children who get the chickenpox vaccine may have a lower risk of developing shingles later on—and those who do get shingles often have a milder case than someone who has had chickenpox.

Getting vaccinated is the best way to prevent chickenpox. And when enough people get vaccinated against chickenpox, the entire community is less likely to get it. So when you and your family get vaccinated, you help keep yourselves and your community healthy.

Who Needs to Get the Chickenpox Vaccine

All children, adolescents, and adults who are not immune to (protected from) chickenpox need two doses of the chickenpox vaccine.

People who have only had one dose of chickenpox vaccine need to get a second dose.

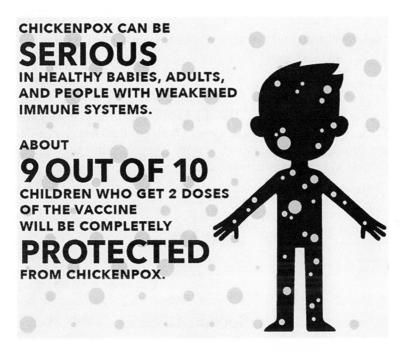

CHICKENPOX CAN BE
SERIOUS
IN HEALTHY BABIES, ADULTS, AND PEOPLE WITH WEAKENED IMMUNE SYSTEMS.

ABOUT
9 OUT OF 10
CHILDREN WHO GET 2 DOSES OF THE VACCINE WILL BE COMPLETELY
PROTECTED
FROM CHICKENPOX.

Figure 12.1. *Facts about Chickenpox Vaccine Shots* (Source: "Vaccine (Shot) for Chickenpox (Varicella)," Centers for Disease Control and Prevention (CDC).)

Children

Children age 12 months and older need to get the chickenpox vaccine as part of their routine vaccine schedule.

Children need 2 doses of the vaccine at the following ages:

- **12 through 15 months** for the first dose

- **4 through 6 years** for the second dose (or sooner as long as it is 3 months after the first dose)

Children at the age of 1 through 12 years can get the MMRV vaccine, which is a combination vaccine that protects against chickenpox, measles, mumps, and rubella. Your child's doctor can recommend the vaccine that is right for your child.

If your child missed the chickenpox vaccines, talk with your child's doctor about scheduling a catch-up shot.

What Are the Side Effects of the Chickenpox Vaccine?

Side effects are usually mild and go away in a few days. They may include:

- Pain, swelling, and redness where the shot was given

- Mild rash

- Low fever

Serious side effects from the chickenpox vaccine are very rare.

Like any medicine, there is a very small chance that the chickenpox vaccine could cause a serious reaction. Keep in mind that getting the chickenpox vaccine is much safer than getting chickenpox.

Section 12.3

Common Cold

This section contains text excerpted from the following sources: Text in this section begins with excerpts from "Common Colds: Protect Yourself and Others," Centers for Disease Control and Prevention (CDC), February 11, 2019; Text beginning with the heading "Causes of Common Cold" is excerpted from "Common Cold and Runny Nose," Centers for Disease Control and Prevention (CDC), September 26, 2017.

Sore throat and runny nose are usually the first signs of a cold, followed by coughing and sneezing. Most people recover in about 7 to 10 days. You can help reduce your risk of getting a cold: wash your hands often, avoid close contact with sick people, and do not touch your face with unwashed hands.

Common colds are the main reason that children miss school and adults miss work. Each year in the United States, there are millions of cases of the common cold. Adults have an average of 2 to 3 colds per year, and children have even more.

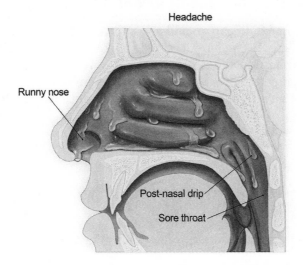

Figure 12.2. *Colds* (Source: "Common Cold and Runny Nose," Centers for Disease Control and Prevention (CDC).)

When you have a cold, mucus fills your nose, causing a runny nose, congestion, and mucus to drip down your throat (postnasal drip), which can cause a sore throat and cough.

Causes of Common Cold

More than 200 viruses can cause the common cold, and infections can spread from person to person through the air and close personal contact. Antibiotics do not work against these viruses and do not help you feel better if you have a cold. Rhinovirus is the most common type of virus that causes colds.

Risk Factors of Common Cold

There are many things that can increase your risk for the common cold, including:

- Exposure to someone with the common cold
- Age (infants and young children are at higher risk for colds)
- A weakened immune system or taking drugs that weaken the immune system
- Season (colds are more common during the fall and winter)

Signs and Symptoms of Common Cold

When germs that cause colds first infect the nose and sinuses (air-filled pockets in the face), the nose makes clear mucus. This helps wash the germs from the nose and sinuses. After two or three days, mucus may change to a white, yellow, or green color. This is normal and does not mean you or your child needs antibiotics. Other signs and symptoms of the common cold can include:

- Sneezing
- Stuffy nose
- Sore throat
- Coughing
- Postnasal drip (mucus dripping down your throat)
- Watery eyes
- Mild headache
- Mild body aches

These symptoms usually peak within 2 to 3 days but can last for up to 10 to 14 days.

When to Seek Medical Care

See a healthcare professional if you or your child has any of the following symptoms:

- Symptoms that last more than 10 days without improvement
- Symptoms that are severe or unusual

If your child is younger than three months of age and has a fever, it is important to call your healthcare professional right away.

Diagnosis and Treatment of Common Cold

Antibiotics are not needed to treat a cold or runny nose, which almost always gets better on its own. Your healthcare professional will determine what type of illness you or your child has by asking about symptoms and doing a physical examination. Sometimes they will also swab the inside of your nose or mouth.

Since the common cold is caused by viruses, antibiotics will not help it get better and may even cause harm in children. Your healthcare professional can give you tips to help with symptoms, such as fever and coughing.

Symptom Relief

Rest, over-the-counter (OTC) medicines and other self-care methods may help you or your child feel better. Remember, always use OTC products as directed. Many OTC products are not recommended for children of certain ages.

Prevention of Common Cold

There are steps you can take to help prevent getting a cold, including:

- Practice good hand hygiene.

- Avoid close contact with people who have colds or other upper respiratory infections.

Section 12.4

Croup

This section includes text excerpted from "Croup," MedlinePlus, National Institutes of Health (NIH), December 31, 2016. Reviewed September 2019.

What Is Croup?

Croup is an inflammation of the vocal cords (larynx) and windpipe (trachea). It causes difficulty breathing, a barking cough, and a hoarse voice. It is also known by the names "spasmodic croup" and "viral croup."

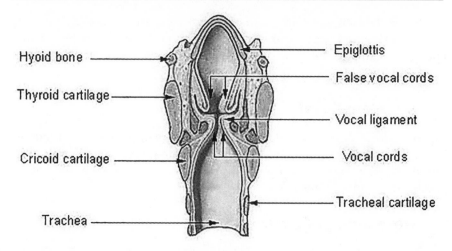

Hyoid bone

Thyroid cartilage

Cricoid cartilage

Trachea

Epiglottis

False vocal cords

Vocal ligament

Vocal cords

Tracheal cartilage

Figure 12.3. *Larynx* (Source: "Larynx and Trachea," Surveillance, Epidemiology, and End Results Program (SEER), National Cancer Institute (NCI).)

The larynx plays an essential role in human speech. During sound production, the vocal cords close together and vibrate as the air expelled from the lungs passes between them.

What Causes Croup

The cause is usually a virus, often parainfluenza virus. Other causes include:

- Allergies
- Reflux

What Are the Symptoms of Croup?

Croup often starts out such as a cold. But then the vocal cords and windpipe become swollen, causing the hoarseness and cough. There may also be a fever and high-pitched noisy sounds when breathing.

The symptoms are usually worse at night and last for about three to five days. Croup is more common in the fall and winter.

Who Are at Risk of Croup?

Children between the ages of six months and three years have the highest risk of getting croup. They may also have more severe symptoms.

How Is Croup Treated?

Most cases of viral croup are mild and can be treated at home. Rarely, croup can become serious and interfere with your child's breathing. If you are worried about your child's breathing, call your healthcare provider right away.

Managing Recurrent Croup in Children*

Presently children who experience recurring croup symptoms receive a variety of treatments. This is because it is not clear which treatments may be best. Some children are given inhaled steroids (similar to what children with asthma use). Others are carefully watched and cautioned to avoid potential triggers (certain foods, environmental allergens, etc), and should episodes of croup recur they are treated with a short course of oral steroids.

*Text excerpted from "Management of Recurrent Croup," ClinicalTrials.gov, National Institutes of Health (NIH), November 13, 2017.

Section 12.5

Fifth Disease

This section includes text excerpted from "Fifth Disease," Centers for Disease Control and Prevention (CDC), November 2, 2015. Reviewed September 2019.

What Is Fifth Disease?

Fifth disease is a mild rash illness caused by *Parvovirus B19*. It is more common in children than adults. A person usually gets sick with fifth disease within four to 14 days after getting infected with *Parvovirus B19*. This disease, also called "erythema infectiosum," got its name because it was fifth in a list of historical classifications of common skin rash illnesses in children.

Signs and Symptoms of Fifth Disease

The symptoms of fifth disease are usually mild and may include:

- Fever
- Runny nose
- Headache
- Rash

You Can Get a Rash on Your Face and Body

You may get a red rash on your face called "slapped cheek" rash. This rash is the most recognized feature of fifth disease. It is more common in children than adults.

Some people may get a second rash a few days later on their chest, back, buttocks, or arms and legs. The rash may be itchy, especially on the soles of the feet. It can vary in intensity and usually goes away in seven to 10 days, but it can come and go for several weeks. As it starts to go away, it may look lacy.

Complications of Fifth Disease

Fifth disease is usually mild for children who are otherwise healthy. But for some people, fifth disease can cause serious health complications, such as chronic anemia that requires medical treatment.

You may be at risk for serious complications from fifth disease if you have a weakened immune system caused by leukemia, cancer, organ transplants, or human immunodeficiency virus (HIV) infection.

Transmission of Fifth Disease

Parvovirus B19—which causes fifth disease—spreads through respiratory secretions, such as saliva, sputum, or nasal mucus, when an infected person coughs or sneezes. You are most contagious when it seems as if you have "just a fever and/or cold" and before you get the rash or joint pain and swelling. After you get the rash you are not likely to be contagious, so then it is usually safe for you or your child to go back to work or school.

People with fifth disease who have weakened immune systems may be contagious for a longer amount of time.

Parvovirus B19 can also spread through blood or blood products. A pregnant woman who is infected with *Parvovirus B19* can pass the virus to her baby.

Once you recover from fifth disease, you develop immunity that generally protects you from *Parvovirus B19* infection in the future.

Diagnosis of Fifth Disease

Healthcare providers can often diagnose fifth disease just by seeing "slapped cheek" rash on a patient's face. They can also do a blood test to determine if you are susceptible or immune to *Parvovirus B19* infection or if you were recently infected. This is not a routine test but can be performed in special circumstances. Talk to your healthcare provider. The blood test may be particularly helpful for pregnant women who may have been exposed to *Parvovirus B19* and are suspected to have fifth disease.

Prevention of Fifth Disease

There is no vaccine or medicine that can prevent *Parvovirus B19* infection. You can reduce your chance of being infected or infecting others by:

- Washing your hands often with soap and water
- Covering your mouth and nose when you cough or sneeze
- Not touching your eyes, nose, or mouth
- Avoiding close contact with people who are sick
- Staying home when you are sick

Once you get the rash, you are probably not contagious. So it is usually then safe for you to go back to work or for your child to return to school or a childcare center.

Healthcare providers who are pregnant should know about potential risks to their baby and discuss this with their doctor.

All healthcare providers and patients should follow strict infection control practices to prevent *Parvovirus B19* from spreading.

Treatment of Fifth Disease

Fifth disease is usually mild and will go away on its own. Children who are otherwise healthy usually recover completely. Treatment usually involves relieving symptoms, such as fever, itching, and joint pain and swelling.

People who have complications from fifth disease should see their healthcare provider for medical treatment.

Section 12.6

Hand, Foot, and Mouth Disease

This section includes text excerpted from "Hand, Foot, and Mouth Disease (HFMD)," Centers for Disease Control and Prevention (CDC), February 22, 2019.

What Is Hand, Foot, and Mouth Disease?

Hand, foot, and mouth disease (HFMD) is a common viral illness that usually affects infants and children younger than five years old. However, it can sometimes occur in older children and adults. Typical symptoms of HFMD include fever, mouth sores, and a skin rash.

Signs and Symptoms of Hand, Foot, and Mouth Disease

The signs and symptoms of HFMD usually start with:

- A fever
- Reduced appetite
- Sore throat
- A feeling of being unwell (malaise)

One or two days after the fever starts, painful sores can develop in the mouth (herpangina). They usually begin as small red spots, often in the back of the mouth, that blister and can become painful.

A skin rash on the palms of the hands and soles of the feet may also develop over one or two days as flat, red spots, sometimes with blisters. It may also appear on the knees, elbows, buttocks, or genital area.

Some people, especially young children, may get dehydrated if they are not able to swallow enough liquids because of painful mouth sores. You should seek medical care in these cases.

Complications of Hand, Foot, and Mouth Disease

Health complications from HFMD are not common:

- Viral or "aseptic" meningitis can occur with HFMD, but it is rare. It causes fever, headache, stiff neck, or back pain and may require the infected person to be hospitalized for a few days.

- Encephalitis (inflammation of the brain) or polio-like paralysis can occur, but this is even rarer.

- Fingernail and toenail loss have been reported, occurring mostly in children within a few weeks after having HFMD. At this time, it is not known whether nail loss was a result of the disease in reported cases. However, in the reports reviewed, the nail loss was temporary, and the nail grew back without medical treatment.

Causes of Hand, Foot, and Mouth Disease

Hand, foot, and mouth disease is caused by viruses that belong to the Enterovirus genus (group), which includes polioviruses, coxsackieviruses, echoviruses, and other enteroviruses.

- Coxsackievirus A16 is typically the most common cause of HFMD in the United States, but other coxsackieviruses can also cause the illness.

- Enterovirus 71 has also been associated with cases and outbreaks of HFMD, mostly in children in East and Southeast Asia. Less often, enterovirus 71 has been associated with severe diseases, such as encephalitis.

Several types of enteroviruses may be identified in outbreaks of hand, foot and mouth disease, but most of the time, only one or two enteroviruses are identified.

Transmission of Hand, Foot, and Mouth Disease

The viruses that cause HFMD can be found in an infected person's:

- Nose and throat secretions (such as saliva, sputum, or nasal mucus)

- Blister fluid

- Feces (poop)

You can get exposed to the viruses that cause HFMD through:

- Close personal contact, such as hugging an infected person

- The air when an infected person coughs or sneezes

- Contact with feces, such as changing diapers of an infected person, then touching your eyes, nose, or mouth before washing your hands

- Contact with contaminated objects and surfaces, such as touching a doorknob that has viruses on it, then touching your eyes, mouth, or nose before washing your hands

It is also possible to get infected with the viruses that cause HFMD if you swallow recreational water, such as water in swimming pools. However, this is not very common. This can happen if the water is not properly treated with chlorine and becomes contaminated with feces from a person who has HFMD.

Generally, a person with HFMD is most contagious during the first week of illness. People can sometimes be contagious for days or weeks after symptoms go away. Some people, especially adults, may become infected and not develop any symptoms, but they can still spread the virus to others. This is why people should always try to maintain good hygiene, such as frequent handwashing, so they can minimize their chance of spreading or getting infections.

You should stay home while you are sick with HFMD. Talk with your healthcare provider if you are not sure when you should return to work or school. The same applies to children returning to daycare.

Hand, foot, and mouth disease is not transmitted to or from pets or other animals.

Diagnosis of Hand, Foot, and Mouth Disease

Hand, foot, and mouth disease is one of the many infections that causes mouth sores. Healthcare providers can usually identify mouth sores caused by HFMD by considering:

- How old the patient is

- What symptoms the patient has

- How the rash and mouth sores look

A healthcare professional may sometimes collect samples from the patient's throat or feces (poop), then send them to a laboratory to test for the virus.

Prevention of Hand, Foot, and Mouth Disease

There is no vaccine in the United States to protect against the viruses that cause HFMD. But researchers are working to develop vaccines to help prevent HFMD in the future.

You can lower your risk of being infected by doing the following:

- Wash your hands often with soap and water for at least 20 seconds, especially after changing diapers and using the toilet.

- Clean and disinfect frequently touched surfaces and soiled items, including toys.

- Avoid close contact, such as kissing, hugging, or sharing eating utensils or cups with people with HFMD.

Treatment of Hand, Foot, and Mouth Disease

There is no specific treatment for HFMD. However, you can do some things to relieve symptoms:

- Take over-the-counter (OTC) medications to relieve pain and fever (aspirin should not be given to children).

- Use mouthwashes or sprays that numb mouth pain.

If a person has mouth sores, it might be painful for them to swallow. However, it is important for people with HFMD to drink enough liquids to prevent dehydration (loss of body fluids). If a person cannot swallow enough liquids to avoid dehydration, they may need to receive them through an IV in their veins.

If you are concerned about your or your child's symptoms you should contact your healthcare provider.

Section 12.7

Infectious Mononucleosis

This section includes text excerpted from "About Infectious Mononucleosis," Centers for Disease Control and Prevention (CDC), May 8, 2018.

What Is Infectious Mononucleosis?

Infectious mononucleosis, also called "mono," is a contagious disease. Epstein-Barr virus (EBV) is the most common cause of infectious mononucleosis, but other viruses can also cause this disease. It is common among teenagers and young adults, especially college students. At least one out of four teenagers and young adults who get infected with EBV will develop infectious mononucleosis.

Symptoms of Infectious Mononucleosis

The symptoms of infectious mononucleosis include:

- Extreme fatigue
- Fever
- Sore throat
- Head and body aches
- Swollen lymph nodes in the neck and armpits
- Swollen liver or spleen or both
- Rash

Enlarged spleen and a swollen liver are less common symptoms. For some people, their liver or spleen or both may remain enlarged even after their fatigue ends.

Most people get better in two to four weeks; however, some people may feel fatigued for several more weeks. Occasionally, the symptoms of infectious mononucleosis can last for six months or longer.

Transmission of Infectious Mononucleosis

Epstein-Barr virus is the most common cause of infectious mononucleosis, but other viruses can cause this disease. Typically, these viruses spread most commonly through bodily fluids, especially saliva.

However, these viruses can also spread through blood during blood transfusion and organ transplantation.

Prevention of Infectious Mononucleosis

There is no vaccine to protect against infectious mononucleosis. You can help protect yourself by not kissing or sharing drinks, food, or personal items, such as toothbrushes, with people who have infectious mononucleosis.

You can help relieve symptoms of infectious mononucleosis by:

- Drinking fluids to stay hydrated

- Getting plenty of rest

- Taking over-the-counter (OTC) medications for pain and fever

If you have infectious mononucleosis, you should not take penicillin antibiotics, such as ampicillin or amoxicillin. Based on the severity of the symptoms, a healthcare provider may recommend treatment of specific organ systems affected by infectious mononucleosis.

Because your spleen may become enlarged as a result of infectious mononucleosis, you should avoid contact sports until you fully recover. Participating in contact sports can be strenuous and may cause the spleen to rupture.

Treatment of Infectious Mononucleosis

Healthcare providers typically diagnose infectious mononucleosis based on symptoms.

Laboratory tests are not usually needed to diagnose infectious mononucleosis. However, specific laboratory tests may be needed to identify the cause of illness in people who do not have a typical case of infectious mononucleosis.

The blood work of patients who have infectious mononucleosis due to EBV infection may show:

- More white blood cells (lymphocytes) than normal

- Unusual looking white blood cells (atypical lymphocytes)

- Fewer than normal neutrophils or platelets

- Abnormal liver function

Section 12.8

Influenza

This section includes text excerpted from "Flu Information for Parents with Young Children," Centers for Disease Control and Prevention (CDC), October 24, 2018.

Flu is more dangerous than the common cold for children. Each year, the flu places a large burden on the health and well-being of children and their families. Annual influenza vaccination is the best method for preventing flu and its potentially severe complications in children.

Children and Influenza

Children younger than five years of age—especially those younger than two years old—are at high risk of serious flu-related complications. A flu vaccine offers the best defense against getting the flu and spreading it to others. Getting vaccinated can reduce flu illnesses, doctor's visits, missed work and school days, and prevent flu-related hospitalizations and deaths in children.

Influenza Is Dangerous for Children

Flu illness is more dangerous than the common cold for children. Each year, millions of children get sick with seasonal flu; thousands of children are hospitalized and some children die from the flu. Children commonly need medical care because of the flu, especially children younger than five years old who become sick with the flu.

- Complications from flu among children in this age group can include:

  - Pneumonia: an illness where the lungs get infected and inflamed

  - Dehydration: when a child's body loses too much water and salts, often because fluid losses are greater than from fluid intake)

  - Worsening of long-term medical problems, such as heart disease or asthma

  - Brain dysfunction such as encephalopathy

- Sinus problems and ear infections

- In rare cases, flu complications can lead to death.

- Flu seasons vary in severity, however, every year children are at risk:

  - The Centers for Disease Control and Prevention (CDC) estimates that since 2010, flu-related hospitalizations among children younger than 5 years ranged from 7,000 to 26,000 in the United States.

  - While relatively rare, some children die from the flu each year. Since 2004 to 2005, flu-related deaths in children reported to the CDC during regular flu seasons have ranged from 37 deaths to 186 deaths.

Some Children Are at Especially High Risk

Children at greatest risk of serious flu-related complications include the following:

- **Children younger than 6 months old.** These children are too young to be vaccinated. The best way to protect them is to make sure people around them are vaccinated.

- **Children aged 6 months up to their 5th birthday.** Since 2010, the CDC estimates that flu-related hospitalizations among children younger than 5 years ranged from 7,000 to 26,000 in the United States. Even children in this age group who are otherwise healthy are at risk simply because of their age. Additionally, children 2 years of age up to their 5th birthday are more likely than healthy older children to be taken to a doctor, an urgent care center, or the emergency room because of the flu. To protect their health, all children 6 months and older should be vaccinated against flu each year. Vaccinating young children, their families, and other caregivers can also help protect them from getting sick.

- **American Indian and Alaskan Native children.** These children are more likely to have severe flu illness that results in hospitalization or death.

- **Children aged 6 months old through 18 years old with chronic health problems, including:**

  - Asthma

- Neurologic and neurodevelopment conditions [including disorders of the brain, spinal cord, peripheral nerve, and muscle such as cerebral palsy, epilepsy (seizure disorders), stroke, intellectual disability (mental retardation), moderate to severe developmental delay, muscular dystrophy, or spinal cord injury

- Chronic lung disease (such as chronic obstructive pulmonary disease (COPD) and cystic fibrosis (CF))

- Heart disease (such as congenital heart disease, congestive heart failure and coronary artery disease (CAD))

- Blood disorders (such as sickle cell disease (SCD))

- Endocrine disorders (such as diabetes mellitus (DM))

- Kidney disorders

- Liver disorders

- Metabolic disorders (such as inherited metabolic disorders and mitochondrial disorders)

- Weakened immune system due to disease or medication (such as people with human immunodeficiency virus (HIV) or acquired immunodeficiency syndrome (AIDS), or cancer, or those on chronic steroids)

- Children who are taking aspirin or salicylate-containing medicines

- Extreme obesity, which has been associated with severe influenza illness in some studies of adults, may also be a risk factor for children. Childhood obesity is defined as a body mass index (BMI) at or above the 95th percentile, for age and sex.

Vaccination Is the Best Protection against Flu

The best way to prevent the flu is with a flu vaccine. The CDC recommends that everyone 6 months of age and older get a seasonal flu vaccine each year by the end of October. However, as long as flu viruses are circulating, vaccination should continue throughout the flu season, even in January or later. Keep in mind that vaccination is especially important for certain people who are at high risk or who are in close contact with high-risk persons. This includes children at high risk for developing complications from flu illness and adults who are close contacts of those children.

Flu vaccines are updated each season if necessary to protect against the influenza viruses that research indicates will be most common during the upcoming season. The 2018 to 2019 vaccine has been updated from last season's vaccine to better match circulating viruses. Immunity from vaccination sets in after about two weeks.

Types of Flu Vaccines for Children

Children six months and older should get an annual influenza (flu) vaccine. For the 2018 to 2019 flu season, the CDC recommends annual influenza vaccination for everyone 6 months and older with any licensed, age-appropriate flu vaccine (inactivated influenza vaccine (IIV) for children aged six months and older or live attenuated influenza vaccine (LAIV4) for children two years of age and older) with no preference expressed for any one vaccine over another.

Flu shots (IIV), vaccines given as an injection and made with inactivated (killed) flu virus are approved for use in people six months and older.

The nasal spray vaccine (LAIV4) is approved for use in people 2 through 49 years of age. However, there is a precaution against the use of nasal spray flu vaccine (LAIV) in people with certain underlying medical conditions.

Your child's healthcare provider will know which vaccines are right for your child.

Special Vaccination Instructions for Children Aged Six Months through Eight Years of Age

- Some children six months through eight years of age require two doses of influenza vaccine. Children six months through eight years getting vaccinated for the first time, and those who have only previously gotten one dose of vaccine, should get two doses of vaccine this season. All children who have previously gotten two doses of vaccine (at any time) only need one dose of vaccine this season. The first dose should be given as soon as vaccine becomes available.

- The second dose should be given at least 28 days after the first dose. The first dose "primes" the immune system; the second dose provides immune protection. Children who only get one dose but need two doses can have reduced or no protection from a single dose of flu vaccine.

- If your child needs the two doses, begin the process early. This will ensure that your child is protected before influenza starts circulating in your community.

- Be sure to get your child a second dose if she or he needs one. It usually takes about two weeks after the second dose for protection to begin

Children Should Be Vaccinated Every Flu Season

Children should be vaccinated every flu season for the best protection against the flu. For children who will need two doses of flu vaccine, the first dose should be given as early in the season as possible. For other children, it is good practice to get them vaccinated by the end of October. However, getting vaccinated later can still be protective, as long as flu viruses are circulating. While seasonal influenza outbreaks can happen as early as October, in most seasons influenza activity peaks between December and February. Since it takes about two weeks after vaccination for antibodies to develop in the body that protects against influenza virus infection, it is best that people get vaccinated so they are protected before influenza begins spreading in their community.

Section 12.9

Measles

This section includes text excerpted from "Top 4 Things Parents Need to Know about Measles," Centers for Disease Control and Prevention (CDC), May 16, 2019.

You may be hearing a lot about measles lately. And all of this news on TV, social media, the Internet, newspapers, and magazines may leave you wondering what you as a parent really need to know about this disease.

Measles Can Be Serious

Some people think of measles as just a little rash and fever that clears up in a few days, but measles can cause serious health complications, especially in children younger than five years of age. There is no way to tell in advance the severity of the symptoms your child will experience.

- About 1 in 5 people in the United States who get measles will be hospitalized

- Every 1 out of 1,000 people with measles will develop brain swelling, which could lead to brain damage

- Every 1 to 3 out of 1,000 people with measles will die, even with the best care

Some of the more common measles symptoms include:

- High fever (may spike to more than 104°F)

- Cough

- Runny nose (coryza)

- Red, watery eyes (conjunctivitis)

- Rash (3 to 5 days after symptoms begin)

Signs and Symptoms of Measles
Symptoms of a Measles Infection after 7 to 14 Days

Measles is not just a little rash. Measles can be dangerous, especially for babies and young children. Measles typically begins with:

- High fever (may spike to more than 104°F)

- Cough

- Runny nose (coryza)

- Red, watery eyes

2 to 3 Days after Symptoms Begin: Koplik Spots

Tiny white spots (Koplik spots) may appear inside the mouth two to three days after symptoms begin.

3 to 5 Days after Symptoms Begin: Measles Rash

Three to five days after symptoms begin, a rash breaks out. It usually begins as flat red spots that appear on the face at the hairline and spread downward to the neck, trunk, arms, legs, and feet.

- Small raised bumps may also appear on top of the flat red spots.

- The spots may become joined together as they spread from the head to the rest of the body.

- When the rash appears, a person's fever may spike to more than 104°F.

Transmission of Measles

Measles spreads through the air when an infected person coughs or sneezes. It is so contagious that if one person has it, up to 9 out of 10 people around her or him will also become infected if they are not protected. Your child can get measles just by being in a room where a person with measles has been, even up to 2 hours after that person has left. An infected person can spread measles to others even before knowing she/he has the disease—from 4 days before developing the measles rash through 4 days afterward.

Measles is a highly contagious virus that lives in the nose and throat mucus of an infected person. It can spread to others through coughing and sneezing. Also, measles virus can live for up to two hours in an airspace where the infected person coughed or sneezed.

If other people breathe the contaminated air or touch the infected surface, then touch their eyes, noses, or mouths, they can become infected. Measles is so contagious that if one person has it, up to 90 percent of the people close to that person who are not immune will also become infected.

Infected people can spread measles to others from four days before through four days after the rash appears.

Measles is a disease of humans; measles virus is not spread by any other animal species.

Your Child Can Still Get Measles in the United States

Measles was declared eliminated from the United States in 2000 thanks to a highly effective vaccination program. Eliminated means that the disease is no longer constantly present in this country. However, measles is still common in many parts of the world. Each year around the world, an estimated 10 million people get measles, and about 110,000 of them die from it.

Even if your family does not travel internationally, you could come into contact with measles anywhere in your community. Every year, measles is brought into the United States by unvaccinated travelers (mostly Americans and sometimes foreign visitors) who get measles while they are in other countries. Anyone who is not protected against measles is at risk.

Plan for Travel
Which Travelers Are at Risk?

You are at risk of measles infection when you travel to areas where measles is spreading and have not been fully vaccinated against measles or have not had measles in the past. The best way to protect yourself and your loved ones from measles is by getting vaccinated.

Before International Travel: Make Sure You are Protected against Measles

The best way to protect yourself and your loved ones from measles is by getting vaccinated. You should plan to be fully vaccinated at least 2 weeks before you depart. If your trip is less than 2 weeks away and you are not protected against measles, you should still get a dose of measles-mumps-rubella (MMR) vaccine. The MMR vaccine protects against all 3 diseases. Two doses of MMR vaccine provides 97 percent protection against measles; one dose provides 93 percent protection.

Call your healthcare provider, your local health department, or locate a pharmacy or clinic near you to schedule an appointment for an MMR vaccine. The CDC does not recommend measles vaccine for infants younger than 6 months of age.

Infants under 12 Months Old

- Get an early dose at 6 to 11 months
- Follow the recommended schedule and get another dose at 12 to 15 months and a final dose at 4 to 6 years

Children over 12 Months Old

- Get first dose immediately
- Get second dose 28 days after first dose

Teens and Adults with No Evidence of Immunity*

- Get first dose immediately
- Get second dose 28 days after first dose

*Acceptable presumptive evidence of immunity against measles includes at least one of the following: written documentation of adequate vaccination, laboratory evidence of immunity, laboratory confirmation of measles, or birth in the United States before 1957.

How Do Measles Outbreaks Start in the United States?

In the United States, most of the measles cases result from international travel. The disease is brought into the United States by unvaccinated people who get infected in other countries. Typically 2 out of 3 of these unvaccinated travelers are Americans. They can spread measles to other people who are not protected against measles, which sometimes leads to outbreaks.

Since measles is still common in many countries, unvaccinated travelers bring measles to the United States and it can spread. Protect yourself, your family, and your community with the MMR vaccine, especially before traveling internationally.

Do not travel if you are sick. Call your doctor immediately if you think you or your child has been exposed to measles.

After International Travel: Watch for Measles

Measles is highly contagious and can spread to others through coughing and sneezing. Measles is so contagious that if one person has it, 90 percent of the people close to that person who are not immune will also become infected. An infected person can spread measles to others 4 days before the rash even develops.

Watch your health for 3 weeks after you return. Measles symptoms typically include:

- High fever (may spike to more than 104°F)
- Cough
- Runny nose (coryza)
- Red, watery eyes (conjunctivitis)
- Rash (3 to 5 days after symptoms begin)

If you or your child gets sick with a rash and fever, call your doctor. Be sure to tell your doctor that you traveled abroad, and whether you have received MMR vaccine.

You Have the Power to Protect Your Child against Measles with a Safe and Effective Vaccine

The best protection against measles is the MMR vaccine. MMR vaccine provides long-lasting protection against all strains of measles. Your child needs two doses of MMR vaccine for best protection:

- The first dose at 12 through 15 months of age

- The second dose at 4 through 6 years of age

If your family is traveling overseas, the vaccine recommendations are a little different:

- If your baby is 6 through 11 months old, she or he should receive 1 dose of MMR vaccine before leaving.

- If your child is 12 months of age or older, she or he will need 2 doses of MMR vaccine (separated by at least 28 days) before departure.

Section 12.10

Mumps

This section includes text excerpted from "Mumps," Centers for Disease Control and Prevention (CDC), March 8, 2019.

Mumps is a contagious disease that is caused by a virus. It typically starts with a few days of fever, headache, muscle aches, tiredness, and loss of appetite. Then most people will have swelling of their salivary glands. This is what causes the puffy cheeks and a tender, swollen jaw.

Signs and Symptoms of Mumps

Mumps is best known for the puffy cheeks and tender, swollen jaw that it causes. This is a result of swollen salivary glands under the ears on one or both sides, often referred to as "parotitis."

Other symptoms that might begin a few days before parotitis include:

- Fever

- Headache

- Muscle aches

- Tiredness

- Loss of appetite

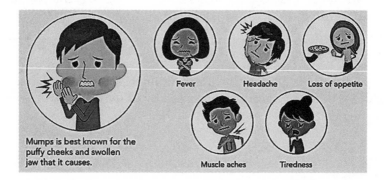

Figure 12.4. *Signs and Symptoms of Mumps* (Source: "Protect Yourself against Mumps," Centers for Disease Control and Prevention (CDC).)

Symptoms typically appear 16 to 18 days after infection, but this period can range from 12 to 25 days after infection.

Some people who get mumps have very mild symptoms (like a cold), or no symptoms at all and may not know they have the disease. In rare cases, mumps can cause more severe complications.

Most people with mumps recover completely within two weeks.

Transmission of Mumps

Mumps is a contagious disease caused by a virus. It spreads through direct contact with saliva or respiratory droplets from the mouth, nose, or throat. An infected person can spread the virus by:

- Coughing, sneezing, or talking

- Sharing items that may have saliva on them, such as water bottles or cups

- Participating in close-contact activities with others, such as playing sports, dancing, or kissing

- Touching objects or surfaces with unwashed hands that are then touched by others

An infected person can likely spread mumps from a few days before their salivary glands begin to swell to up to five days after the swelling begins. A person with mumps should limit their contact with others during this time. For example, stay home from school and do not attend social events.

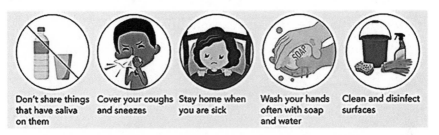

Don't share things that have saliva on them   Cover your coughs and sneezes   Stay home when you are sick   Wash your hands often with soap and water   Clean and disinfect surfaces

Figure 12.5. *Keep from Spreading Mumps* (Source: "Protect Yourself against Mumps," Centers for Disease Control and Prevention (CDC).)

Mumps Virus Still Around

Mumps occurs in the United States, and the MMR vaccine is the best way to prevent the disease.

- Check your child's immunization record or contact the doctor to see whether your child has already received the MMR vaccine.

- Get your child vaccinated on time; visit the immunization scheduler for newborn to 6-year-old children.

- Remember that some preteens and teens also need MMR vaccine; review the preteens and teens schedule.

- Get an additional vaccine dose if your health department recommends it to a group you are part of during an outbreak.

- Recognize the signs and symptoms of mumps.

- Let your doctor know right away if you think you or someone in your family may have mumps.

Complications of Mumps

Mumps can occasionally cause complications.

Complications can include:

- Inflammation of the testicles (orchitis) in males who have reached puberty; this may lead to a decrease in testicular size (testicular atrophy)

- Inflammation of the ovaries (oophoritis) and/or breast tissue (mastitis)

- Inflammation in the pancreas (pancreatitis)

- Inflammation of the brain (encephalitis)

- Inflammation of the tissue covering the brain and spinal cord (meningitis)

- Deafness

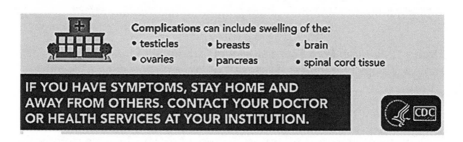

Figure 12.6. *Vaccination Helps Prevent Mumps Complications* (Source: "Protect Yourself against Mumps," Centers for Disease Control and Prevention (CDC).)

Neither inflammation of the testicles nor inflammation of the ovaries caused by mumps has been shown to lead to infertility.

Vaccine to Prevent Mumps

The best way to protect against mumps is to get the measles-mumps-rubella shot (called the "MMR shot"). Doctors recommend that all children get the MMR shot.

Why Should My Child Get the Measles-Mumps-Rubella Shot?

The MMR shot:

- Protects your child from mumps, a potentially serious disease, as well as measles and rubella.

- Prevents your child from getting a fever and swollen glands under the ears or jaw from mumps.

- Keeps your child from missing school or childcare (and keeps you from missing work to care for your sick child)

Is the Measles-Mumps-Rubella Shot Safe?

Yes. The MMR shot is very safe and effective at preventing mumps (as well as measles and rubella). Vaccines, like any medicine, can have side effects. But most children who get the MMR shot have no side effects.

What Are the Side Effects?

Most children do not have any side effects from the shot. The side effects that do occur are usually very mild, such as a fever, rash, soreness or swelling where the shot was given, or temporary pain and stiffness in the joints (mostly in teens and adults). More serious side effects are rare. These may include high fever that could cause a seizure.

Is There a Link between the Measles-Mumps-Rubella Shot and Autism?

No. Scientists in the United States and other countries have carefully studied the MMR shot. None has found a link between autism and the MMR shot.

Section 12.11

Rabies

This section contains text excerpted from the following sources:
Text in this section begins with excerpts from "Rabies," Centers for
Disease Control and Prevention (CDC), June 11, 2019; Text under
the heading "Treatment of Rabies" is excerpted from "Rabies,"
Centers for Disease Control and Prevention (CDC), January 2018.

Rabies is a fatal but preventable viral disease. It can spread to people and pets if they are bitten or scratched by a rabid animal. In the United States, rabies is mostly found in wild animals, such as bats, raccoons, skunks, and foxes. However, in many other countries dogs still carry rabies, and most rabies deaths in people around the world are caused by dog bites.

The rabies virus infects the central nervous system (CNS). If a person does not receive the appropriate medical care after a potential rabies exposure, the virus can cause disease in the brain, ultimately resulting in death. Rabies can be prevented by vaccinating pets, staying away from wildlife, and seeking medical care after potential exposures before symptoms start.

What Are the Signs and Symptoms of Rabies?

This time between the exposure and the appearance of symptoms is called the "incubation period," and it may last for weeks to months. The incubation period may vary based on the location of the exposure site (how far away it is from the brain), the type of rabies virus, and any existing immunity.

The first symptoms of rabies may be very similar to those of the flu including general weakness or discomfort, fever, or headache. These symptoms may last for days.

There may be also discomfort or a prickling or itching sensation at the site of the bite, progressing within days to acute symptoms of cerebral dysfunction, anxiety, confusion, and agitation. As the disease progresses, the person may experience delirium, abnormal behavior, hallucinations, hydrophobia (fear of water), and insomnia. The acute period of disease typically ends after 2 to 10 days. Once clinical signs of rabies appear, the disease is nearly always fatal, and treatment is typically supportive. To date, less than 20 cases of human survival from clinical rabies have been documented, and only a few survivors had no history of pre- or postexposure prophylaxis.

The signs, symptoms, and outcome of rabies in animals can vary but are often similar to those in humans, including early nonspecific symptoms, acute neurologic symptoms, and ultimately death.

How Is Rabies Transmitted?

Rabies virus is transmitted through direct contact (such as through broken skin or mucous membranes in the eyes, nose, or mouth) with saliva or brain/nervous system tissue from an infected animal.

People usually get rabies from the bite of a rabid animal. It is also possible, but rare, for people to get rabies from nonbite exposures, which can include scratches, abrasions, or open wounds that are exposed to saliva or other potentially infectious material from a rabid animal. Other types of contact, such as petting a rabid animal or contact with the blood, urine or feces of a rabid animal, are not associated with risk for infection and are not considered to be exposures of concern for rabies.

Other modes of transmission—aside from bites and scratches—are uncommon. Inhalation of aerosolized rabies virus is one potential nonbite route of exposure, but except for laboratory workers, most people will not encounter an aerosol of rabies virus. Rabies transmission through corneal and solid organ transplants have been recorded, but they are also very rare. There has only been two known solid organ donor with rabies in the United States since 2008. Many organ procurement organizations have added a screening question about rabies exposure to their procedures for evaluating the suitability of each donor.

Bite and nonbite exposures from an infected person could theoretically transmit rabies, but no such cases have been documented. Casual contact, such as touching a person with rabies or contact with noninfectious fluid or tissue (urine, blood, feces), is not associated with risk for infection. Contact with someone who is receiving rabies vaccination does not constitute rabies exposure, does not pose a risk for infection, and does not require postexposure prophylaxis.

Rabies virus becomes noninfectious when it dries out and when it is exposed to sunlight. Different environmental conditions affect the rate at which the virus becomes inactive, but in general, if the material containing the virus is dry, the virus can be considered noninfectious.

How Is Rabies Diagnosed?

In animals, rabies is diagnosed using the direct fluorescent antibody (DFA) test, which looks for the presence of rabies virus antigens in brain tissue. In humans, several tests are required.

Rapid and accurate laboratory diagnosis of rabies in humans and other animals is essential for the timely administration of postexposure prophylaxis. Within a few hours, a diagnostic laboratory can determine whether or not an animal is rabid and inform the responsible medical personnel. The laboratory results may save a patient from unnecessary physical and psychological trauma, and financial burdens, if the animal is not rabid.

In addition, laboratory identification of positive rabies cases may aid in defining current epidemiologic patterns of disease and provide appropriate information for the development of rabies control programs.

The nature of rabies disease dictates that laboratory tests be standardized, rapid, sensitive, specific, economical, and reliable.

When Should You Seek Medical Attention?

If you have been in contact with any wildlife or unfamiliar animals, particularly if you have been bitten or scratched, you should talk with a healthcare or public-health professional to determine your risk for rabies or other illnesses. Wash any wounds immediately with soap and water and then plan to see a healthcare provider. (It is important to know that, unlike most other animals that carry rabies, many types of bats have very small teeth which may leave marks that disappear quickly. If you are unsure, seek medical advice to be safe.)

Remember that rabies is a medical urgency but not an emergency. Decisions should not be delayed.

See your doctor for attention for any trauma due to an animal attack before considering the need for rabies vaccination. After any wounds have been addressed, your doctor—possibly in consultation with your state or local health department—will help you decide if you need treatment known as "rabies postexposure prophylaxis" (PEP). Decisions to start PEP will be based on your type of exposure, the animal you were exposed to, whether the animal is available for testing, and laboratory and surveillance information for the geographic area where the exposure occurred.

In the United States, PEP consists of a regimen of one dose of immune globulin and four doses of rabies vaccine over a 14-day period. Rabies immune globulin and the first dose of rabies vaccine should be given by your healthcare provider as soon as possible after exposure. Current vaccines are relatively painless and are given in your arms, such as the flu or tetanus vaccine; rabies vaccines are not given in the stomach.

Rabies Prevention
How Can You Prevent Rabies in People?

Understanding your rabies risk and knowing what to do after contact with animals can save lives. Any mammal can get rabies, but the most commonly affected animals in the United States are raccoons, skunks, bats, and foxes. The best way to avoid rabies in the United States is to stay away from wildlife. Leave all wildlife alone, including injured animals. If you find an injured animal, do not touch it; contact local authorities for assistance.

Rabies in dogs is still common in many countries outside the United States, so find out if rabies is present in dogs or wildlife at your destination before international travel.

Because pets can get rabies from wildlife and then could spread it to humans, preventing rabies in pets is also an important step in preventing human rabies cases.

If you do come into contact with a rabid animal, rabies in humans is 100 percent preventable through prompt appropriate medical care. If you are bitten, scratched, or unsure, talk to a healthcare provider about whether you need PEP.

Preventing Rabies around the Globe

Although dog rabies is no longer a problem in the United States, the most important global source of rabies in humans is from uncontrolled rabies in dogs. Children are often at greatest risk from rabies. They are more likely to be bitten by dogs and are also more likely to be severely exposed through multiple bites in high-risk sites on the body. Severe exposures make it more difficult to prevent rabies unless access to good medical care is immediately available.

This major source of rabies in humans can be eliminated through ensuring adequate animal vaccination and control, educating those at risk, and enhancing access of those bitten to appropriate medical care. The annual World Rabies Day campaign, first observed in 2007, brings together researchers and partners to accomplish these goals by mobilizing awareness and resources in support of human rabies prevention and animal rabies control around the world.

Treatment of Rabies
Vaccination after an Animal Bite

If you are bitten by an animal that could have rabies, you can get the rabies vaccine to keep you from developing the disease. A doctor can help decide if you need the vaccine.

If you have not been vaccinated for rabies before, you will need four doses of the vaccine. You will get the first dose right away, followed by additional doses:

- Three days after the first dose

- One week after the first dose

- Two weeks after the first dose

People who have a weakened immune system need another dose four weeks after the first dose.

You will also get a shot called "Rabies Immune Globulin" with the first dose to help your body fight the virus faster.

If you have already had the rabies vaccine, you will need two doses after an animal bite—you will get the first dose right away, followed by a second dose three days after the first. You would not need the Rabies Immune Globulin shot.

If you think you or someone in your family needs the rabies vaccine, talk with a doctor.

Who Should Not Get the Rabies Vaccine

Some people should not get the rabies vaccine—or may need to wait to get it. Be sure to tell your doctor before getting vaccinated if you:

- Have had an allergic reaction to the rabies vaccine in the past

- Have other severe allergies

- Have HIV/AIDS

- Have cancer

- Are taking medicines that can affect your immune system

If you have already come in contact with rabies—such as if you have been bitten by an animal that could have rabies—you will need to get the vaccine even if you have any of these conditions.

Section 12.12

Rubella

This section includes text excerpted from documents published by two public domain sources. Text under the headings marked 1 are excerpted from "Rubella (German Measles, Three-Day Measles)," Centers for Disease Control and Prevention (CDC), September 15, 2017; Text under the headings marked 2 are excerpted from "Rubella: Make Sure Your Child Gets Vaccinated," Centers for Disease Control and Prevention (CDC), February 19, 2019.

What Is Rubella?[1]

Rubella is a contagious disease caused by a virus. Most people who get rubella usually have a mild illness, with symptoms that can include a low-grade fever, sore throat, and a rash that starts on the face and spreads to the rest of the body. Rubella can cause a miscarriage or serious birth defects in a developing baby if a woman is infected while she is pregnant. The best protection against rubella is the measles-mumps-rubella (MMR) vaccine.

Signs and Symptoms of Rubella[1]

In children, rubella is usually mild, with few noticeable symptoms. For children who do have symptoms, a red rash is typically the first sign. The rash generally first appears on the face and then spreads to the rest of the body, and lasts about three days.

Other symptoms that may occur one to five days before the rash appears include:

- A low-grade fever

- Headache

- Mild pink eye (redness or swelling of the white of the eye)

- General discomfort

- Swollen and enlarged lymph nodes

- Cough

- Runny nose

Transmission of Rubella[1]

Rubella spreads when an infected person coughs or sneezes. Also, if a woman is infected with rubella while she is pregnant, she can pass it to her developing fetus and cause serious harm.

A person with rubella may spread the disease to others up to one week before the rash appears, and remain contagious up to 7 days after. However, 25 to 50 percent of people infected with rubella do not develop a rash or have any symptoms.

People infected with rubella should tell friends, family, and people they work with, especially pregnant women, if they have rubella. If your child has rubella, it is important to tell your child's school or day-care provider.

Complications of Rubella[2]

Rubella is a contagious disease caused by a virus. For some people—especially pregnant women and their unborn babies—rubella can be serious. Make sure you and your child are protected from rubella by getting vaccinated on schedule.

Young children who get rubella usually have a mild illness, with symptoms that can include a low-grade fever, sore throat, and a rash that starts on the face and spreads to the rest of the body. Older children and adults are more likely to have a headache, pink eye, and general discomfort before the rash appears.

Rubella Is Dangerous for Pregnant Women and Unborn Babies

The most serious complication from rubella infection is the harm it can cause a pregnant woman's unborn baby. If an unvaccinated pregnant woman gets infected with rubella virus she can have a miscarriage (the loss of a pregnancy during the first 23 weeks), or her baby can die just after birth. Also, she can pass the virus to her unborn baby who can develop serious birth defects, such as:

- Heart problems

- Loss of hearing and eyesight

- Intellectual disability

- Liver or spleen damage

Serious birth defects are more common if a woman is infected early in her pregnancy, especially in the first trimester (first 12 weeks). In fact, women infected with rubella early in pregnancy have a 1 in 5 chance of having problems with the pregnancy.

Children should be vaccinated on schedule to protect them from rubella infection and to prevent them from spreading rubella to a pregnant woman and her unborn baby.

Treatment of Rubella[1]

There is no specific medicine to treat rubella or make the disease go away faster. In many cases, symptoms are mild. For others, mild symptoms can be managed with bed rest and medicines for fever, such as acetaminophen.

If you are concerned about your symptoms or your child's symptoms, contact your doctor.

Prevention of Rubella[2]
Protect Your Child, and Others, with Rubella Vaccine

The best way to protect your child from rubella is to get her or him vaccinated on schedule. Children should be vaccinated against rubella to protect them from infection and to prevent them from spreading rubella to a pregnant woman and her unborn baby, as well those who cannot get vaccinated because they have a health condition or are too young.

Rubella vaccine is usually given as part of a combination vaccine called "MMR," which protects against three diseases: measles, mumps, and rubella. MMR vaccine is safe and effective and has been widely used in the United States for more than 30 years.

Children should get 2 doses of MMR vaccine:

- The first dose at 12 through 15 months of age

- The second dose at 4 through 6 years of age, before entering school

Your child's doctor may also offer the MMRV vaccine, which protects against four diseases: measles, mumps, rubella, and varicella (chickenpox).

Talk to your child's healthcare professional for help deciding which vaccine to use.

Chapter 13

Parasitic and Fungal Infections

Chapter Contents

Section 13.1

Ascariasis and Hookworm Infection

This section contains text excerpted from the following sources: Text under the heading "About Ascariasis" is excerpted from "Ascariasis FAQs," Centers for Disease Control and Prevention (CDC), January 10, 2013. Reviewed September 2019; Text under the heading "About Hookworm" is excerpted from "Hookworm FAQs," Centers for Disease Control and Prevention (CDC), December 16, 2014. Reviewed September 2019.

About Ascariasis

Ascaris is an intestinal parasite of humans. It is the most common human worm infection. The larvae and adult worms live in the small intestine and can cause intestinal disease.

How Is Ascariasis Spread?

Ascaris lives in the intestine and *Ascaris* eggs are passed in the feces of infected persons. If the infected person defecates outside (near bushes, in a garden, or field), or if the feces of an infected person are used as fertilizer, then eggs are deposited on the soil. They can then mature into a form that is infective. Ascariasis is caused by ingesting infective eggs. This can happen when hands or fingers that have contaminated dirt on them are put in the mouth or by consuming vegetables or fruits that have not been carefully cooked, washed or peeled.

Who Is at Risk for Infection?

Infection occurs worldwide in warm and humid climates, where sanitation and hygiene are poor, including in temperate zones during warmer months. Persons in these areas are at risk if soil contaminated with human feces enters their mouths or if they eat vegetables or fruit that have not been carefully washed, peeled or cooked. Ascariasis is now uncommon in the United States.

What Are the Symptoms of Ascariasis?

People infected with *Ascaris* often show no symptoms. If symptoms do occur they can be light and include abdominal discomfort. Heavy infections can cause intestinal blockage and impair growth in children.

Other symptoms such as cough are due to the migration of the worms through the body.

How Is Ascariasis Diagnosed?

Healthcare providers can diagnose ascariasis by taking a stool sample and using a microscope to look for the presence of eggs. Some people notice infection when a worm is passed in their stool or is coughed up. If this happens, bring in the worm specimen to your healthcare provider for a diagnosis.

How Can I Prevent Infection?

- Avoid contact with soil that may be contaminated with human feces, including with human fecal matter ("night soil") used to fertilize crops.

- Wash your hands with soap and warm water before handling food.

- Teach children the importance of washing hands to prevent infection.

- Wash, peel, or cook all raw vegetables and fruits before eating, particularly those that have been grown in soil that has been fertilized with manure.

Transmission of infection to others can be prevented by:

- Not defecating outdoors
- Effective sewage disposal systems

What Is the Treatment for Ascariasis?

Anthelmintic medications (drugs that rid the body of parasitic worms), such as albendazole and mebendazole, are the drugs of choice for treatment. Infections are generally treated for 1 to 3 days. The recommended medications are effective.

What Is Preventive Treatment?

In developing countries, groups at higher risk for soil-transmitted helminth infections (hookworm, *Ascaris*, and whipworm) are often treated without a prior stool examination. Treating in this way is called "preventive treatment" (or "preventive chemotherapy"). The high-risk groups identified by the WHO are preschool and school-age children, women of childbearing age (including pregnant women in the 2nd and 3rd trimesters and lactating women), and adults in occupations where there is a high risk of heavy infections. School-age children are often treated through school health programs and preschool children and pregnant women at visits to health clinics.

What Is Mass Drug Administration?

The soil-transmitted helminths (hookworm, *Ascaris*, and whipworm) and four other "neglected tropical diseases" (river blindness, lymphatic filariasis, schistosomiasis, and trachoma) are sometimes treated through mass drug administrations. Since the drugs used are safe and inexpensive or donated, entire risk groups are offered preventive treatment. Mass drug administrations (MDAs) are conducted periodically (often annually), commonly with drug distributors who go door-to-door. Multiple neglected tropical diseases are often treated simultaneously using MDAs.

About Hookworm

Hookworm is an intestinal parasite of humans. The larvae and adult worms live in the small intestine can cause intestinal disease. The two main species of hookworm infecting humans are *Ancylostoma duodenale* and *Necator americanus.*

How Is Hookworm Spread?

Hookworm eggs are passed in the feces of an infected person. If an infected person defecates outside (near bushes, in a garden, or field) or if the feces from an infected person are used as fertilizer, eggs are deposited on soil. They can then mature and hatch, releasing larvae (immature worms). The larvae mature into a form that can penetrate the skin of humans. Hookworm infection is transmitted primarily by walking barefoot on contaminated soil. One kind of hookworm (*Ancylostoma duodenale*) can also be transmitted through the ingestion of larvae.

Who Is at Risk for Infection?

People living in areas with warm and moist climates and where sanitation and hygiene are poor are at risk for hookworm infection if they walk barefoot or in other ways allow their skin to have direct contact with contaminated soil. Soil is contaminated by an infected person defecating outside or when human feces ("night soil") are used as fertilizer. Children who play in contaminated soil may also be at risk.

What Are the Signs and Symptoms of Hookworm?

Itching and a localized rash are often the first signs of infection. These symptoms occur when the larvae penetrate the skin. A person with a light infection may have no symptoms. A person with a heavy infection may experience abdominal pain, diarrhea, loss of appetite, weight loss, fatigue, and anemia. The physical and cognitive growth of children can be affected.

How Is Hookworm Diagnosed?

Healthcare providers can diagnose hookworm by taking a stool sample and using a microscope to look for the presence of hookworm eggs.

How Can I Prevent Infection?

Do not walk barefoot in areas where hookworm is common and where there may be fecal contamination of the soil. Avoid other skin-to-soil contact and avoid ingesting such soil. Fecal contamination occurs when people defecate outdoors or use human feces as fertilizer.

The infection of others can be prevented by not defecating outdoors or using human feces as fertilizer, and by effective sewage disposal systems.

What Is the Treatment for Hookworm?

Hookworm infections are generally treated for 1 to 3 days with medication prescribed by your healthcare provider. The drugs are effective and appear to have few side effects. Iron supplements may be prescribed if you have anemia.

What Is Preventive Treatment?

In developing countries, groups at higher risk for soil-transmitted helminth infections (hookworm, *Ascaris*, and whipworm) are often treated without a prior stool examination. Treating in this way is called "preventive treatment" (or "preventive chemotherapy"). The high-risk groups identified by the WHO are preschool and school-age children, women of childbearing age (including pregnant women in the 2nd and 3rd trimesters and lactating women), and adults in occupations where there is a high risk of heavy infections. School-age children are often treated through school health programs and preschool children and pregnant women at visits to health clinics.

What Is Mass Drug Administration?

The soil-transmitted helminths (hookworm, *Ascaris*, and whipworm) and four other "neglected tropical diseases" (river blindness, lymphatic filariasis, schistosomiasis, and trachoma) are sometimes treated through MDAs. Since the drugs used are safe and inexpensive or donated, entire risk groups are offered preventive treatment. Mass drug administrations are conducted periodically (often annually), commonly with drug distributors who go door-to-door. Multiple neglected tropical diseases are often treated simultaneously using MDAs.

Section 13.2

Baylisascaris *Infection*

This section includes text excerpted from "About Baylisascaris," Centers for Disease Control and Prevention (CDC), April 11, 2018.

What Is Baylisascaris*?*

Baylisascaris worms are intestinal parasites found in a wide variety of animals. Different species of *Baylisascaris* are associated with different animal hosts. For example, *Baylisascaris procyonis* is found in raccoons, and *Baylisascaris columnaris* is found in skunks. Cases of *Baylisascaris* infection in people are not frequently reported but can be severe. *Baylisascaris procyonis* is thought to pose the greatest risk to people because of the often close association of raccoons to human dwellings.

How Do People Get Infected?

People become infected by ingesting infectious eggs. Most infections are in children and others who are more likely to put dirt or animal waste in their mouth by mistake.

How Can You Prevent Baylisascaris Infection?

Eggs passed in raccoon feces are not immediately infectious. In the environment, eggs take two to four weeks to become infectious. If raccoons have set up a den or a latrine (places where raccoons defecate) in your yard, raccoon feces and material contaminated with raccoon feces should be removed carefully and burned, buried, or sent to a landfill. Care should be taken to avoid contaminating hands and clothes. Treat decks, patios, and other surfaces with boiling water or a propane flame-gun (exercise proper precautions). Prompt removal and destruction of raccoon feces before the eggs become infectious will reduce the risk for exposure and possible infection.

Do not keep, feed, or adopt wild animals, including raccoons, as pets.

Washing your hands after working or playing outdoors is good practice for preventing a number of diseases.

What Are the Symptoms and Signs of Baylisascaris Infection?

The incubation period (time from exposure to symptoms) is usually one to four weeks. If present, signs and symptoms can include the following:

- Nausea

- Tiredness

- Liver enlargement

- Loss of coordination

- Lack of attention to people and surroundings

- Loss of muscle control

- Blindness

- Coma

223

What Should You Do If You Think You Are Infected with Baylisascaris?

You should discuss your concerns with your healthcare provider, who will examine you and ask you questions (for example, about your interactions with raccoons or other wild animals). *Baylisascaris* infection is difficult to diagnose in humans. There are no widely available tests, so the diagnosis is often made by ruling out other diseases.

How Is Baylisascaris Infection Treated?

A healthcare provider can discuss treatment options with you. No drug has been found to be completely effective against *Baylisascaris* infection in people. Albendazole has been recommended for some cases.

If You Have Baylisascaris Infection, Should Your Family Members Be Tested for the Infection?

Baylisascaris infection is not contagious, so one person cannot give the infection to another. However, if your family may have been exposed the same way you were (such as contact with or exposure to an environment contaminated with a raccoon or exotic pet feces), they should consult with a healthcare provider.

Section 13.3

Cryptosporidiosis

This section includes text excerpted from "Cryptosporidium—
General Information for the Public," Centers for Disease Control and
Prevention (CDC), August 16, 2017.

What Is Cryptosporidium?

Cryptosporidiosis is a disease that causes watery diarrhea. It is caused by microscopic germs—parasites called "*Cryptosporidium.*"

Cryptosporidium, or "Crypto" for short, can be found in water, food, soil, or on surfaces or dirty hands that have been contaminated with the feces of humans or animals infected with the parasite. During 2001 to 2010, Crypto was the leading cause of waterborne disease outbreaks, linked to recreational water use in the United States. The parasite is found in every region of the United States and throughout the world.

How Is Cryptosporidiosis Spread?

Crypto lives in the gut of infected humans or animals. An infected person or animal sheds Crypto parasites in their poop. An infected person can shed 10,000,000 to 100,000,000 Crypto germs in a single bowel movement. Shedding of Crypto in poop begins when symptoms such as diarrhea begin and can last for weeks after symptoms stop. Swallowing as few as 10 Crypto germs can cause infection.

Crypto can be spread by:

- Swallowing recreational water (for example, the water in swimming pools, fountains, lakes, rivers) contaminated with Crypto

  - Crypto's high tolerance to chlorine enables the parasite to survive for long periods of time in chlorinated drinking and swimming-pool water

- Drinking untreated water from a lake or river that is contaminated with Crypto

- Swallowing water, ice, or beverages contaminated with poop from infected humans or animals

- Eating undercooked food or drinking unpasteurized/raw apple cider or milk that is contaminated with Crypto

- Touching your mouth with contaminated hands:

  - Hands can become contaminated through a variety of activities, such as touching surfaces or objects (e.g., toys, bathroom fixtures, changing tables, diaper pails) that have been contaminated by poop from an infected person, changing diapers, caring for an infected person, and touching an infected animal

Crypto is not spread through contact with blood.

What Are the Symptoms of Cryptosporidiosis, When Do They Begin, and How Long Do They Last?

Symptoms of Crypto generally begin 2 to 10 days (average 7 days) after becoming infected with the parasite. Symptoms include:

- Watery diarrhea
- Stomach cramps or pain
- Dehydration
- Nausea
- Vomiting
- Fever
- Weight loss

Symptoms usually last about 1 to 2 weeks (with a range of a few days to 4 or more weeks) in people with healthy immune systems.

The most common symptom of cryptosporidiosis is watery diarrhea. Some people with Crypto will have no symptoms at all.

Who Is Most at Risk for Cryptosporidiosis?

People who are most likely to become infected with *Cryptosporidium* include:

- Children who attend childcare centers, including diaper-aged children
- Childcare workers
- Parents of infected children
- Older adults (ages 75 years and older)
- People who take care of other people with Crypto
- International travelers
- Backpackers, hikers, and campers who drink unfiltered, untreated water
- People who drink from untreated, shallow, unprotected wells
- People, including swimmers, who swallow water from contaminated sources
- People who handle infected calves or other ruminants, such as sheep

Contaminated water might include water that has not been boiled or filtered, as well as contaminated recreational water sources (e.g., swimming pools, lakes, rivers, ponds, and streams). Several community-wide outbreaks have been linked to drinking tap water or recreational water contaminated with *Cryptosporidium*. Crypto's high tolerance to chlorine enables the parasite to survive for long periods of time in chlorinated drinking and swimming-pool water. This means anyone swallowing contaminated water could get ill.

Note: Although Crypto can infect all people, some groups are likely to develop more serious illness:

- Young children and pregnant women may be more likely to get dehydrated because of their diarrhea so they should drink plenty of fluids while ill.

- People with severely weakened immune systems are at risk for more serious disease. Symptoms may be more severe and could lead to serious or life-threatening illnesses. Examples of people with weakened immune systems include those with human immunodeficiency virus (HIV)/acquired immunodeficiency syndrome (AIDS); those with inherited diseases that affect the immune system; and cancer and transplant patients who are taking certain immunosuppressive drugs.

What Should You Do If You Think You Might Have Cryptosporidiosis?

For diarrhea whose cause has not been determined, the following actions may help relieve symptoms:

- Drink plenty of fluids to remain well hydrated and avoid dehydration. Serious health problems can occur if the body does not maintain proper fluid levels. For some people, diarrhea can be severe resulting in hospitalization due to dehydration.

- Maintain a well-balanced diet. Doing so may help speed recovery.

- Avoid beverages that contain caffeine, such as tea, coffee, and many soft drinks.

- Avoid alcohol, as it can lead to dehydration.

Contact your healthcare provider if you suspect that you have cryptosporidiosis.

How Is Cryptosporidiosis Diagnosed?

Cryptosporidiosis is a diarrheal disease that is spread through contact with the stool of an infected person or animal. The disease is diagnosed by examining stool samples. People infected with Crypto can shed the parasite irregularly in their poop (for example, one day they shed parasite, the next day they do not, the third day they do) so patients may need to give three samples collected on three different days to help make sure that a negative test result is accurate and really means they do not have Crypto. Healthcare providers should specifically request testing for Crypto. Routine ova and parasite testing do not normally include Crypto testing.

What Is the Treatment for Cryptosporidiosis?

Most people with healthy immune systems will recover from cryptosporidiosis without treatment. The following actions may help relieve symptoms:

- Drink plenty of fluids to remain well hydrated and avoid dehydration. Serious health problems can occur if the body does not maintain proper fluid levels. For some people, diarrhea can be severe resulting in hospitalization due to dehydration.

- Maintain a well-balanced diet. Doing so may help speed recovery.

- Avoid beverages that contain caffeine, such as tea, coffee, and many soft drinks.

- Avoid alcohol, as it can lead to dehydration.

Over-the-counter (OTC) antidiarrheal medicine might help slow down diarrhea, but a healthcare provider should be consulted before such medicine is taken.

A drug called "nitazoxanide' has been FDA-approved for the treatment of diarrhea caused by *Cryptosporidium* in people with healthy immune systems and is available by prescription. Consult with your healthcare provider for more information about the potential advantages and disadvantages of taking nitazoxanide.

Individuals who have health concerns should talk to their healthcare provider.

Note: Infants, young children, and pregnant women may be more likely than others to suffer from dehydration. Losing a lot of fluids from diarrhea can be dangerous—and especially life-threatening in infants. These people should drink extra fluids when they are sick. Severe dehydration may require hospitalization for treatment with fluids given through your vein (intravenous or IV fluids). If you are pregnant or a parent and you suspect you or your child are severely dehydrated, contact a healthcare provider about fluid replacement options.

How to Keep Your House Clean to Help Prevent the Spread of Cryptosporidiosis

No cleaning method is guaranteed to be completely effective against Crypto. However, you can lower the chance of spreading Crypto by taking the following precautions:

- Wash linens, clothing, dishwasher- or dryer-safe soft toys, etc. soiled with poop or vomit as soon as possible.
  - Flush excess vomit or poop on clothes or objects down the toilet.
  - Use laundry detergent, and wash in hot water: 113°F or hotter for at least 20 minutes or at 122°F or hotter for at least 5 minutes.
  - Machine dry on the highest heat setting.
- For other household objects and surfaces (for example, diaper-change areas):
  - Remove all visible poop.
  - Clean with soap and water.
  - Let dry completely for at least 4 hours.
    - If possible, expose to direct sunlight during the 4 hours.
- Wash your hands with soap and water after cleaning objects or surfaces that could be contaminated with Crypto.

Note: The best way to prevent the spread of *Cryptosporidium* in the home is by practicing good hygiene. Wash your hands frequently with soap and water, especially after using the toilet, after changing diapers, and before eating or preparing food. Alcohol-based hand sanitizers are not effective against Crypto.

How Can You Protect Yourself and Others from Getting Cryptosporidiosis?
Prevention and Control
Practice Good Hygiene Everywhere

- Help keep yourself and your loved ones healthy by washing your hands often with soap and water, especially during key times when you are likely to spread germs.

- Alcohol-based hand sanitizers are not effective against Crypto. Washing hands at key times with soap and water can help prevent infections.

At Childcare Facilities

- Exclude children who are sick with diarrhea from childcare settings until diarrhea has stopped.

- Clean, sanitize, or disinfect toys and surfaces to prevent germs from spreading easily.

- Wash hands regularly with soap and water to keep kids and caregivers healthy.

- Move adults with diarrhea to jobs that minimize opportunities for spreading Crypto (for example, to administrative work instead of food or drink preparation).

At the Pool, Lake, and Other Places We Swim

- If sick with diarrhea, do not swim or let kids swim.
  - If Crypto is diagnosed, wait 2 weeks after diarrhea has stopped to go swimming.
- Do not swallow the water.
- Take young children on bathroom breaks or check their diapers every 60 minutes.
  - Change diapers in the bathroom or diaper-changing area—not waterside—to keep germs and poop out of the water.

Avoid Water That Might Be Contaminated

- Do not drink untreated water or use untreated ice from lakes, rivers, springs, ponds, streams, or shallow wells.

- Follow the advice given during local drinking-water advisories.

- If the safety of drinking water is in doubt (for example, if the water source is unknown), use at least one of the following:

  - Commercially bottled water

  - Water that has been previously boiled for at least 1 minute and left to cool. At elevations above 6,500 feet (1,981 meters), boil for 3 minutes.

  - A filter designed to remove Crypto

    - The label might read "National Sanitation Foundation (NSF) 53" or "NSF 58."

    - Filter labels that read "absolute pore size of 1 micron or smaller" are also effective.

Avoid Food That Might Be Contaminated

- If you drink milk or apple cider, only buy if it has been pasteurized.

- Do not eat fruits and vegetables washed in water that might be contaminated.

Practice Extra Caution While Traveling

- Do not use or drink inadequately treated water or use ice when traveling in countries where the water might be unsafe.

- Avoid eating uncooked foods when traveling in countries where the food supply might be unsafe.

Section 13.4

Giardiasis

This section includes text excerpted from "Giardia—General
Information," Centers for Disease Control and Prevention (CDC),
July 22, 2015. Reviewed September 2019.

What Is Giardiasis?

Giardia is a microscopic parasite that causes the diarrheal illness
known as "giardiasis." *Giardia* (also known as *"Giardia intestinalis,"*
"Giardia lamblia," or *"Giardia duodenalis"*) is found on surfaces or in
soil, food, or water that has been contaminated with feces (poop) from
infected humans or animals.

Giardia is protected by an outer shell that allows it to survive outside the body for long periods of time and makes it tolerant to chlorine
disinfection. While the parasite can be spread in different ways, water
(drinking water and recreational water) is the most common mode of
transmission.

Signs and Symptoms of Giardiasis

Giardiasis is the most frequently diagnosed intestinal parasitic disease in the United States and among travelers with chronic diarrhea.
Signs and symptoms may vary and can last for one to two weeks or
longer. In some cases, people infected with *Giardia* have no symptoms.

Acute symptoms include:

- Diarrhea

- Gas

- Greasy stools that tend to float

- Stomach or abdominal cramps

- Upset stomach or nausea/vomiting

- Dehydration (loss of fluids)

Other, less-common symptoms include itchy skin, hives, and swelling of the eye and joints. Sometimes, the symptoms of giardiasis might
seem to resolve, only to come back again after several days or weeks.
Giardiasis can cause weight loss and failure to absorb fat, lactose,
vitamin A and vitamin B_{12}.

In children, severe giardiasis might delay physical and mental growth, slow development, and cause malnutrition.

Diagnosis and Detection of Giardiasis

Because *Giardia* cysts can be excreted intermittently, multiple stool collections (i.e., three stool specimens collected on separate days) increase test sensitivity. The use of concentration methods and tri-chrome staining might not be sufficient to identify *Giardia* because variability in the concentration of organisms in the stool can make this infection difficult to diagnose. For this reason, fecal immunoassays that are more sensitive and specific should be used.

Rapid immune-chromatographic cartridge assays also are available but should not take the place of routine ova and parasite examination. Only molecular testing (e.g., polymerase chain reaction) can be used to identify the subtypes of *Giardia*.

Sources of Infection and Risk Factors of Giardiasis
General Epidemiology

Giardiasis is a diarrheal illness caused by the parasite *Giardia intestinalis* (also known as "*Giardia lamblia*" or "*Giardia duodenalis*"). A parasite is an organism that feeds off of another to survive.

Giardiasis is a global disease. It infects nearly 2 percent of adults and 6 to 8 percent of children in developed countries worldwide. Nearly 33 percent of people in developing countries have had giardiasis. In the United States, *Giardia* infection is the most common intestinal parasitic disease affecting humans.

People become infected with *Giardia* by swallowing *Giardia* cysts (hard shells containing *Giardia*) found in contaminated food or water. Cysts are instantly infectious once they leave the host through feces (poop). An infected person might shed 1 to 10 billion cysts daily in their feces (poop) and this might last for several months. However, swallowing as few as 10 cysts might cause someone to become ill. *Giardia* may be passed from person-to-person or even from animal-to-person. Also, oral–anal contact during sex has been known to cause infection. Symptoms of giardiasis normally begin 1 to 3 weeks after a person has been infected.

Giardia infection rates have been known to go up in late summer. Between 2006 and 2008 in the United States, known cases of giardiasis were twice as high between June and October as they were between January and March.

Anyone may become infected with *Giardia*. However, those at greatest risk are:

- Travelers to countries where giardiasis is common
- People in childcare settings
- Those who are in close contact with someone who has the disease
- People who swallow contaminated drinking water
- Backpackers or campers who drink untreated water from lakes or rivers
- People who have contact with animals who have the disease
- Men who have sex with men

The risk of humans acquiring *Giardia* infection from dogs or cats is small. The exact type of *Giardia* that infects humans is usually not the same type that infects dogs and cats.

Molecular Characterization

Giardia intestinalis (*G. duodenalis, G. lamblia*) can be subdivided based on molecular analysis into what are known as different genetic assemblages (A, B, C, D, E, F, and G). Some of these assemblages can be classified even further into subtypes like for example A-I, A-II, A-III, A-IV. Each assemblage is capable of infecting certain species, and some assemblages are more commonly seen than others.

Table 13.1. Assemblages of Molecular Characterization

Assemblages	Some Species Commonly Infected
A-I	Humans and animals (cats, dogs, livestock, deer, muskrats, beavers, voles, guinea pigs, ferrets)
A-II	Humans (more common than A-I)
A-III and A-IV	Exclusively animals
B	Humans and animals (livestock, chinchillas, beavers, marmosets, rodents)
C and D	Dogs, coyotes
E	Alpacas, cattle, goats, pigs, sheep
F	Cats

Prevention and Control of Giardiasis
Practice Good Hygiene

- Everywhere

  - Wash hands with soap and clean, running water for at least 20 seconds; rub your hands together to make a lather and be sure to scrub the backs of your hands, between your fingers, and under your nails.

    - Before, during, and after preparing food

    - Before eating food

    - Before and after caring for someone who is sick

    - Before and after treating a cut or wound

    - After using the toilet

    - After changing diapers or cleaning up a child who has used the toilet

    - After blowing your nose, coughing, or sneezing

    - After touching an animal or animal waste

    - After handling pet food or pet treats

    - After touching garbage

  - Help young children and other people you are caring for with handwashing as needed.

- At childcare facilities

  - To reduce the risk of spreading the disease, children with diarrhea should be removed from childcare settings until diarrhea has stopped.

- At recreational water venues (for example, pools, beaches, fountains)

  - Protect others by not swimming if you have diarrhea (this is most important for children in diapers).

  - Shower before entering the water.

  - Wash children thoroughly (especially their bottoms) with soap and water after they use the bathroom or after their diapers are changed and before they enter the water.

- Take children on frequent bathroom breaks and check their diapers often.

- Change diapers in the bathroom, not by the water.

- Around animals

  - Minimize contact with the feces (poop) of all animals, especially young animals.

  - When cleaning up animal feces (poop), wear disposable gloves and always wash hands when finished.

  - Wash hands after any contact with animals or their living areas.

- Outside

  - Wash hands after gardening, even if wearing gloves.

Avoid Water That May Be Contaminated

- Do not swallow water while swimming in pools, hot tubs, interactive fountains, lakes, rivers, springs, ponds, streams, or the ocean.

- Do not drink untreated water from lakes, rivers, springs, ponds, streams, or shallow wells.

- Do not drink poorly treated water or ice made from water during community outbreaks caused by contaminated drinking water.

- Do not use or drink poorly treated water or use ice when traveling in countries where the water supply might be unsafe.

- If the safety of drinking water is in doubt (for example, during or after an outbreak, in a place with poor sanitation or lack of water treatment systems), do one of the following:

  - Drink bottled water.

  - Disinfect tap water by heating it to a rolling boil for 1 minute.

  - Use a filter that has been tested and certified for cyst and oocyst reduction; filtered tap water will need additional treatment to kill or weaken bacteria and viruses.

Avoid Eating Food That May Be Contaminated

- Use safe, uncontaminated water to wash all food that is to be eaten raw.

- After washing vegetables and fruit in safe, uncontaminated water, peel them if you plan to eat them raw.

- Avoid eating raw or uncooked foods when traveling in countries with poor food and water treatment.

Clean Up after Ill Pets and People

Giardia is hard to completely eliminate from the environment, but you can decrease the risk of human infection or of your dog's or cat's reinfection if it has been ill. The risk of acquiring *Giardia* infection from your dog or cat is small, but there are some steps you can take to minimize your exposure.

Clean and disinfect your home in this way:

- **Hard surfaces** (for example: cement and tile floors, pet crates, tables, trash cans, etc.)

  - **Cleaning**

    - Wear gloves.

    - Remove feces and discard in a plastic bag.

    - Clean and scrub surfaces using soap. Rinse the surface thoroughly until no obvious visible contamination is present.

  - **Disinfection**

    - Wear gloves.

    - Disinfect according to manufacturer guidelines using one of the following:

      - Quaternary ammonium compound products (QATS), which are found in some household cleaning products; the active ingredient may be listed as alkyl dimethyl ammonium chloride.

      - Bleach mixed with water (3/4 cup of bleach to 1 gallon of water)

    - Follow product instructions, ensuring the product stays in contact with the surface for the recommended amount of time.

- Rinse with clean water.
- **Carpet/Upholstered furniture**
  - **Cleaning**
    - Wear gloves.
    - If feces are on a carpet or upholstered furniture, remove them with absorbent material (for example, double-layered paper towels).
    - Place and discard the feces in a plastic bag.
    - Clean the contaminated area with regular detergent or carpet cleaning agents.
    - Allow carpet or upholstered furniture to fully dry.
  - **Disinfection**
    - Wear gloves.
    - Steam clean the area at 158°F for 5 minutes or 212°F for 1 minute.
    - Quaternary ammonium compound products are found in some carpet cleaning products and can also be used after cleaning to disinfect. Read the product labels for specifications, and follow all instructions.
- **Other items (toys, clothing, pet bed, etc.)**
  - Household items should be cleaned and disinfected daily while a dog or cat is being treated for *Giardia* infection.
  - **Dishwasher**
    - Dishwasher-safe toys and water and food bowls can be disinfected in a dishwasher that has a dry cycle or a final rinse that exceeds one of the following:
      - 113°F for 20 minutes
      - 122°F for 5 minutes
      - 162°F for 1 minute
      - If a dishwasher is not available, submerge dishwasher-safe items in boiling water for at least 1 minute (at elevations above 6,500 feet, boil for 3 minutes).

- **Washer and dryer**

  - Clothing, some pet items (for example, bedding and cloth toys), and linens (sheets and towels) can be washed in the washing machine and then heat-dried on the highest heat setting for 30 minutes.

  - If a clothes dryer is not available, allow clothes to thoroughly air dry under direct sunlight.

Treatment of Giardiasis

Several drugs can be used to treat *Giardia* infection. Effective treatments include metronidazole, tinidazole, and nitazoxanide. Alternatives to these medications include paromomycin, quinacrine, and furazolidone. Some of these drugs may not be routinely available in the United States.

Different factors may shape how effective a drug regimen will be, including medical history, nutritional status, and condition of the immune system. Therefore, it is important to discuss treatment options with a healthcare provider.

Section 13.5

Head Lice

This section includes text excerpted from "Head Lice,"
MedlinePlus, National Institutes of Health (NIH),
September 9, 2016. Reviewed September 2019.

What Are Head Lice?

Head lice are tiny insects that live on people's heads. Adult lice are about the size of sesame seeds. The eggs, called "nits," are even smaller—about the size of a dandruff flake. Lice and nits are found on or near the scalp, most often at the neckline and behind the ears.

Head lice are parasites, and they need to feed on human blood to survive. They are one of the three types of lice that live on humans. The other two types are body lice and pubic lice. Each type of lice is different, and getting one type does not mean that you will get another type.

How Do Head Lice Spread?

Lice move by crawling because they cannot hop or fly. They spread by close person-to-person contact. Rarely, they can spread through sharing personal belongings such as hats or hairbrushes. Personal hygiene and cleanliness have nothing to do with getting head lice. You also cannot get pubic lice from animals. Head lice do not spread disease.

Who Is at Risk for Head Lice?

Children ages 3 to 11 and their families get head lice most often. This is because young children often have head-to-head contact while playing together.

What Are the Symptoms of Head Lice?

The symptoms of head lice include:

- Tickling feeling in the hair
- Frequent itching, which is caused by an allergic reaction to the bites
- Sores from scratching. Sometimes the sores can become infected with bacteria.
- Trouble sleeping, because head lice are most active in the dark

How Do You Know If You Have Head Lice?

A diagnosis of head lice usually comes from seeing a louse or nit. Because they are very small and move quickly, you may need to use a magnifying lens and a fine-toothed comb to find lice or nits.

What Are the Treatments for Head Lice?

Treatments for head lice include both over-the-counter (OTC) and prescription shampoos, creams, and lotions. If you want to use an OTC treatment and you are not sure which one to use or how to use one, ask your healthcare provider or pharmacist. You should also check with your healthcare provider first if you are pregnant or nursing, or if you want to use a treatment on a young child.

Follow these steps when using a head lice treatment:

- Apply the product according to the instructions. Only apply it to the scalp and the hair attached to the scalp. You should not use it on other body hair.

- Use only one product at a time, unless your healthcare provider tells you to use two different kinds at once.

- Pay attention to what the instructions say about how long you should leave the medicine on the hair and on how you should rinse it out.

- After rinsing, use a fine-toothed comb or special "nit comb" to remove dead lice and nits.

- After each treatment, check the hair for lice and nits. You should comb the hair to remove nits and lice every two to three days. Do this for two to three weeks to be sure that all lice and nits are gone.

All household members and other close contacts should be checked and treated if necessary. If an OTC treatment does not work for you, you can ask your healthcare provider for a prescription product.

Can Head Lice Be Prevented?

There are steps you can take to prevent the spread of lice. If you already have lice, besides treatment, you should:

- Wash your clothes, bedding, and towels with hot water, and dry them using the hot cycle of the dryer

- Soak your combs and brushes in hot water for 5 to 10 minutes

- Vacuum the floor and furniture, particularly where you sat or lay

- If there are items that you cannot wash, seal them in a plastic bag for two weeks.

To prevent your children from spreading lice:

- Teach children to avoid head-to-head contact during play and other activities

- Teach children not to share clothing and other items that they put on their head, such as headphones, hair ties, and helmets

- If your child has lice, be sure to check the policies at school and/ or daycare. Your child may not be able to go back until the lice have been completely treated.

There is no clear scientific evidence that lice can be suffocated by home remedies, such as mayonnaise, olive oil, or similar substances. You also should not use kerosene or gasoline; they are dangerous and flammable.

Section 13.6

Hymenolepis *Infection*

This section includes text excerpted from "Hymenolepiasis— Hymenolepiasis FAQs," Centers for Disease Control and Prevention (CDC), January 10, 2012. Reviewed September 2019.

What Is Hymenolepis nana *Infection?*

The dwarf tapeworm, or *Hymenolepis nana*, is found worldwide. Infection is most common in children, in persons living in institutional settings, and in people who live in areas where sanitation and personal hygiene are inadequate.

How Did You Get Infected?

One becomes infected by accidentally ingesting dwarf tapeworm eggs. This can happen by ingesting fecally contaminated food or water, by touching your mouth with contaminated fingers, or by ingesting contaminated soil. People can also become infected if they accidentally ingest an infected arthropod (intermediate host, such as a small beetle or mealworm) that have gotten into the food.

Adult dwarf tapeworms are very small in comparison with other tapeworms and may reach 15 to 40 mm (up to 2 inches) in length. The adult dwarf tapeworm is made up of many small segments called "proglottids." As the dwarf tapeworm matures inside the intestine, these segments break off and pass into the stool. An adult dwarf tapeworm can live for 4 to 6 weeks. However, once you are infected, the dwarf tapeworm may reproduce inside the body (autoinfection) and continue the infection.

What Are the Symptoms of a Dwarf Tapeworm Infection?

Most people who are infected do not have any symptoms. Those who have symptoms may experience nausea, weakness, loss of appetite, diarrhea, and abdominal pain. Young children, especially those with a heavy infection, may develop a headache, itchy bottom, or have difficulty sleeping. Sometimes the infection is misdiagnosed as a pinworm infection.

Contrary to popular belief, a dwarf tapeworm infection does not generally cause weight loss. You cannot feel the dwarf tapeworm inside your body.

How Is Dwarf Tapeworm Infection Diagnosed?

Diagnosis is made by identifying dwarf tapeworm eggs in the stool. Your healthcare provider will ask you to submit stool specimens collected over several days to see if you are infected.

Is a Dwarf Tapeworm Infection Serious?

No. Infection with the dwarf tapeworm is generally not serious. However, a prolonged infection can lead to more severe symptoms; therefore, medical attention is needed to eliminate the dwarf tapeworm.

How Is a Dwarf Tapeworm Infection Treated?

Treatment is available. A prescription drug called "praziquantel" is given. The medication causes the dwarf tapeworm to dissolve within the intestine. Praziquantel is generally well tolerated. Sometimes more than one treatment is necessary.

Can Infection Be Spread to Other Family Members?

Yes. Eggs are infectious (meaning they can reinfect you or infect others) immediately after being shed in feces.

What Should You Do If You Think You Have a Dwarf Tapeworm Infection?

See your healthcare provider for diagnosis and treatment.

How Can Dwarf Tapeworm Infection Be Prevented?

To reduce the likelihood of infection you should:

- Wash your hands with soap and warm water after using the toilet, changing diapers, and before preparing food.

- Teach children the importance of washing hands to prevent infection.

- When traveling in countries where food is likely to be contaminated, wash, peel, or cook all raw vegetables and fruits with safe water before eating.

Section 13.7

Pinworm Infection

This section includes text excerpted from "Pinworm Infections—
Pinworm Infection FAQs," Centers for Disease Control and
Prevention (CDC), January 10, 2013. Reviewed September 2019.

What Is a Pinworm?

A pinworm ("threadworm") is a small, thin, white roundworm (nematode) called *"Enterobius vermicularis"* that sometimes lives in the colon and rectum of humans. Pinworms are about the length of a staple. While an infected person sleeps, female pinworms leave the intestine through the anus and deposit their eggs on the surrounding skin.

What Are the Symptoms of Pinworm Infection?

Pinworm infection (called "enterobiasis" or "oxyuriasis") causes itching around the anus which can lead to difficulty sleeping and restlessness. Symptoms are caused by the female pinworm laying her eggs. Symptoms of pinworm infection usually are mild and some infected people have no symptoms.

Who Is at Risk for Pinworm Infection?

Pinworm infection occurs worldwide and affects people of all ages and socioeconomic levels. It is the most common worm infection in the United States. Pinworm infection occurs most commonly among:

- School-aged and preschool-aged children

- Institutionalized persons

- Household members and caretakers of persons with pinworm infection

Pinworm infection often occurs in more than one person in the household and institutional settings. Childcare centers often are the site of cases of pinworm infection.

How Is Pinworm Infection Spread?

Pinworm infection is spread by the fecal–oral route, that is by the transfer of infective pinworm eggs from the anus to someone's mouth, either directly by hand or indirectly through contaminated clothing, bedding, food, or other articles.

Pinworm eggs become infective within a few hours of being deposited on the skin around the anus and can survive for two to three weeks on clothing, bedding, or other objects. People become infected, usually unknowingly, by swallowing (ingesting) infective pinworm eggs that are on fingers, under fingernails, or on clothing, bedding, and other contaminated objects and surfaces. Because of their small size, pinworm eggs sometimes can become airborne and ingested while breathing.

Can Your Family Become Infected with Pinworms from Swimming Pools?

Pinworm infections are rarely spread through the use of swimming pools. Pinworm infections occur when a person swallows pinworm eggs picked up from contaminated surfaces or fingers. Although chlorine levels found in pools are not high enough to kill pinworm eggs, the presence of a small number of pinworm eggs in thousands of gallons of water (the amount typically found in pools) makes the chance of infection unlikely.

Does Co-Bathing *Lead to Infection?*

During this treatment time and two weeks after the final treatment, it is a good idea to avoid co-bathing and the reuse or sharing of washcloths. Showering may be preferred to avoid possible contamination of bathwater. Careful handling and frequent changing of underclothing, nightclothes, towels, and bedding can help reduce infection, reinfection, and environmental contamination with pinworm eggs. These items should be laundered in hot water, especially after each treatment of the infected person and after each usage of washcloths until the infection is cleared.

Did Your Pets Give You Pinworms/Can You Give Pinworms to Your Pets?

No. Humans are considered to be the only hosts of *E. vermicularis*, which is also known as the "human pinworm."

How Is Pinworm Infection Diagnosed?

Itching during the night in a child's perianal area strongly suggests pinworm infection. Diagnosis is made by identifying the worm or its eggs. Worms can sometimes be seen on the skin near the anus or on underclothing, pajamas, or sheets about two to three hours after falling asleep.

Pinworm eggs can be collected and examined using the "tape test" as soon as the person wakes up. This "test" is done by firmly pressing the adhesive side of clear, transparent cellophane tape to the skin around the anus. The eggs stick to the tape and the tape can be placed on a slide and looked at under a microscope. Because washing/bathing or having a bowel movement can remove eggs from the skin, this test should be done as soon as the person wakes up in the morning before they wash, bathe, go to the toilet, or get dressed. The "tape test" should be done on three consecutive mornings to increase the chance of finding pinworm eggs.

Because itching and scratching of the anal area are common in pinworm infection, samples taken from under the fingernails may also contain eggs. Pinworm eggs are rarely found in routine stool or urine samples.

How Is Pinworm Infection Treated?

Pinworm can be treated with either prescription or over-the-counter (OTC) medications. A healthcare provider should be consulted before treating a suspected case of pinworm infection.

Treatment involves two doses of medication with the second dose being given two weeks after the first dose. All household contacts and caretakers of the infected person should be treated at the same time. Reinfection can occur easily so strict observance of good hand hygiene is essential (e.g., proper handwashing, maintaining clean short fingernails, avoiding nail-biting, avoiding scratching the peri-anal area).

Daily morning bathing and daily changing of underwear help remove a large proportion of eggs. Showering may be preferred to avoid possible contamination of bathwater. Careful handling and frequent changing of underclothing, nightclothes, towels, and bedding can help reduce infection, reinfection, and environmental contamination with pinworm eggs. These items should be laundered in hot water, especially after each treatment of the infected person and after each usage of washcloths until the infection is cleared.

Should Family and Other Close Contacts of Someone with Pinworm Also Be Treated for Pinworm?

Yes. The infected person and all household contacts and caretakers of the infected person should be treated at the same time.

What Should Be Done If the Pinworm Infection Occurs Again?

Reinfection occurs easily. Prevention should always be discussed at the time of treatment. Good hand hygiene is the most effective means of prevention. If pinworm infection occurs again, the infected person should be re-treated with the same two-dose treatment. The infected person's household contacts and caretakers also should be treated. If pinworm infection continues to occur, the source of the infection should be sought and treated. Playmates, schoolmates, close contacts outside the home, and household members should be considered possible sources of infection. Each infected person should receive the recommended two-dose treatment.

How Can Pinworm Infection and Reinfection Be Prevented?

Strict observance of good hand hygiene is the most effective means of preventing pinworm infection. This includes washing hands with soap and warm water after using the toilet, changing diapers, and before handling food. Keep fingernails clean and short, avoid fingernail-biting, and avoid scratching the skin in the perianal area. Teach children the importance of washing hands to prevent infection.

Daily morning bathing and changing of underclothes helps remove a large proportion of pinworm eggs and can help prevent infection and reinfection. Showering may be preferred to avoid possible contamination of bathwater. Careful handling (avoid shaking) and frequent laundering of underclothes, nightclothes, towels, and bedsheets using hot water also help reduce the chance of infection and reinfection by reducing environmental contamination with eggs.

Control can be difficult in childcare centers and schools because the rate of reinfection is high. In institutions, mass and simultaneous treatment, repeated in two weeks, can be effective. Hand hygiene is the most effective method of prevention. Trimming and scrubbing the fingernails and bathing after treatment is important to help prevent reinfection and spread of pinworms.

Section 13.8

Scabies

This section includes text excerpted from "Scabies," Centers for Disease Control and Prevention (CDC), October 31, 2017.

What Is Scabies?

Scabies is a skin condition caused by mites. It commonly leads to intense itching and a pimple-like skin rash that may affect various areas of the body. Scabies is contagious and can spread quickly in areas where people are in close physical contact.

How Can You Get Scabies?

- Scabies usually is spread by skin-to-skin contact with a person who has scabies.

- Scabies sometimes is spread indirectly by sharing items such as clothing, towels, or bedding used by an infested person.

- Scabies can spread easily under crowded conditions where close body and skin contact is common.

How Can You Prevent Getting Scabies?

Prevent scabies by avoiding skin-to-skin contact with a person who has scabies and contact with items such as clothing or bedding used by a person infested with scabies mites.

An indirect spread can occur more easily when a person has crusted scabies.

What Are the Symptoms of Scabies?

Common symptoms of itching and a pimple-like skin rash may affect much of the body or be limited to common places such as:

- Between the fingers
- Wrist
- Elbow
- Armpit
- Genitals
- Nipple
- Waist
- Buttocks
- Shoulder blades

Symptoms affect the head, face, neck, palms, and soles in infants and very young children, but usually not adults and older children.

When a person is first infested with scabies mites, it usually takes two to six weeks for symptoms to appear after being infested. If a person has had scabies before, symptoms appear one to four days after exposure.

An infested person can transmit scabies, even if they do not have symptoms until they are successfully treated and the mites and eggs are destroyed.

How Can Scabies Be Treated?

Scabies should be treated with topical creams that can kill the mites, which are available by prescription from your healthcare provider. In addition to the infested person, the treatment also is recommended for people with whom they have been in contact.

Bedding, clothing, and towels used by infested persons and people they are in close contact with should be decontaminated. To disinfest items:

- Wash them in hot water and dry in a hot dryer or dry-clean

- Store items that cannot be washed in a sealed plastic bag for at least 72 hours

- Thoroughly clean and vacuum rooms

Section 13.9

Swimmer's Itch

This section includes text excerpted from "Swimmer's Itch FAQs,"
Centers for Disease Control and Prevention (CDC), October 22, 2018.

What Is Swimmer's Itch?

Swimmer's itch, also called "cercarial dermatitis," appears as a skin rash caused by an allergic reaction to certain microscopic parasites that infect some birds and mammals. These parasites are released from infected snails into fresh and saltwater (such as lakes, ponds, and oceans). While the parasite's preferred host is the specific bird or mammal, if the parasite comes into contact with a swimmer, it burrows into the skin and causes an allergic reaction and rash. Swimmer's itch is found throughout the world and is more frequent during the summer months.

How Does Water Become Infested with the Parasite?

The adult parasite lives in the blood of infected animals, such as ducks, geese, gulls, swans, and certain mammals such as muskrats and raccoons. The parasites produce eggs that are passed in the feces of infected birds or mammals.

If the eggs land in or are washed into the water, the eggs hatch, releasing small, free-swimming microscopic larvae. These larvae swim in the water in search of a certain species of aquatic snail.

If the larvae find one of these snails, they infect the snail, multiply, and undergo further development. Infected snails release a different type of microscopic larvae (or cercariae, hence the name cercarial dermatitis) into the water. This larval form then swims about searching for a suitable host (bird, muskrat) to continue the life cycle. Although humans are not suitable hosts, the microscopic larvae burrow into the swimmer's skin, and may cause an allergic reaction and rash. Because these larvae cannot develop inside a human, they soon die.

What Are the Signs and Symptoms of Swimmer's Itch?

Symptoms of swimmer's itch may include:

- Tingling, burning, or itching of the skin

- Small reddish pimples

- Small blisters

Within minutes to days after swimming in contaminated water, you may experience tingling, burning, or itching of the skin. Small reddish pimples appear within twelve hours. Pimples may develop into small blisters. Scratching the areas may result in secondary bacterial infections. Itching may last up to a week or more, but will gradually go away.

Because swimmer's itch is caused by an allergic reaction to infection, the more often you swim or wade in contaminated water, the more likely you are to develop more serious symptoms. The greater the number of exposures to contaminated water, the more intense and immediate symptoms of swimmer's itch will be.

Be aware that swimmer's itch is not the only rash that may occur after swimming in fresh or saltwater.

Do You Need to See Your Healthcare Provider for Treatment?

Most cases of swimmer's itch do not require medical attention. If you have a rash, you may try the following for relief:

- Use corticosteroid cream
- Apply cool compresses to the affected areas
- Bathe in Epsom salts or baking soda
- Soak in colloidal oatmeal baths
- Apply baking soda paste to the rash (made by stirring water into baking soda until it reaches a paste-like consistency)
- Use an anti-itch lotion

Though difficult, try not to scratch. Scratching may cause the rash to become infected. If itching is severe, your healthcare provider may suggest prescription-strength lotions or creams to lessen your symptoms.

Can Swimmer's Itch Be Spread from Person-to-Person?

Swimmer's itch is not contagious and cannot be spread from one person to another.

Who Is at Risk for Swimmer's Itch?

Anyone who swims or wades in infested water may be at risk. Larvae are more likely to be present in shallow water by the shoreline. Children are most often affected because they tend to swim, wade, and play in shallow water more than adults. Also, they are less likely to towel dry themselves when leaving the water.

Once an Outbreak of Swimmer's Itch Has Occurred in Water, Will the Water Always Be Unsafe?

No. Many factors must be present for swimmer's itch to become a problem in water. Since these factors change (sometimes within a swim season), swimmer's itch will not always be a problem. However, there is no way to know how long water may be unsafe. Larvae generally survive for 24 hours once they are released from the snail. However, an infected snail will continue to produce cercariae throughout the remainder of its life. For future snails to become infected, migratory birds or mammals in the area must also be infected so the life cycle can continue.

Is It Safe to Swim in Your Swimming Pool?

Yes. As long as your swimming pool is well maintained and chlorinated, there is no risk of swimmer's itch. The appropriate snails must be present in order for the swimmer's itch to occur.

What Can Be Done to Reduce the Risk of Swimmer's Itch?

To reduce the likelihood of developing swimmer's itch:

- Do not swim in areas where swimmer's itch is a known problem or where signs have been posted warning of unsafe water.

- Do not swim near or wade in marshy areas where snails are commonly found.

- Towel dry or shower immediately after leaving the water.

- Do not attract birds (e.g., by feeding them) to areas where people are swimming.

- Encourage health officials to post signs on shorelines where swimmer's itch is a current problem.

Section 13.10

Tinea and Ringworm

This section includes text excerpted from "Fungal Diseases—Ringworm," Centers for Disease Control and Prevention (CDC), August 6, 2018.

What Is Ringworm?

Ringworm is a common infection of the skin and nails that is caused by fungus. The infection is called "ringworm" because it can cause an itchy, red, circular rash. Ringworm is also called "tinea" or "dermatophytosis." The different types of ringworm are usually named for the location of the infection on the body.

Areas of the body that can be affected by ringworm include:

- Feet (tinea pedis, commonly called "athlete's foot")

- Groin, inner thighs, or buttocks (tinea cruris, commonly called "jock itch")

- Scalp (tinea capitis)

- Beard (tinea barbae)

- Hands (tinea manuum)

- Toenails or fingernails (tinea unguium, also called "onychomycosis")

- Other parts of the body such as arms or legs (tinea corporis)

Approximately 40 different species of fungi can cause ringworm; the scientific names for the types of fungi that cause ringworm are *Trichophyton, Microsporum*, and *Epidermophyton*.

Symptoms of Ringworm Infections

Ringworm can affect the skin on almost any part of the body as well as the fingernails and toenails. The symptoms of ringworm often depend on which part of the body is infected, but they generally include:

- Itchy skin

- Ring-shaped rash

- Red, scaly, cracked skin

- Hair loss

Symptoms typically appear between 4 and 14 days after the skin comes in contact with the fungi that cause ringworm.

- **Feet (tinea pedis or "athlete's foot"):** The symptoms of ringworm on the feet include red, swollen, peeling, itchy skin between the toes (especially between the pinky toe and the one next to it). The sole and heel of the foot may also be affected. In severe cases, the skin on the feet can blister.

- **Scalp (tinea capitis):** Ringworm on the scalp usually looks like a scaly, itchy, red, circular bald spot. The bald spot can grow in size and multiple spots might develop if the infection spreads. Ringworm on the scalp is more common in children than it is in adults.

- **Groin (tinea cruris or "jock itch"):** Ringworm on the groin looks like scaly, itchy, red spots, usually on the inner sides of the skin folds of the thigh.

- Beard (tinea barbae): Symptoms of ringworm on the beard include scaly, itchy, red spots on the cheeks, chin, and upper neck. The spots might become crusted over or filled with pus, and the affected hair might fall out.

Ringworm Risk and Prevention
Who Gets Ringworm

Ringworm is very common. Anyone can get ringworm, but people who have weakened immune systems may be especially at risk for infection and may have problems fighting off a ringworm infection. People who use public showers or locker rooms, athletes (particularly those who are involved in contact sports such as wrestling), people who wear tight shoes and have excessive sweating, and people who have close contact with animals may also be more likely to come in contact with the fungi that cause ringworm.

How Can I Prevent Ringworm?

- Keep your skin clean and dry.

- Wear shoes that allow air to circulate freely around your feet.

- Do not walk barefoot in areas such as locker rooms or public showers.

- Clip your fingernails and toenails short and keep them clean.

- Change your socks and underwear at least once a day.

- Do not share clothing, towels, sheets, or other personal items with someone who has ringworm.

- Wash your hands with soap and running water after playing with pets. If you suspect that your pet has ringworm, take it to see a veterinarian. If your pet has ringworm, follow the steps below to prevent spreading the infection.

- If you are an athlete involved in close contact sports, shower immediately after your practice session or match, and keep all of your sports gear and uniform clean. Do not share sports gear (helmet, etc.) with other players.

My Pet Has Ringworm and I Am Worried about Ringworm in My House. What Should I Do?

Ringworm can easily transfer from animals to humans. You can take the following steps to protect yourself and your pet:

For People

- Do:

  - Wash your hands with soap and running water after playing with or petting your pet.

  - Wear gloves and long sleeves if you must handle animals with ringworm, and always wash your hands after handling the animals.

  - Vacuum the areas of the home that the infected pet commonly visits. This will help to remove infected fur or flakes of skin.

  - Disinfect areas the pet has spent time in, including surfaces and bedding.

    - The spores of this fungus can be killed with common disinfectants, such as diluted chlorine bleach (1/4 cup per gallon water), benzalkonium chloride, or strong detergents.

    - Never mix cleaning products. This may cause harmful gases.

- Do not handle animals with ringworm if your immune system is weak in any way (if you have human immunodeficiency virus (HIV)/acquired immunodeficiency syndrome (AIDS), are undergoing cancer treatment, or are taking medications that suppress the immune system, for example).

For Pets

- Protect your pet's health by:
    - If you suspect that your pet has ringworm, make sure it is seen by a veterinarian for treatment.
    - If one of your pets has ringworm, make sure you have every pet in the household checked for ringworm infection.

There Is a Ringworm Outbreak in My Child's School/ Day-care Center. What Should I Do?

- Contact your local health department for more information.
- Tell your child not to share personal items, such as clothing, hairbrushes, and hats, with other people.
- Take your child to see a pediatrician if she or he develops ringworm symptoms.
- Check with your child's school or daycare to see if she or he can still attend classes or participate in athletics.

Sources of Infection

The fungi that cause ringworm can live on the skin and in the environment. There are three main ways that ringworm can spread:

- **From a person who has ringworm.** People can get ringworm after contact with someone who has the infection. To avoid spreading the infection, people with ringworm should not share clothing, towels, combs, or other personal items with other people.

- **From an animal that has ringworm.** People can get ringworm after touching an animal that has ringworm. Many different kinds of animals can spread ringworm to people, including dogs and cats, especially kittens and puppies. Other animals such as cows, goats, pigs, and horses can also spread ringworm to people.

- **From the environment.** The fungi that cause ringworm can live on surfaces, particularly in damp areas, such as locker rooms and public showers. For that reason, it is a good idea not to walk barefoot in these places.

Diagnosis of Ringworm

Your healthcare provider can usually diagnose ringworm by looking at the affected skin and asking questions about your symptoms. She or he may also take a small skin scraping to be examined under a microscope or sent to a laboratory for a fungal culture.

Treatment of Ringworm

The treatment for ringworm depends on its location on the body and how serious the infection is. Some forms of ringworm can be treated with nonprescription ("over-the-counter") medications, but other forms of ringworm need treatment with prescription antifungal medication.

- Ringworm on the skin, like athlete's foot (tinea pedis) and jock itch (tinea cruris), can usually be treated with nonprescription antifungal creams, lotions, or powders applied to the skin for two to four weeks. There are many nonprescription products available to treat ringworm, including:

  - Clotrimazole (Lotrimin, Mycelex®)

  - Miconazole (Aloe Vesta® Antifungal, Azolen™, Baza® Antifungal, Carrington® Antifungal, Critic Aid® Clear, Cruex® Prescription Strength, DermaFungal, Desenex®, Fungoid Tincture, Micaderm, Micatin®, Micro-Guard™, Miranel, Mitrazol, Podactin, Remedy® Antifungal, Secura® Antifungal)

  - Terbinafine (Lamisil®)

  - Ketoconazole (Xolegel®)

For nonprescription creams, lotions, or powders, follow the directions on the package label. Contact your healthcare provider if your infection does not go away or gets worse.

- Ringworm on the scalp (tinea capitis) usually needs to be treated with prescription antifungal medication taken by mouth for one to three months. Creams, lotions, or powders do not work for ringworm on the scalp. Prescription antifungal medications used to treat ringworm on the scalp include:

- Griseofulvin (Grifulvin V, Gris-PEG)
- Terbinafine
- Itraconazole (Onmel®, Sporanox®)
- Fluconazole (Diflucan®)

You should contact your healthcare provider if:

- Your infection gets worse or does not go away after using nonprescription medications.
- You or your child has ringworm on the scalp. Ringworm on the scalp needs to be treated with prescription antifungal medication.

Section 13.11

Toxoplasmosis

This section includes text excerpted from "Parasites—Toxoplasmosis (Toxoplasma Infection)," Centers for Disease Control and Prevention (CDC), August 29, 2018.

Toxoplasmosis is considered to be a leading cause of death attributed to foodborne illness in the United States. More than 40 million men, women, and children in the U.S. carry the *Toxoplasma* parasite, but very few have symptoms because the immune system usually keeps the parasite from causing illness. However, women newly infected with *Toxoplasma* during or shortly before pregnancy and anyone with a compromised immune system should be aware that toxoplasmosis can have severe consequences.

Toxoplasmosis is considered one of the neglected parasitic infections of the United States, a group of five parasitic diseases that have been targeted by the Centers for Disease Control and Prevention (CDC) for public-health action.

What Is Toxoplasmosis?

Toxoplasmosis is an infection caused by a single-celled parasite called "*Toxoplasma gondii.*" While the parasite is found throughout the world, more than 40 million people in the United States may be infected with the *Toxoplasma* parasite. The *Toxoplasma* parasite can persist for long periods of time in the bodies of humans (and other animals), possibly even for a lifetime. Of those who are infected, however, very few have symptoms because a healthy person's immune system usually keeps the parasite from causing illness. However, pregnant women and individuals who have compromised immune systems should be cautious; for them, a *Toxoplasma* infection could cause serious health problems.

How Do People Get Toxoplasmosis?

A *Toxoplasma* infection occurs in one of the following:

- Eating undercooked, contaminated meat (especially pork, lamb, and venison) or shellfish (for example, oysters, clams, or mussels).

- Accidental ingestion of undercooked, contaminated meat or shellfish after handling them and not washing hands thoroughly. (*Toxoplasma* cannot be absorbed through intact skin).

- Eating food that was contaminated by knives, utensils, cutting boards, and other foods that have had contact with raw, contaminated meat or shellfish.

- Drinking water contaminated with *Toxoplasma gondii.*

- Accidentally swallowing the parasite through contact with cat feces that contain *Toxoplasma*. This might happen by:

  - Cleaning a cat's litter box when the cat has shed *Toxoplasma* in its feces

  - Touching or ingesting anything that has come into contact with cat feces that contain *Toxoplasma*

  - Accidentally ingesting contaminated soil (e.g., not washing hands after gardening or eating unwashed fruits or vegetables from a garden)

- Mother-to-child (congenital) transmission.

- Receiving an infected organ transplant or infected blood via transfusion, though this is rare.

What Are the Signs and Symptoms of Toxoplasmosis?

Symptoms of the infection vary.

- Most people who become infected with *Toxoplasma gondii* are not aware of it because they have no symptoms at all.

- Some people who have toxoplasmosis may feel as if they have the "flu" with swollen lymph glands or muscle aches and pains that may last for a month or more.

- Severe toxoplasmosis, causing damage to the brain, eyes, or other organs, can develop from an acute *Toxoplasma* infection or one that had occurred earlier in life and is now reactivated. Severe *toxoplasmosis* is more likely in individuals who have weak immune systems, though occasionally, even persons with healthy immune systems may experience eye damage from toxoplasmosis.

- Signs and symptoms of ocular toxoplasmosis can include reduced vision, blurred vision, pain (often with bright light), redness of the eye, and sometimes tearing. Ophthalmologists sometimes prescribe medicine to treat active disease. Whether or not the medication is recommended depends on the size of the eye lesion, the location, and the characteristics of the lesion (acute active, versus chronic not progressing). An ophthalmologist will provide the best care for ocular toxoplasmosis.

- Most infants who are infected while still in the womb have no symptoms at birth, but they may develop symptoms later in life. A small percentage of infected newborns have serious eye or brain damage at birth.

Who Is at Risk for Developing Severe Toxoplasmosis?

People who are most likely to develop severe toxoplasmosis include:

- Infants born to mothers who are newly infected with *Toxoplasma gondii* during or just before pregnancy.

- Persons with severely weakened immune systems, such as individuals with AIDS, those taking certain types of chemotherapy, and those who have recently received an organ transplant.

What Should You Do If You Think You at Risk for Severe Toxoplasmosis?

If you are planning to become pregnant, your healthcare provider may test you for *Toxoplasma gondii*. If the test is positive it means you have already been infected sometime in your life. There usually is little need to worry about passing the infection to your baby. If the test is negative, take the necessary precautions to avoid infection.

If you are already pregnant, you and your healthcare provider should discuss your risk for toxoplasmosis. Your healthcare provider may order a blood sample for testing.

If you have a weakened immune system, ask your doctor about having your blood tested for *Toxoplasma*. If your test is positive, your doctor can tell you if and when you need to take medicine to prevent the infection from reactivating. If your test is negative, it means you need to take precautions to avoid infection.

What Should I Do If I Think I May Have Toxoplasmosis?

If you suspect that you may have toxoplasmosis, talk to your healthcare provider. Your provider may order one or more varieties of blood tests specific for toxoplasmosis. The results from the different tests can help your provider determine if you have a *Toxoplasma gondii* infection and whether it is a recent (acute) infection.

What Is the Treatment for Toxoplasmosis?

Once a diagnosis of toxoplasmosis is confirmed, you and your healthcare provider can discuss whether treatment is necessary. In an otherwise healthy person who is not pregnant, treatment usually is not needed. If symptoms occur, they typically go away within a few weeks to months. For pregnant women or persons who have weakened immune systems, medications are available to treat toxoplasmosis.

How Can I Prevent Toxoplasmosis?

There are several steps you can take to reduce your chances of becoming infected with *Toxoplasma gondii*.

Cook food to safe temperatures. A food thermometer should be used to measure the internal temperature of cooked meat. Color is not a reliable indicator that meat has been cooked to a temperature high enough to kill harmful pathogens such as *Toxoplasma*. Do not sample meat until it is cooked. The U.S. Department of Agriculture (USDA) recommends the following for meat preparation:

- **For Whole Cuts of Meat (excluding poultry)**

Cook to at least 145°F (63°C) as measured with a food thermometer placed in the thickest part of the meat, then allow the meat to rest for three minutes before carving or consuming. According to USDA, "A 'rest time' is the amount of time the product remains at the final temperature after it has been removed from a grill, oven, or other heat sources. During the three minutes after meat is removed from the heat source, its temperature remains constant or continues to rise, which destroys pathogens."

- **For Ground Meat (excluding poultry)**

Cook to at least 160°F (71°C); ground meats do not require a rest time.

- **For All Poultry (whole cuts and ground)**

Cook to at least 165°F (74°C). The internal temperature should be checked in the innermost part of the thigh, the innermost part of the wing, and the thickest part of the breast. Poultry does not require a rest time.

- Freeze meat for several days at sub-zero (0°F) temperatures before cooking to greatly reduce the chance of infection. Freezing does not reliably kill other parasites that may be found in meat (such as certain species of *Trichinella*) or harmful bacteria. Cooking meat to USDA-recommended internal temperatures is the safest method to destroy all parasites and other pathogens.

- Peel or wash fruits and vegetables thoroughly before eating.

- Do not drink unpasteurized goat's milk.

- Do not eat raw or undercooked oysters, mussels, or clams (these may be contaminated with *Toxoplasma* that has washed into seawater).

- Wash cutting boards, dishes, counters, utensils, and hands with soapy water after contact with raw meat, poultry, seafood, or unwashed fruits or vegetables.

- Wear gloves when gardening and during any contact with soil or sand because it might be contaminated with cat feces that contain *Toxoplasma*. Wash hands with soap and water after gardening or contact with soil or sand.

- Ensure that the cat litter box is changed daily. The *Toxoplasma* parasite does not become infectious until 1 to 5 days after it is shed in a cat's feces.

- Wash hands with soap and water after cleaning out a cat's litter box.

- Teach children the importance of washing hands to prevent infection.

If I Am at Risk, Can I Keep My Cat?

Yes, you may keep your cat if you are a person at risk for a severe infection (e.g., you have a weakened immune system or are pregnant); however, there are several safety precautions you should take to avoid being exposed to *Toxoplasma gondii,* including the following:

- Ensure the cat litter box is changed daily. The *Toxoplasma* parasite does not become infectious until 1 to 5 days after it is shed in a cat's feces.

- If you are pregnant or immunocompromised:

  - Avoid changing cat litter if possible. If no one else can perform the task, wear disposable gloves and wash your hands with soap and water afterward.

  - Keep cats indoors. This is because cats become infected with *Toxoplasma* through hunting and eating rodents, birds, or other small animals that are infected with the parasite.

  - Do not adopt or handle stray cats, especially kittens. Do not get a new cat while you are pregnant or immunocompromised.

- Feed cats only canned or dried commercial food or well-cooked table food, not raw or undercooked meats.

- Keep your outdoor sandboxes covered.

- Your veterinarian can answer any other questions you may have regarding your cat and risk for toxoplasmosis.

Once Infected with Toxoplasma Is My Cat Always Be Able to Spread the Infection to Me?

No, cats only spread *Toxoplasma* in their feces for one to three weeks following infection with the parasite. Like humans, cats rarely have symptoms when infected, so most people do not know if their cat has been infected. Your veterinarian can answer any other questions you may have regarding your cat and risk for toxoplasmosis.

Chapter 14

Other Diseases Associated with Infections

Chapter Contents

Section 14.1

Encephalitis and Meningitis

This section includes text excerpted from "Meningitis and Encephalitis Fact Sheet," National Institute of Neurological Disorders and Stroke (NINDS), May 13, 2019.

What Are Meningitis and Encephalitis?

Infections and other disorders affecting the brain and spinal cord can activate the immune system, which leads to inflammation. These diseases, and the resulting inflammation can produce a wide range of symptoms, including fever, headache, seizures, and changes in behavior or confusion. In extreme cases, these can cause brain damage, stroke, or even death.

Inflammation of the meninges, the membranes that surround the brain and spinal cord, is called "meningitis;" inflammation of the brain itself is called "encephalitis." Myelitis refers to inflammation of the spinal cord. When both the brain and the spinal cord are involved, the condition is called "encephalomyelitis."

What Causes Meningitis and Encephalitis

Infectious causes of meningitis and encephalitis include bacteria, viruses, fungi, and parasites. For some individuals, environmental exposure (such as a parasite), recent travel, or an immunocompromised state (such as HIV, diabetes, steroids, chemotherapy treatment) are important risk factors. There are also noninfectious causes such as autoimmune/rheumatological diseases and certain medications.

Meningitis

Bacterial meningitis is a rare but potentially fatal disease. Several types of bacteria can first cause an upper respiratory tract infections and then travel through the bloodstream to the brain. The disease can also occur when certain bacteria invade the meninges directly. Bacterial meningitis can cause stroke, hearing loss, and permanent brain damage.

- **Pneumococcal meningitis** is the most common form of meningitis and is the most serious form of bacterial meningitis. Some 6,000 cases of pneumococcal meningitis are reported in the

United States each year. The disease is caused by the bacterium *Streptococcus pneumoniae,* which also causes pneumonia, blood poisoning (septicemia), and ear and sinus infections. At particular risk are children under age 2 and adults with a weakened immune system. People who have had pneumococcal meningitis often suffer neurological damage ranging from deafness to severe brain damage. Immunizations are available for certain strains of the pneumococcal bacteria.

- **Meningococcal meningitis** is caused by the bacterium *Neisseria meningitides.* Each year in the United States about 2,600 people get this highly contagious disease. High-risk groups include infants under the age of 1 year, people with suppressed immune systems, travelers to foreign countries where the disease is endemic, and college students (freshmen in particular), military recruits, and others who reside in dormitories. Between 10 and 15 percent of cases are fatal, with another 10 and 15 percent causing brain damage and other serious side effects. If meningococcal meningitis is diagnosed, people in close contact with an infected individual should be given preventative antibiotics.

- *Haemophilus influenzae* **meningitis** was at one time the most common form of bacterial meningitis. Fortunately, the *Haemophilus influenzae* B vaccine has greatly reduced the number of cases in the United States. Those most at risk of getting this disease are children in child-care settings and children who do not have access to the vaccine.

Other forms of bacterial meningitis include *Listeria monocytogenes* meningitis (in which certain foods such as unpasteurized dairy or deli meats are sometimes implicated); *Escherichia coli (E. coli)* meningitis, which is most common in elderly adults and newborns and may be transmitted to a baby through the birth canal; and Mycobacterium tuberculosis meningitis, a rare disease that occurs when the bacterium that causes tuberculosis attacks the meninges.

Viral, or aseptic, meningitis is usually caused by enteroviruses— common viruses that enter the body through the mouth and travel to the brain and surrounding tissues where they multiply. Enteroviruses are present in mucus, saliva, and feces, and can be transmitted through direct contact with an infected person or an infected object or surface. Other viruses that cause meningitis include *varicella-zoster* (the virus that causes chickenpox and can appear decades later as shingles), influenza, mumps, HIV, and *herpes simplex type 2* (genital herpes).

Fungal infections can affect the brain. The most common form of fungal meningitis is caused by the fungus *Cryptococcus neoformans* (*C. neoformans*) (found mainly in dirt and bird droppings). Cryptococcal meningitis mostly occurs in immunocompromised individuals, such as those with AIDS but can also occur in healthy people. Some of these cases can be slow to develop and smolder for weeks. Although treatable, fungal meningitis often recurs in nearly half of affected persons.

Parasitic causes include cysticercosis (a tapeworm infection in the brain), which is common in other parts of the world, as well as cerebral malaria.

There are rare cases of amoebic meningitis, sometimes related to freshwater swimming, which can be rapidly fatal.

Encephalitis

Encephalitis, usually viral, can be caused by some of the same infections listed above. However, up to 60 percent of cases remain undiagnosed. Several thousand cases of encephalitis are reported each year, but many more may occur since the symptoms may be mild to nonexistent in most individuals.

Most diagnosed cases of encephalitis in the United States are caused by *herpes simplex virus types 1* (HSV-1) and 2, arboviruses (such as West Nile virus), which are transmitted from infected animals to humans through the bite of an infected tick, mosquito, or other bloodsucking insects, or enteroviruses. Lyme disease, a bacterial infection spread by tick bite, occasionally causes meningitis, and very rarely encephalitis. Rabies virus, which is transmitted by bites of rabid animals, is an extremely rare cause of human encephalitis.

Herpes simplex encephalitis (HSE) is responsible for about 10 percent of all encephalitis cases, with a frequency of about 2 cases per million persons per year. More than half of untreated cases are fatal. About 30 percent of cases result from the initial infection with the HSV; the majority of cases are caused by reactivation of an earlier infection. Most people acquire HSV-1 (the cause of cold sores or fever blisters) in childhood.

Herpes simplex encephalitis due to HSV-1 can affect any age group but is most often seen in persons under age 20 or over age 40. This rapidly progressing disease is the single most important cause of fatal sporadic encephalitis in the United States. Symptoms can include headache and fever for up to five days, followed by personality and behavioral changes, seizures, hallucinations, and altered levels of consciousness. Brain damage in adults and in children beyond the first month of life is usually seen in the frontal lobes (leading to behavioral and personality changes) and temporal lobes (leading to memory and speech problems) and can be severe.

An infected mother can transmit the disease to her child at birth, through contact with genital secretions. In newborns, symptoms such as lethargy, irritability, tremors, seizures, and poor feeding generally develop between 4 and 11 days after delivery.

Four common forms of mosquito-transmitted viral encephalitis are seen in the United States:

- **Equine encephalitis** affects horses and humans.

  - *Eastern equine encephalitis* also infects birds that live in freshwater swamps of the eastern U.S. seaboard and along the Gulf Coast. In humans, symptoms are seen 4 to 10 days following transmission and include sudden fever, general flu-like muscle pains, and headache of increasing severity, followed by coma and death in severe cases. About half of infected individuals die from the disorder. Fewer than 10 human cases are seen annually in the United States.

  - *Western equine encephalitis* is seen in farming areas in the western and central plains states. Symptoms begin 5 to 10 days following infection. Children, particularly those under 12 months of age, are affected more severely than adults and may have permanent neurologic damage. Death occurs in about 3 percent of cases.

  - *Venezuelan equine encephalitis* is very rare in this country. Children are at greatest risk of developing severe complications, while adults generally develop flu-like symptoms. Epidemics in South and Central America have killed thousands of people and left others with permanent, severe neurologic damage.

- **LaCrosse encephalitis** occurs most often in the upper midwestern states (Illinois, Wisconsin, Indiana, Ohio, Minnesota, and Iowa) but also has been reported in the southeastern and mid-Atlantic regions of the country. Most cases are seen in children under age 16. Symptoms such as vomiting, headache, fever, and lethargy appear 5 to 10 days following infection. Severe complications include seizures, coma, and permanent neurologic damage. About 100 cases of LaCrosse encephalitis are reported each year.

- **St. Louis encephalitis** is most prevalent in temperate regions of the United States but can occur throughout most of the country. The disease is generally milder in children than in adults, with elderly adults at highest risk of severe disease or death. Symptoms typically appear 7 to 10 days following infection and include headache and fever. In more severe cases, confusion and disorientation, tremors, convulsions (especially in the very young), and coma may occur.

- **West Nile encephalitis** is usually transmitted by a bite from an infected mosquito, but can also occur after transplantation of an infected organ or transfusions of infected blood or blood products. Symptoms are flu-like and include fever, headache, and joint pain. Some individuals may develop a skin rash and swollen lymph glands, while others may not show any symptoms. At highest risk are older adults and people with weakened immune systems.

Who Is at Risk for Encephalitis and Meningitis?

Anyone—from infants to older adults—can get encephalitis or meningitis. People with weakened immune systems, including those persons with HIV or those taking immunosuppressant drugs, are at increased risk.

How Are These Disorders Transmitted?

Some forms of bacterial meningitis and encephalitis are contagious and can be spread through contact with saliva, nasal discharge, feces, or respiratory and throat secretions (often spread through kissing, coughing, or sharing drinking glasses, eating utensils, or such personal items as toothbrushes, lipstick, or cigarettes). For example, people sharing a household, daycare center, or classroom with an infected person can become infected. College students living in dormitories—in particular, college freshmen—have a higher risk of contracting meningococcal meningitis than college students overall. Children who have not been given routine vaccines are at increased risk of developing certain types of bacterial meningitis.

Because these diseases can occur suddenly and progress rapidly, anyone who is suspected of having either meningitis or encephalitis should immediately contact a doctor or go to the hospital.

What Are the Signs and Symptoms?

The hallmark signs of meningitis include some or all of the following: sudden fever, severe headache, nausea or vomiting, double vision, drowsiness, sensitivity to bright light, and a stiff neck. Encephalitis can be characterized by fever, seizures, change in behavior, and confusion and disorientation. Related neurological signs depend on which part of the brain is affected by the encephalitic process as some of these are quite localized while others are more widespread.

Meningitis often appears with flu-like symptoms that develop over one to two days. Distinctive rashes are typically seen in some forms of the disease. Meningococcal meningitis may be associated with kidney and adrenal gland failure and shock.

How Are Meningitis and Encephalitis Diagnosed?

Following a physical exam and medical history to review activities of the past several days or weeks (such as recent exposure to insects, ticks or animals, any contact with ill persons, or recent travel; preexisting medical conditions and medications), the doctor may order various diagnostic tests to confirm the presence of infection or inflammation. Early diagnosis is vital, as symptoms can appear suddenly and escalate to brain damage, hearing and/or speech loss, blindness, or even death.

Diagnostic tests include:

- A neurological examination involves a series of physical examination tests designed to assess motor and sensory function, nerve function, hearing and speech, vision, coordination and balance, mental status, and changes in mood or behavior.

- Laboratory screening of blood, urine, and body secretions can help detect and identify brain and/or spinal cord infection and determine the presence of antibodies and foreign proteins. Such tests can also rule out metabolic conditions that may have similar symptoms.

- Analysis of the cerebrospinal fluid that surrounds and protects the brain and spinal cord can detect infections in the brain and/or spinal cord, acute and chronic inflammation, and other diseases. A small amount of cerebrospinal fluid is removed by a special needle that is inserted into the lower back and the fluid is tested to detect the presence of bacteria, blood, and viruses. The testing can also measure glucose levels (a low glucose level can be seen in bacterial or fungal meningitis) and white blood cells (elevated white blood cell counts are a sign of inflammation), as well as protein and antibody levels.

Brain imaging can reveal signs of brain inflammation, internal bleeding or hemorrhage, or other brain abnormalities. Two painless, noninvasive imaging procedures are routinely used to diagnose meningitis and encephalitis.

- **Computed tomography (CT) scan** combines x-rays and computer technology to produce rapid, clear, two-dimensional images of organs, bones, and tissues. Occasionally a contrast dye is injected into the bloodstream to highlight the different tissues in the brain and to detect signs of encephalitis or inflammation of the meninges.

- **Magnetic resonance imaging (MRI)** uses computer-generated radio waves and a strong magnet to produce detailed images of body structures, including tissues, organs, bones, and nerves. An MRI can help identify brain and spinal cord inflammation, infection, tumors, and other conditions. A contrast dye may be injected prior to the test to reveal more detail.

Additionally, electroencephalography, or EEG, can identify abnormal brain waves by monitoring electrical activity in the brain noninvasively through the skull. Among its many functions, EEG is used to help diagnose patterns that may suggest specific viral infections, such as herpes virus and to detect seizures that do not show any clinical symptoms but may contribute to an altered level of consciousness in critically ill individuals.

Individuals with encephalitis often show mild flu-like symptoms. In more severe cases, people may experience problems with speech or hearing, double vision, hallucinations, personality changes, and loss of consciousness. Other severe complications include loss of sensation in some parts of the body, muscle weakness, partial paralysis in the arms and legs, impaired judgment, seizures, and memory loss.

How Are These Infections Treated?

People who are suspected of having meningitis or encephalitis should receive immediate, aggressive medical treatment. Both diseases can progress quickly and have the potential to cause severe, irreversible neurological damage.

Meningitis

Early treatment of bacterial meningitis involves antibiotics that can cross the blood–brain barrier (a lining of cells that keeps harmful microorganisms and chemicals from entering the brain). Appropriate antibiotic treatment for most types of meningitis can greatly reduce the risk of dying from the disease. Anticonvulsants to prevent seizures and corticosteroids to reduce brain inflammation may be prescribed.

Infected sinuses may need to be drained. Corticosteroids such as prednisone may be ordered to relieve brain pressure and swelling and to prevent hearing loss that is common in *Haemophilus influenza* meningitis. Lyme disease is treated with antibiotics.

Antibiotics, developed to kill bacteria, are not effective against viruses. Fortunately, viral meningitis is rarely life-threatening and no specific treatment is needed. Fungal meningitis is treated with intravenous antifungal medications.

Encephalitis

Antiviral drugs used to treat viral encephalitis include acyclovir and ganciclovir. For most encephalitis-causing viruses, no specific treatment is available.

Autoimmune causes of encephalitis are treated with additional immunosuppressant drugs and screening for underlying tumors when appropriate. Acute disseminated encephalomyelitis, noninfectious inflammatory brain disease is mostly seen in children, is treated with steroids.

Anticonvulsants may be prescribed to stop or prevent seizures. Corticosteroids can reduce brain swelling. Affected individuals with breathing difficulties may require artificial respiration.

Once the acute illness is under control, comprehensive rehabilitation should include cognitive rehabilitation and physical, speech, and occupational therapy.

Important signs of meningitis or encephalitis to watch for in an infant include fever, lethargy, not waking for feedings, vomiting, body stiffness, unexplained/unusual irritability, and a full or bulging fontanel (the soft spot on the top of the head).

Can Meningitis and Encephalitis Be Prevented?

People should avoid sharing food, utensils, glasses, and other objects with someone who may be exposed to or have the infection. People should wash their hands often with soap and rinse under running water.

Effective vaccines are available to prevent *Haemophilus influenza*, pneumococcal and meningococcal meningitis.

People who live, work, or go to school with someone who has been diagnosed with bacterial meningitis may be asked to take antibiotics for a few days as a preventive measure.

To lessen the risk of being bitten by an infected mosquito or other arthropod, people should limit outdoor activities at night, wear long-sleeved clothing when outdoors, use insect repellents that are most effective for that particular region of the country, and rid lawn and outdoor areas of freestanding pools of water, in which mosquitoes breed. Repellants should not be overapplied, particularly on young children and especially infants, as chemicals such as N, N-Diethyl-meta-toluamide (DEET) may be absorbed through the skin.

What Is the Prognosis for These Infections?

The outcome generally depends on the particular infectious agent involved, the severity of the illness, and how quickly treatment is given. In most cases, people with very mild encephalitis or meningitis can make a full recovery, although the process may be slow.

Individuals who experience only headache, fever, and stiff neck may recover in 2 to 4 weeks. Individuals with bacterial meningitis typically show some relief 48 to 72 hours following initial treatment but are more likely to experience complications caused by the disease. In more serious cases, these diseases can cause hearing and/or speech loss, blindness, permanent brain and nerve damage, behavioral changes, cognitive disabilities, lack of muscle control, seizures, and memory loss. These individuals may need long-term therapy, medication, and supportive care.

The recovery from encephalitis is variable depending on the cause of the disease and the extent of brain inflammation.

Section 14.2

Pneumonia

This section includes text excerpted from "Pneumonia," Centers for Disease Control and Prevention (CDC), October 22, 2018.

What Is Pneumonia?

Pneumonia is an infection of the lungs that can cause mild to severe illness in people of all ages. Depending on the cause, doctors often treat pneumonia with medicine. In addition, vaccines can prevent some types of pneumonia. However, it is still the leading infectious cause of death in children younger than five years old worldwide. Common signs of pneumonia include cough, fever, and difficulty breathing. You can help prevent pneumonia and other respiratory infections by following good hygiene practices. These practices include washing your hands regularly and disinfecting frequently touched surfaces. Making healthy choices, like quitting smoking and managing ongoing medical conditions, can also help prevent pneumonia.

Causes of Pneumonia

Viruses, bacteria, and fungi can all cause pneumonia. In the United States, common causes of viral pneumonia are influenza and respiratory syncytial virus (RSV). A common cause of bacterial pneumonia is *Streptococcus pneumoniae* (pneumococcus). However, clinicians are not always able to find out which germ caused someone to get sick with pneumonia.

Community-acquired pneumonia is when someone develops pneumonia in the community (not in a hospital). Healthcare-associated pneumonia is when someone develops pneumonia during or following a stay in a healthcare facility. Healthcare facilities include hospitals, long-term care facilities, and dialysis centers. Ventilator-associated pneumonia is when someone gets pneumonia after being on a ventilator, a machine that supports breathing. The bacteria and viruses that most commonly cause pneumonia in the community are different from those in healthcare settings.

Risk of Pneumonia

Pneumonia is an infection of the lungs that can cause mild to severe illness in people of all ages. Children younger than five years old are more likely to get pneumonia. Common signs of pneumonia can include cough, fever, and trouble breathing.

Prevention of Pneumonia

Each year in the United States, about 1 million people have to seek care in a hospital due to pneumonia. Unfortunately, about 50,000 people die from the disease each year in the United States. Vaccines and appropriate treatment (such as antibiotics and antivirals) could prevent many of these deaths. These vaccines are safe, but side effects can occur. Most side effects are mild and go away on their own within a few days. Encourage friends and loved ones to make sure they are up to date with their vaccines.

Section 14.3

Reye Syndrome

This section includes text excerpted from "Reye's Syndrome Information Page," National Institute of Neurological Disorders and Stroke (NINDS), Mar 27, 2019.

What Is Reye Syndrome?

Reye syndrome (RS) is primarily a children's disease, although it can occur at any age. It affects all organs of the body but is most harmful to the brain and the liver—causing an acute increase of pressure within the brain and, often, massive accumulations of fat in the liver and other organs. RS is defined as a two-phase illness because it generally occurs in conjunction with a previous viral infection, such as the flu or chickenpox. The disorder commonly occurs during recovery from a viral infection, although it can also develop three to five days after the onset of the viral illness. RS is often misdiagnosed as encephalitis, meningitis, diabetes, drug overdose, poisoning, sudden infant death syndrome, or psychiatric illness.

Symptoms of Reye Syndrome

Symptoms of RS include persistent or recurrent vomiting, listlessness, personality changes, such as irritability or combativeness, disorientation or confusion, delirium, convulsions, and loss of consciousness. If these symptoms are present during or soon after a viral illness, medical attention should be sought immediately. The symptoms of RS in infants do not follow a typical pattern; for example, vomiting does not always occur. Epidemiologic evidence indicates that aspirin (salicylate) is the major preventable risk factor for RS. The mechanism by which aspirin and other salicylates trigger RS is not completely understood. A "Reye-like" illness may occur in children with genetic metabolic disorders and other toxic disorders. A physician should be consulted before giving a child any aspirin or anti-nausea medicines during a viral illness, which can mask the symptoms of RS.

Treatment of Reye Syndrome

There is no cure for RS. Successful management, which depends on early diagnosis, is primarily aimed at protecting the brain against irreversible damage by reducing brain swelling, reversing the metabolic injury, preventing complications in the lungs, and anticipating cardiac arrest. It has been learned that several inborn errors of metabolism mimic RS in that the first manifestation of these errors may be an encephalopathy with liver dysfunction. These disorders must be considered in all suspected cases of RS. Some evidence suggests that treatment in the end stages of RS with hypertonic IV glucose solutions may prevent the progression of the syndrome.

Prognosis of Reye Syndrome

Recovery from RS is directly related to the severity of the swelling of the brain. Some people recover completely, while others may sustain varying degrees of brain damage. Those cases in which the disorder progresses rapidly and the patient lapses into a coma have a poorer prognosis than those with a less severe course. Statistics indicate that when RS is diagnosed and treated in its early stages, chances of recovery are excellent. When diagnosis and treatment are delayed, the chances for successful recovery and survival are severely reduced. Unless RS is diagnosed and treated successfully, death is common, often within a few days.

Part Three

Medical Conditions
Appearing in Childhood

Chapter 15

Allergies in Children

Chapter Contents

Section 15.1

Allergy and Relief in Kids

This section contains text excerpted from the following
sources: Text in this section begins with excerpts from "Allergy,"
MedlinePlus, National Institutes of Health (NIH), May 16, 2018;
Text under the heading "Allergy Relief for Your Child" is excerpted
from "Allergy Relief for Your Child," U.S. Food and Drug
Administration (FDA), January 6, 2017.

An allergy is a reaction by your immune system to something that does not bother most other people. People who have allergies often are sensitive to more than one thing. Substances that often cause reactions are:

- Pollen

- Dust mites

- Mold spores

- Pet dander

- Food

- Insect stings

- Medicines

Normally, your immune system fights germs. It is your body's defense system. In most allergic reactions, however, it is responding to a false alarm. Genes and the environment probably both play a role.

Allergies can cause a variety of symptoms, such as a runny nose, sneezing, itching, rashes, swelling, or asthma. Allergies can range from minor to severe. Anaphylaxis is a severe reaction that can be life-threatening. Doctors use skin and blood tests to diagnose allergies. Treatments include medicines, allergy shots, and avoiding the substances that cause reactions.

Allergy Relief for Your Child

Children are magnets for colds. But when the sniffles and sneezing would not go away for weeks, the culprit may be allergies.

Long-lasting sneezing, with a stuffy or runny nose, may signal the presence of allergic rhinitis—the collection of symptoms that affect the nose when you have an allergic reaction to something you breathe in and that lands on the lining inside the nose.

Allergies may be seasonal or can strike year-round (perennial). In most parts of the United States, plant pollen are often the cause of seasonal allergic rhinitis—more commonly called "hay fever." Indoor substances, such as mold, dust mites, and pet dander, may cause the perennial kind.

Up to 40 percent of children suffer from allergic rhinitis. And children are more likely to develop allergies if one or both parents have allergies.

The U.S. Food and Drug Administration (FDA) regulates over-the-counter (OTC) and prescription medicines that offer allergy relief as well as allergen extracts used to diagnose and treat allergies. Take care to read and follow the directions provided when giving any medicine to children, including these products.

Immune System Reaction

An allergy is the body's reaction to a specific substance or allergen. Our immune system responds to the invading allergen by releasing histamine and other chemicals that typically trigger symptoms in the nose, lungs, throat, sinuses, ears, eyes, skin, or stomach lining.

In some children, allergies can also trigger symptoms of asthma—a disease that causes wheezing or difficulty breathing. If a child has allergies and asthma, "not controlling the allergies can make asthma worse," says Anthony Durmowicz, M.D., a pediatric pulmonary doctor at the FDA.

Avoid Pollen, Mold and Other Allergy Triggers

If your child has seasonal allergies, pay attention to pollen counts and try to keep your child inside when the levels are high.

- In the late summer and early fall, during ragweed pollen season, pollen levels are highest in the morning.

- In the spring and summer, during the grass pollen season, pollen levels are highest in the evening.

- Some molds, another allergy trigger, may also be seasonal. For example, leaf mold is more common in the fall.

- Sunny, windy days can be especially troublesome for pollen allergy sufferers.

It may also help to keep windows closed in your house and car and run the air conditioner.

Allergy Medicines for Children

For most children, symptoms may be controlled by avoiding the allergen, if known, and using OTC medicines. But if a child's symptoms are persistent and not relieved by OTC medicines, see a healthcare professional.

Although some allergy medicines are approved for use in children as young as six months, the FDA cautions that simply because a product's box says that it is intended for children does not mean it is intended for children of all ages. Always read the label to make sure the product is right for your child's age.

When your child is taking more than one medication, read the label to be sure that the active ingredients are not the same. Although the big print may say the product is to treat a certain symptom, different products may have the same medicine (active ingredient). It might seem that you are buying different products to treat different symptoms, but in fact, the same medicine could be in all the products. The result: You might accidentally be giving too much of one type of medicine to your child.

Children are more sensitive than adults to many drugs. For example, some antihistamines can have adverse effects at lower doses on young patients, causing excitability or excessive drowsiness.

Allergy Shots and Children

Jay E. Slater, M.D., a pediatric allergist at the FDA, says that children who do not respond to either OTC or prescription medications, or who suffer from frequent complications of allergic rhinitis, may be candidates for allergen immunotherapy—commonly known as "allergy shots."

After allergy testing, typically by skin testing to detect what allergens your child may react to, a healthcare professional injects the child with "extracts"—small amounts of the allergens that trigger a reaction. The doses are gradually increased so that the body builds up immunity to these allergens. Allergen extracts are manufactured from natural substances, such as pollen, insect venoms, animal hair, and foods. More than 1,200 extracts are licensed by the FDA.

In 2014, the FDA approved three new immunotherapy products that are taken under the tongue for treatment of hay fever caused by certain pollen, two of them for use in children. All of them are intended for daily use, before and during the pollen season. They are not meant for immediate symptom relief. Although they are intended for at-home use, these are prescription medications, and first doses are taken in the presence of a healthcare provider. The products are Oralair, Grastek, and Ragwitek (which is approved for use in adults only).

In 2017, the FDA approved Odactra, the first immunotherapy product administered under the tongue for treatment of house dust mite-induced allergic rhinitis (nasal inflammation) with or without conjunctivitis (eye inflammation). Odactra is approved for use only in adults.

"Allergy shots are never appropriate for food allergies," adds Slater, "but it's common to use extracts to test for food allergies so the child can avoid those foods."

"In the last 20 years, there has been a remarkable transformation in allergy treatments," says Slater. "Kids used to be miserable for months out of the year, and drugs made them incredibly sleepy. But today's products offer proven approaches for relief of seasonal allergy symptoms."

Section 15.2

Food Allergies

This section includes text excerpted from "Food Allergies in Schools," Centers for Disease Control and Prevention (CDC), February 14, 2018.

Food Allergy Facts

Food allergies are growing food safety and public-health concerns that affect an estimated four to six percent of children in the United States. There is no cure for food allergies and reactions can be life-threatening. Strict avoidance of the food allergen is the only way to prevent a reaction. However, since it is not always easy or possible to avoid certain foods, staff in schools, out-of-school time and early care and education programs (ECE) should develop plans for preventing an allergic reaction and responding to a food allergy emergency, including anaphylaxis. Early and quick recognition and treatment can prevent serious health problems or death.

What Is a Food Allergy?

A food allergy occurs when the body has a specific and reproducible immune response to certain foods. The body's immune response can be severe and life-threatening, such as anaphylaxis. Although the immune system normally protects people from germs, in people with food allergies, the immune system mistakenly responds to food as if it were harmful.

Eight foods or food groups account for 90 percent of serious allergic reactions in the United States: milk, eggs, fish, crustacean shellfish, wheat, soy, peanuts, and tree nuts.

The symptoms and severity of allergic reactions to food can be different between individuals, and can also be different for one person over time. Anaphylaxis is a sudden and severe allergic reaction that may cause death. Not all allergic reactions will develop into anaphylaxis.

Children with food allergies are two to four times more likely to have asthma or other allergic conditions than those without food allergies.

The prevalence of food allergies among children increased 18 percent from 1997 to 2007, and allergic reactions to foods have become the most common cause of anaphylaxis in community health settings.

Although difficult to measure, research suggests that approximately four percent of children and adolescents are affected by food allergies.

Managing Food Allergies at School
Voluntary Guidelines for Managing Food Allergies in Schools and Early Care and Education Programs

The Centers for Disease Control and Prevention (CDC) in consultation with the U.S. Department of Education (ED), several federal agencies, and many stakeholders, provide practical information and recommendations for each of the five priority areas that should be addressed in each school's or ECE program's Food Allergy Management Prevention Plan:

- Ensure the daily management of food allergies in individual children

- Prepare for food allergy emergencies

- Provide professional development on food allergies for staff members

- Educate children and family members about food allergies

- Create and maintain a healthy and safe educational environment

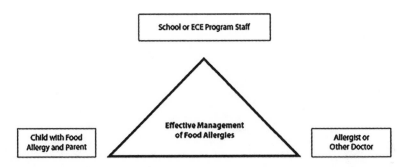

Figure 15.1. *Food Allergy Management in Schools and Early Care* (Source: "Voluntary Guidelines for Managing Food Allergies in Schools and Early Care and Education Programs," Centers for Disease Control and Prevention (CDC).)

The management of any chronic health condition should be based on a partnership among school or early care and education (ECE) program staff, children and their families, and the family's allergist or other doctor.

Chapter 16

Blood and Circulatory Disorders in Children

Chapter Contents

Section 16.1

Iron-Deficiency Anemia

This section includes text excerpted from "Iron-Deficiency
Anemia," National Heart, Lung, and Blood
Institute (NHLBI), January 18, 2019.

What Is Iron-Deficiency Anemia?

Iron-deficiency anemia is a common type of anemia that occurs in children if they do not have enough iron in their body. Children with mild or moderate iron-deficiency anemia may not have any signs or symptoms. More severe iron-deficiency anemia may cause fatigue or tiredness, shortness of breath, or chest pain.

If your child's doctor diagnoses her or him with iron-deficiency anemia, their treatment will depend on the cause and severity of the condition. The doctor may recommend healthy eating changes, iron supplements, intravenous iron therapy for mild to moderate iron-deficiency anemia, or red blood cell (RBC) transfusion for severe iron-deficiency anemia. You may need to address the cause of iron deficiency in your child, such as any underlying bleeding.

If undiagnosed or untreated, iron-deficiency anemia can cause serious complications, including heart failure and development delays in children.

What Causes Iron-Deficiency Anemia among Children

Your child's body needs iron to make healthy RBCs. Iron-deficiency anemia usually develops over time because your body's intake of iron is too low. Low intake of iron can happen because of blood loss, consuming less than the recommended daily amount of iron, and medical conditions that make it hard for your body to absorb iron from the gastrointestinal (GI) tract.

Blood Loss

When your child loses blood, she or he loses iron. Certain conditions or medicines can cause blood loss and lead to iron-deficiency anemia. Common causes of blood loss that lead to iron-deficiency anemia include:

- Bleeding in the GI tract, from an ulcer, colon cancer, or regular use of medicines such as aspirin or nonsteroidal anti-inflammatory drugs (NSAIDs), such as ibuprofen and naproxen

- Certain rare genetic conditions such as hereditary hemorrhagic telangiectasia, which causes bleeding in the bowels

- Frequent blood tests

- Injury or surgery

- Heavy menstrual periods

- Urinary-tract bleeding

Consuming Less than Recommended Daily Amounts of Iron

Iron-deficiency anemia can be caused by getting less than the recommended daily amounts of iron. The recommended daily amounts of iron will depend on your child's age or sex.

Table 16.1. Recommended Daily Iron Intake for Children

Age	Male	Female
Birth to 6 Months	0.27 mg	0.27 mg
7 to 12 Months	11 mg	11 mg
1 to 3 Years	7 mg	7 mg
4 to 8 Years	10 mg	10 mg
9 to 13 Years	8 mg	8 mg
14 to 18 Years	11 mg	15 mg

Table 16.1 lists the recommended amounts of iron, in milligrams (mg) at different ages and stages of children. Until the teen years, the recommended amount of iron is the same for boys and girls. From birth to 6 months, babies need 0.27 mg of iron. This number goes up to 11 mg for children ages 7 to 12 months, and down to 7 mg for children ages 1 to 3. From ages 4 to 8, children need 10 mg, and from ages 9 to 13, 8 mg. From ages 14 to 18, boys need 11 mg, while girls need 15 mg.

Problems Absorbing Iron

Even if your child consumes the recommended daily amount of iron, your child's body may not be able to absorb the iron. Certain conditions or medicines can decrease ability of child's body to absorb iron and lead to iron-deficiency anemia. These conditions include:

- **Intestinal and digestive conditions**, such as celiac disease; inflammatory bowel diseases (IBD), including ulcerative colitis and Crohn disease; and *Helicobacter pylori* infection

- **Certain rare genetic conditions**, such as a *TMRPSS6* gene mutation that causes the child's body to make too much of a hormone called "hepcidin." Hepcidin blocks the intestine from absorbing iron.

What Are the Risk Factors of Iron-Deficiency Anemia among Children?

Age

Children may be at increased risk for iron deficiency at certain ages:

- Infants between 6 and 12 months, especially if they are fed only breast milk or are fed formula that is not fortified with iron. The iron that full-term infants have stored in their bodies is used up in the first 4 to 6 months of life. Babies who were born prematurely may be at an even higher risk, as most of a new-borns' iron stores are developed only during the third trimester of pregnancy.

- Children between ages one and two, especially if they drink a lot of cow's milk. Cow's milk is low in iron.

- Teens, who have increased need for iron during growth spurts

Unhealthy Environments

Lead in children's blood. Lead may accumulate in children's blood from their environment or water. It interferes with the body's ability to make hemoglobin.

Family History and Genetics

Von Willebrand disease is an inherited bleeding disorder that affects the blood's ability to clot. This makes it harder to stop bleeding and can increase the risk of iron-deficiency anemia from trauma, surgery, or heavy menstrual periods.

Teenage girls with a gene for hemophilia, including symptomatic female carriers who have heavy menstrual periods, may be at risk for iron-deficiency anemia.

Lifestyle Habits

Certain lifestyle habits may increase your risk for iron-deficiency anemia, including:

- **Vegetarian or vegan eating patterns.** Not eating enough iron-rich foods, such as meat and fish, may result in your children getting less than the recommended daily amount of iron.

- **Endurance activities and athletes.** Athletes, especially young females, are at risk for iron deficiency. Endurance athletes lose iron through their gastrointestinal tracts. They also lose iron through the breakdown of RBC, called "hemolysis." Hemolysis, in this case, is caused by strong muscle contractions and the impact of feet repeatedly striking the ground, such as with marathon runners.

Sex

Girls above the age of 14 years need more iron than boys of the same age.

What Are the Signs, Symptoms, and Complications Associated with Iron-Deficiency Anemia among Children?

Common signs of iron-deficiency anemia include:

- Brittle nails or spooning of the nails
- Cracks at the sides of the mouth
- Pale skin
- Swelling or soreness of the tongue

Common symptoms of iron-deficiency anemia include:

- Chest pain
- Coldness in the hands and feet
- Difficulty concentrating
- Dizziness
- Fatigue, or feeling tired

- Headache

- Irregular heartbeat, a sign of more serious iron-deficiency anemia

- Pica, which are unusual cravings for nonfood items, such as ice, dirt, paint, or starch

- Restless legs syndrome (RLS)

- Shortness of breath

- Weakness

Undiagnosed or untreated iron-deficiency anemia may cause the following complications:

- Depression

- Heart problems

- Increased risk of infections

- Motor or cognitive development delays

How Iron-Deficiency Anemia Is Diagnosed

Iron-deficiency anemia may be detected during routine blood tests during a pediatric checkup. To diagnose iron-deficiency anemia, your child's doctor may ask questions about the risk factors, do a physical exam, or order blood tests or other diagnostic tests.

What Is the Treatment for Iron-Deficiency Anemia?

Treatment for iron-deficiency anemia will depend on its cause and severity. Treatments may include iron supplements, procedures, surgery, and dietary changes. Severe iron-deficiency anemia may require intravenous (IV) iron therapy or a blood transfusion.

Section 16.2

Sickle Cell Disease

This section includes text excerpted from "Sickle Cell Disease," MedlinePlus, National Institutes of Health (NIH), June 7, 2018.

What Is Sickle Cell Disease?

Sickle cell disease (SCD) is a group of inherited red blood cell (RBC) disorders. If you have SCD, there is a problem with your hemoglobin. Hemoglobin is a protein in RBCs that carries oxygen throughout the body. With SCD, the hemoglobin forms into stiff rods within the RBCs. This changes the shape of the RBCs. The cells are supposed to be disc-shaped, but this changes them into a crescent, or sickle, shape.

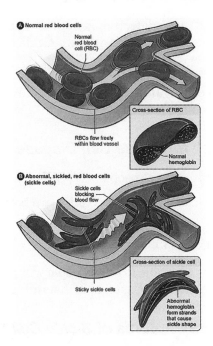

Figure 16.1. *Normal Red Blood Cells and Sickle Red Blood Cells* (Source: "Sickle Cell Disease," National Heart, Lung, and Blood Institute (NHLBI).)

Figure A shows normal red blood cells flowing freely in a blood vessel. The inset image shows a cross-section of a normal red blood cell with normal hemoglobin. Figure B shows abnormal, sickled red blood cells blocking blood flow in a blood vessel. The inset image shows a cross-section of a sickle cell with abnormal (sickle) hemoglobin forming abnormal stiff rods.

The sickle-shaped cells are not flexible and cannot change shape easily. Many of them burst apart as they move through your blood vessels. The sickle cells usually only last 10 to 20 days, instead of the normal 90 to 120 days. Your body may have trouble making enough new cells to replace the ones that you lost. Because of this, you may not have enough RBCs. This is a condition called "anemia," and it can make you feel tired.

The sickle-shaped cells can also stick to vessel walls, causing a blockage that slows or stops the flow of blood. When this happens, oxygen cannot reach nearby tissues. The lack of oxygen can cause attacks of sudden, severe pain, called "pain crises." These attacks can occur without warning. If you get one, you might need to go to the hospital for treatment.

What Causes Sickle Cell Disease

The cause of SCD is a defective gene, called a "sickle cell gene." People with the disease are born with two sickle cell genes, one from each parent.

If you are born with one sickle cell gene, it is called "sickle cell trait." People with sickle cell trait are generally healthy, but they can pass the defective gene on to their children.

Who Is at Risk for Sickle Cell Disease?

In the United States, most people with SCD are African Americans:

- About 1 in 13 African American babies are born with sickle cell trait

- About 1 in every 365 black children is born with SCD

Sickle cell disease also affects some people who come from Hispanic, Southern European, Middle Eastern, or Asian Indian backgrounds.

What Are the Symptoms of Sickle Cell Disease?

People with SCD start to have signs of the disease during the first year of life, usually around five months of age. Early symptoms of SCD may include:

- Painful swelling of the hands and feet

- Fatigue or fussiness from anemia

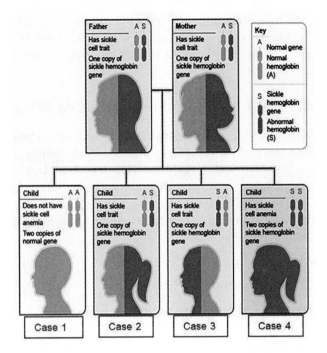

Figure 16.2. *Inheritance Pattern for Sickle Cell Disease* (Source: "Sickle Cell Disease," National Heart, Lung, and Blood Institute (NHLBI).)

The image shows how hemoglobin S genes are inherited. A person inherits two hemoglobin genes—one from each parent. A normal hemoglobin A gene will make normal hemoglobin. A hemoglobin S gene will make abnormal hemoglobin.

- A yellowish color of the skin (jaundice) or the whites of the eyes (icterus)

The effects of SCD vary from person to person and can change over time. Most of the signs and symptoms of SCD are related to complications of the disease. They may include severe pain, anemia, organ damage, and infections.

How Is Sickle Cell Disease Diagnosed?

A blood test can show if your child have SCD or sickle cell trait. All states now test newborns as part of their screening programs, so treatment can begin early.

People who are thinking about having children can have a test to find out how likely it is that their children will have SCD.

Doctors can also diagnose SCD before a baby is born. That test uses a sample of amniotic fluid (the liquid in the sac surrounding the baby) or tissue taken from the placenta (the organ that brings oxygen and nutrients to the baby).

What Are the Treatments for Sickle Cell Disease?

The only cure for SCD is bone marrow or stem cell transplantation. Because these transplants are risky and can have serious side effects, they are usually only used in children with severe SCD. For the transplant to work, the bone marrow must be a close match. Usually, the best donor is a sibling.

There are treatments that can help relieve symptoms, lessen complications, and prolong life:

- Antibiotics to try to prevent infections in younger children

- Pain relievers for acute or chronic pain

- Childhood immunizations to prevent infections

Section 16.3

Thalassemia

This section contains text excerpted from the following sources:
Text under the heading "What Is Thalassemia?" is excerpted
from "Thalassemia," Centers for Disease Control and Prevention
(CDC), April 23, 2019; Text beginning with the heading "Causes of
Thalassemia" is excerpted from "Thalassemias," National Heart,
Lung, and Blood Institute (NHLBI), December 9, 2014. Reviewed
September 2019.

What Is Thalassemia?

Thalassemia is an inherited (i.e., passed from parents to children through genes) blood disorder caused when the body does not make enough of a protein called "hemoglobin," an important part of red blood cells (RBCs). When there is not enough hemoglobin, the body's RBCs do not function properly and they last shorter periods of time, so there are fewer healthy RBCs traveling in the bloodstream.

Red blood cells carry oxygen to all the cells of the body. Oxygen is a sort of food that cells use to function. When there are not enough healthy RBCs, there is also not enough oxygen delivered to all the other cells of the body, which may cause a person to feel tired, weak or short of breath. This is a condition called "anemia." People with thalassemia may have mild or severe anemia. Severe anemia can damage organs and lead to death.

The various types of thalassemia have specific names related to the severity of the disorder.

Alpha-Thalassemias

- Alpha-thalassemia silent carrier

- Alpha-thalassemia minor also called "alpha-thalassemia trait"

- Hemoglobin H disease

- Alpha-thalassemia major also called "hydrops fetalis"

Beta-Thalassemias

- Beta-thalassemia minor also called "beta-thalassemia trait"

- Beta-thalassemia intermedia

- Beta-thalassemia major, also called "Cooley anemia" or "beta-zero" (ß0) thalassemia

- Beta-plus (ß+) thalassemia

- Mediterranean anemia

Causes of Thalassemia

Your body makes three types of blood cells: RBCs, white blood cells (WBCs), and platelets. RBCs contain hemoglobin, an iron-rich protein that carries oxygen from your lungs to all parts of your body. Hemoglobin also carries carbon dioxide (CO_2) (a waste gas) from your body to your lungs, where it is exhaled.

Hemoglobin has two kinds of protein chains: alpha-globin and beta-globin. If your body does not make enough of these protein chains or they are abnormal, RBCs will not form correctly or carry enough oxygen. Your body will not work well if your RBCs do not make enough healthy hemoglobin.

Genes control how the body makes hemoglobin protein chains. When these genes are missing or altered, thalassemias occur.

Thalassemias are inherited disorders—that is, they are passed from parents to children through genes. People who inherit faulty hemoglobin genes from one parent but normal genes from the other are called "carriers." Carriers often have no signs of illness other than mild anemia. However, they can pass the faulty genes on to their children.

People who have moderate to severe forms of thalassemia have inherited faulty genes from both parents.

Alpha-Thalassemias

You need four genes (two from each parent) to make enough alpha-globin protein chains. If one or more of the genes is missing, you will have alpha-thalassemia trait or disease. This means that your body does not make enough alpha-globin protein.

- If you are only missing one gene, you are a "silent" carrier. This means you will not have any signs of illness.

- If you are missing two genes, you have alpha-thalassemia trait (also called "alpha-thalassemia minor"). You may have mild anemia.

- If you are missing three genes, you are likely to have hemoglobin H disease (which a blood test can detect). This form of thalassemia causes moderate to severe anemia.

Very rarely, a baby is missing all four genes. This condition is called "alpha-thalassemia major" or "hydrops fetalis." Babies who have hydrops fetalis usually die before or shortly after birth.

Beta-Thalassemias

You need two genes (one from each parent) to make enough beta globin protein chains. If one or both of these genes are altered, you will have beta-thalassemia. This means that your body will not make enough beta globin protein.

- If you have one altered gene, you are a carrier. This condition is called "beta-thalassemia trait" or "beta-thalassemia minor." It causes mild anemia.

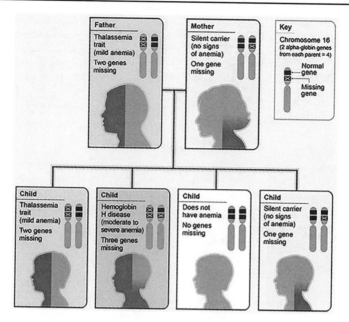

Figure 16.3. *Inheritance Pattern for Alpha Thalassemia*

The picture shows one example of how alpha-thalassemia is inherited. The alpha-globin genes are located on chromosome 16. A child inherits four alpha-globin genes (two from each parent). In this example, the father is missing two alpha-globin genes and the mother is missing one alpha-globin gene. Each child has a 25 percent chance of inheriting two missing genes and two normal genes (thalassemia trait), three missing genes and one normal gene (hemoglobin H disease), four normal genes (no anemia), or one missing gene and three normal genes (silent carrier).

- If both genes are altered, you will have beta-thalassemia intermedia or beta-thalassemia major (also called "Cooley anemia"). The intermediate form of the disorder causes moderate anemia. The major form causes severe anemia.

Risk Factors of Thalassemia

Family history and ancestry are the two risk factors for thalassemias.

- **Family history.** Thalassemias are inherited—that is, the genes for the disorders are passed from parents to their children. If your parents have missing or altered hemoglobin-making genes, you may have thalassemia.

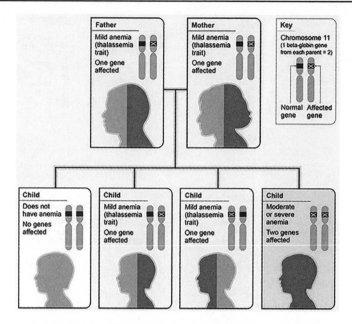

Figure 16.4. *Inheritance Pattern for Beta Thalassemia*

The picture shows one example of how beta-thalassemia is inherited. The beta-globin gene is located on chromosome 11. A child inherits two beta-globin genes (one from each parent). In this example, each parent has one altered beta-globin gene. Each child has a 25 percent chance of inheriting two normal genes (no anemia), a 50 percent chance of inheriting one altered gene and one normal gene (beta-thalassemia trait), or a 25 percent chance of inheriting two altered genes (beta-thalassemia major).

- **Ancestry.** Thalassemias occur most often among people of Italian, Greek, Middle Eastern, Southern Asian, and African descent.

Signs, Symptoms, and Complications of Thalassemia

A lack of oxygen in the bloodstream causes the signs and symptoms of thalassemias. The lack of oxygen occurs because the body does not make enough healthy RBCs and hemoglobin. The severity of symptoms depends on the severity of the disorder.

No Symptoms

Alpha-thalassemia silent carriers generally have no signs or symptoms of the disorder. The lack of alpha-globin protein is so minor that the body's hemoglobin works normally.

Mild Anemia

People who have alpha- or beta-thalassemia trait can have mild anemia. However, many people who have these types of thalassemia have no signs or symptoms.

Mild anemia can make you feel tired. Mild anemia caused by alpha-thalassemia trait might be mistaken for iron-deficiency anemia.

Mild to Moderate Anemia and Other Signs and Symptoms

People who have beta-thalassemia intermedia have mild to moderate anemia. They also may have other health problems, such as:

- **Slowed growth and delayed puberty.** Anemia can slow down a child's growth and development.

- **Bone problems.** Thalassemia may cause bone marrow to expand. When bone marrow expands, the bones become wider than normal. They may become brittle and break easily.

- **An enlarged spleen.** The spleen is an organ that helps your body fight infection and remove unwanted material. When a person has thalassemia, the spleen has to work very hard. As a result, the spleen becomes larger than normal. This makes anemia worse. If the spleen becomes too large, it must be removed.

Screening and Prevention of Thalassemia

You cannot prevent thalassemias because they are inherited (passed from parents to children through genes). However, prenatal tests can detect these blood disorders before birth.

Family genetic studies may help find out whether people have missing or *altered-hemoglobin* genes that cause thalassemias.

If you know of family members who have thalassemias and you are thinking of having children, consider talking with your doctor and a genetic counselor. They can help determine your risk for passing the disorder to your children.

Diagnosis of Thalassemia

Doctors diagnose thalassemias using blood tests, including a complete blood count (CBC) and special hemoglobin tests.

Moderate and severe thalassemias usually are diagnosed in early childhood. This is because signs and symptoms, including severe anemia, often occur within the first two years of life.

People who have milder forms of thalassemia may be diagnosed after a routine blood test shows they have anemia. Doctors might suspect thalassemia if a person has anemia and is a member of an ethnic group that is at increased risk for thalassemias.

Doctors also test the amount of iron in the blood to find out whether the anemia is due to iron deficiency or thalassemia. Iron-deficiency anemia occurs if the body does not have enough iron to make hemoglobin. The anemia in thalassemia occurs because of a problem with either the alpha-globin or beta-globin chains of hemoglobin, not because of a lack of iron.

Because thalassemias are passed from parents to children through genes, family genetic studies also can help diagnose the disorder. These studies involve taking a family medical history and doing blood tests on family members. The tests will show whether any family members have missing or altered hemoglobin genes.

If you know of family members who have thalassemias and you are thinking of having children, consider talking with your doctor and a genetic counselor. They can help determine your risk for passing the disorder to your children.

If you are expecting a baby and you and your partner are thalassemia carriers, you may want to consider prenatal testing.

Prenatal testing involves taking a sample of amniotic fluid or tissue from the placenta. (Amniotic fluid is the fluid in the sac surrounding a growing embryo. The placenta is the organ that attaches the umbilical cord to the mother's womb.) Tests done on the fluid or tissue can show whether your baby has thalassemia and how severe it might be.

Treatment of Thalassemia

Treatments for thalassemias depend on the type and severity of the disorder. People who are carriers or who have alpha- or beta-thalassemia trait have mild or no symptoms. They will likely need little or no treatment.

Doctors use three standard treatments for moderate and severe forms of thalassemia. These treatments include blood transfusions, iron chelation therapy, and folic acid supplements. Other treatments have been developed or are being tested, but they are used much less often.

Section 16.4

Hemophilia

This section includes text excerpted from "Hemophilia,"
Centers for Disease Control and Prevention (CDC),
September 6, 2018.

What Is Hemophilia?

Hemophilia is usually an inherited bleeding disorder in which the blood does not clot properly. This can lead to spontaneous bleeding as well as bleeding following injuries or surgery. Blood contains many proteins called "clotting factors" that can help to stop bleeding. Children with hemophilia have low levels of either factor VIII or factor IX. The severity of hemophilia that a child has is determined by the amount of factor in the blood. The lower the amount of the factor, the more likely it is that bleeding will occur which can lead to serious health problems.

Causes of Hemophilia

Hemophilia is caused by a mutation or change, in one of the genes, that provides instructions for making the clotting factor proteins needed to form a blood clot. This change or mutation can prevent the clotting protein from working properly or to be missing altogether. These genes are located on the X chromosome. Males have one X and one Y chromosome (XY) and females have two X chromosomes (XX). Males inherit the X chromosome from their mothers and the Y chromosome from their fathers. Females inherit one X chromosome from each parent.

The X chromosome contains many genes that are not present on the Y chromosome. This means that males only have one copy of most of the genes on the X chromosome, whereas females have two copies. Thus, males can have a disease such as hemophilia if they inherit an affected X chromosome that has a mutation in either the factor VIII or factor IX gene. Females can also have hemophilia, but this is much rarer. In such cases, both X chromosomes are affected or one is affected and the other is missing or inactive. In these females, bleeding symptoms may be similar to males with hemophilia.

A female with one affected X chromosome is a "carrier" of hemophilia. Sometimes a female who is a carrier can have symptoms of hemophilia. In addition, she can pass the affected X chromosome with the clotting factor gene mutation on to her children.

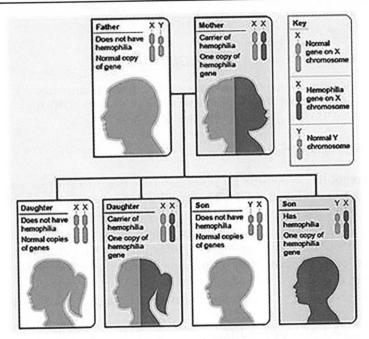

Figure 16.5. *Inheritance Pattern for Hemophilia: Example 1* (Source: "Hemophilia," National Heart, Lung, and Blood Institute (NHLBI).)

The image shows one example of how the hemophilia gene is inherited. In this example, the father does not have hemophilia (that is, he has two normal chromosomes—X and Y). The mother is a carrier of hemophilia (that is, she has one hemophilia gene on one X chromosome and one normal X chromosome).

Even though hemophilia runs in families, some families have no prior history of family members with hemophilia. Sometimes, there are carrier females in the family, but no affected boys, just by chance. However, about one-third of the time, the baby with hemophilia is the first one in the family to be affected with a mutation in the gene for the clotting factor.

Hemophilia can result in:

- Bleeding within joints that can lead to chronic joint disease and pain

- Bleeding in the head and sometimes in the brain which can cause long-term problems, such as seizures and paralysis

- Death can occur if the bleeding cannot be stopped or if it occurs in a vital organ, such as the brain

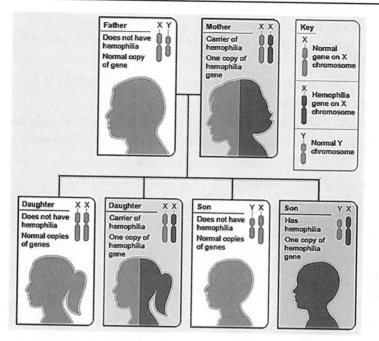

Figure 16.6. *Inheritance Pattern for Hemophilia: Example 2* (Source: "Hemophilia," National Heart, Lung, and Blood Institute (NHLBI).)

The image shows one example of how the hemophilia gene is inherited. In this example, the father has hemophilia (that is, he has the hemophilia gene on the X chromosome). The mother is not a hemophilia carrier (that is, she has two normal X chromosomes).

Types of Hemophilia

There are several different types of hemophilia. The following two are the most common:

- **Hemophilia A (classic hemophilia).** This type is caused by a lack or decrease of clotting factor VIII.

- **Hemophilia B (Christmas disease).** This type is caused by a lack or decrease of clotting factor IX.

Signs and Symptoms of Hemophilia

Common signs of hemophilia include:

- Bleeding into the joints. This can cause swelling and pain or tightness in the joints; it often affects the knees, elbows, and ankles.

- Bleeding into the skin (which is bruising) or muscle and soft tissue causing a buildup of blood in the area (called a "hematoma")

- Bleeding of the mouth and gums, and bleeding that is hard to stop after losing a tooth

- Bleeding after circumcision (surgery performed on male babies to remove the hood of skin, called the "foreskin," covering the head of the penis)

- Bleeding after having shots, such as vaccinations

- Bleeding in the head of an infant after a difficult delivery

- Blood in the urine or stool

- Frequent and hard-to-stop nosebleeds

Who Is Affected by Hemophilia?

Hemophilia occurs in about 1 of every 5,000 male births. Hemophilia A is about 4 times as common as hemophilia B, and about half of those affected have a severe form. Hemophilia affects children from all racial and ethnic groups.

Diagnosis of Hemophilia

Many people who have or have had family members with hemophilia will ask that their baby boys get tested soon after birth. About one-third of babies who are diagnosed with hemophilia have a new mutation not present in other family members. In these cases, a doctor might check for hemophilia if a newborn is showing certain signs of hemophilia.

To make a diagnosis, doctors would perform certain blood tests to show if the blood is clotting properly. If it does not, then they would do clotting factor tests, also called "factor assays," to diagnose the cause of the bleeding disorder. These blood tests would show the type of hemophilia and severity.

Families with a History of Hemophilia

Any family history of bleeding, such as following surgery or injury, or unexplained deaths among brothers, sisters, or other male relatives, such as maternal uncles, grandfathers, or cousins should be discussed with a doctor to see if hemophilia was a cause. A doctor often will get a thorough family history to find out if a bleeding disorder exists in the family.

Many people who have or have had family members with hemophilia will ask that their baby boys get tested soon after birth. In the best of cases, testing for hemophilia is planned before the baby's delivery so that a sample of blood can be drawn from the umbilical cord (which connects the mother and baby before birth) immediately after birth and tested to determine the level of the clotting factors. Umbilical cord blood testing is better at finding low levels of factor VIII (8) than it is at finding low levels of factor IX (9). This is because factor IX (9) levels take more time to develop and are not at a normal level until a baby is at least 6 months of age. Therefore, a mildly low level of factor IX (9) at birth does not necessarily mean that the baby has hemophilia B. A repeat test when the baby is older might be needed in some cases.

Families with No Previous History of Hemophilia

About one-third of babies who are diagnosed with hemophilia have no other family members with the disorder. A doctor might check for hemophilia in a newborn if:

- Bleeding after the circumcision of the penis goes on for a long time.

- Bleeding goes on for a long time after drawing blood and heel sticks (pricking the infant's heel to draw blood for newborn screening tests).

- Bleeding in the head (scalp or brain) after a difficult delivery or after using special devices or instruments to help deliver the baby (e.g., vacuum or forceps).

- Unusual raised bruises or large numbers of bruises. If a child is not diagnosed with hemophilia during the newborn period, the family might notice unusual bruising once the child begins standing or crawling.

Those with severe hemophilia can have serious bleeding problems right away. Thus, they often are diagnosed during the first year of life. People with milder forms of hemophilia might not be diagnosed until later in life.

Screening Tests

Screening tests are blood tests that show if the blood is clotting properly. Some of the types of screening tests are discussed below.

Complete Blood Count

This common test measures the amount of hemoglobin (the red pigment inside red blood cells that carries oxygen), the size and number of red blood cells and the number of different types of white blood cells and platelets found in the blood. The Complete Blood Count (CBC) is normal in people with hemophilia. However, if a person with hemophilia has unusually heavy bleeding or bleeds for a long time, the hemoglobin and the red blood cell count can be low.

Activated Partial Thromboplastin Time Test

This test measures how long it takes for blood to clot. It measures the clotting ability of factors VIII, IX, XI, and XII. If any of these clotting factors are too low, it takes longer than normal for the blood to clot. The results of this test will show a longer clotting time among people with hemophilia A or B.

Prothrombin Time Test

This test also measures the time it takes for blood to clot. It measures primarily the clotting ability of factors I, II, V, VII, and X. If any of these factors are too low, it takes longer than normal for the blood to clot. The results of this test will be normal among most people with hemophilia A and B.

Fibrinogen Test

This test also helps doctors assess a patient's ability to form a blood clot. This test is ordered either along with other blood clotting tests or when a patient has an abnormal PT or APTT test result, or both. Fibrinogen is another name for clotting factor I.

Clotting Factor Tests

Clotting factor tests, also called "factor assays," are required to diagnose a bleeding disorder. This blood test shows the type of hemophilia and the severity. It is important to know the type and severity in order to create the best treatment plan.

Table 16.2. Type of Hemophilia and the Severity

Severity	Levels of Factor VIII or IX in the Blood
Normal (person who does not have hemophilia)	50 to 100%
Mild hemophilia	Greater than 5% but less than 50%
Moderate hemophilia	1 to 5%
Severe hemophilia	Less than 1%

Treatment of Hemophilia

The best way to treat hemophilia is to replace the missing blood clotting factor so that the blood can clot properly. This is typically done by injecting treatment products, called "clotting factor concentrates," into a person's vein. Clinicians typically prescribe treatment products for episodic care or prophylactic care. Episodic care is used to stop a patient's bleeding episodes; prophylactic care is used to prevent bleeding episodes from occurring. It is now possible for people with hemophilia, and their families, to learn how to give their own clotting factor treatment products at home. Giving factor treatment products at home means that bleeds can be treated quicker, resulting in less serious bleeding and fewer side effects.

Treatment Centers

Hemophilia is a complex disorder. Good quality medical care from doctors and nurses who know a lot about the disorder can help people with hemophilia prevent some serious problems. Often the best choice for care is at a comprehensive hemophilia treatment center (HTC). An HTC provides patients with the care and education to address all issues related to the disorder. The team consists of physicians (hematologists or blood specialists), nurses, social workers, physical therapists, and other healthcare providers who are specialized in the care of people with bleeding disorders.

Treatment Medications
Clotting Factor Products

There are two main types of clotting factor concentrates available.

- **Plasma-derived factor concentrates.** Plasma is the liquid part of blood. It is pale yellow or straw-colored and contains proteins, such as antibodies, albumin, and clotting factors.

Several factors concentrate treatment products are available that are made from human plasma proteins. All blood and parts of blood, such as plasma, are routinely tested for viruses. The plasma is collected from many people, and then it goes through several processes to separate it into components, such as clotting factors. The clotting proteins are then made into a freeze-dried product, which is tested and treated to kill any potential viruses before it is packaged for use.

- **Recombinant factor concentrates.** Until 1992, all factor replacement products were made from human plasma. In 1992, the U.S. Food and Drug Administration (FDA) approved recombinant factor VIII concentrate, which does not come from human plasma. This concentrate is genetically engineered using DNA technology. Commercially prepared factor concentrates are treated to remove or inactivate blood-borne viruses. Additionally, recombinant factors VIII and IX do not contain any plasma or albumin, and therefore, cannot spread any bloodborne viruses.

Some people who infuse with clotting factor concentrates may develop an inhibitor. Inhibitors make it more difficult to stop a bleeding episode because they prevent the treatment from working.

Other Treatment Products
Hemlibra®

Hemlibra® works by replacing the function of factor VIII, rather than replacing the missing clotting factor VIII directly. It can be used to either prevent or reduce the frequency of bleeding episodes in people with hemophilia A. This treatment product can be given by injection under the skin. Patients who use Hemlibra® for prophylaxis and use clotting factor concentrates to treat breakthrough bleeds, can still develop an inhibitor. Traditional laboratory inhibitor testing methods do not work when testing for inhibitors in patients on Hemlibra®; as such, a specialized testing method called the "chromogenic Bethesda assay" is needed.

DDAVP® or Stimate® (Desmopressin Acetate)

DDAVP® and Stimate® are medications that are similar to a hormone that occurs naturally in the body. The medications release factor VIII from where it is stored in the body tissues. For people with mild, as well as some cases of moderate, hemophilia, this can work to increase the person's own factor VIII levels so that they do not have to use clotting factors to stop bleeding episodes. DDAVP® can be given through a vein and Stimate® via a nasal spray.

Amicar® (Epsilon Amino Caproic Acid)

Amicar® is a medication that can be given through a vein or by mouth (as a pill or a liquid). It prevents blood clots from breaking down, resulting in a firmer clot, and is often used for bleeding in the mouth or after a tooth has been removed because it blocks a substance found in the saliva (spit) that breaks down clots.

Cryoprecipitate

Cryoprecipitate is a substance that comes from thawing fresh frozen plasma. It is rich in factor VIII and was commonly used to control serious bleeding in the past. However, because there is no method to kill viruses, such as HIV and hepatitis, in cryoprecipitate, it is no longer used as the current standard of treatment in the United States.

Section 16.5

Thrombophilia

"Thrombophilia (Excessive Blood Clotting),"
© 2017 Omnigraphics. Reviewed September 2019.

What Is Thrombophilia?

Thrombophilia, also known as "hypercoagulation," is a medical disorder in which excessive blood clotting occurs. In healthy people, a wound that causes bleeding triggers an immediate response in the body. Blood platelets begin to stick together in masses called "blood clots." This process is known as "coagulation" and is the body's primary means of stopping blood loss. Thrombophilia means that the body has an abnormal blood-clotting response. Thrombophilia can manifest as an overactive blood-clot response, in which blood clots form too easily or too often. It can also refer to persistent blood clots that are not dissolved by the body, or blood clots that form inside blood vessels or arteries.

Causes of Thrombophilia

Excessive blood-clotting disorders can be inherited or acquired. Acquired clotting disorders can result from traumatic injury, surgery, long-term bed rest, obesity, severe dehydration, certain chronic health conditions, and the use of certain medications. Excessive blood clotting can also be caused by sitting for long periods of time during car or airplane trips. Certain medical history factors can also indicate a person's likelihood of having an excessive blood-clotting disorder, primarily family members who have been diagnosed with an excessive blood-clotting disorder. The majority of pediatric thrombophilia cases occur in children who have a combination of multiple risk factors.

Symptoms and Risks of Thrombophilia

Symptoms of excessive blood-clotting disorders vary depending on where excessive blood clots form in the body.

Chest pain, shortness of breath, and pain in the upper arms, back, neck, or jaw can be symptoms of a blood clot in the heart or lungs. This type of blood clot can result in a heart attack, which restricts or blocks blood flow to part of the heart. An undiagnosed or untreated heart attack can result in serious long-term complications, including death.

Persistent headaches, changes in ability to speak, difficulty understanding others talking, dizziness, or paralysis can indicate a blood clot in the brain. This type of blood clot can result in a stroke. A stroke causes restricted blood flow to the brain, which can result in serious complications including death if left undiagnosed or untreated.

Swelling, pain, redness, or warm skin on the arms or legs can indicate a type of blood clot known as a "deep vein thrombosis." These types of blood clots can travel through the bloodstream and cause serious complications if they reach the brain, heart, or lungs.

Diagnosis of Thrombophilia

Excessive blood-clotting disorders are diagnosed through physical exam, medical history interview, and diagnostic blood tests. Blood tests for excessive clotting measure the levels of various blood components such as red and white blood cells, platelets, and blood-clotting protein factors. Blood tests also analyze the clotting behavior of the blood samples to identify normal or abnormal clotting function. Medical history factors are evaluated to assess a person's risk for excessive blood-clotting disorder. Some factors that indicate a possible blood-clotting disorder diagnosis include frequent unexplained bruising and/or family members who have been diagnosed with a blood-clotting disorder.

Treatment and Prevention of Thrombophilia

There is no course of prevention for inherited thrombophilia. To reduce the risk of acquired thrombophilia, it is important to follow prescribed treatments for diseases that can result in excessive blood clotting, such as diabetes and certain heart and vascular disorders. Most cases of thrombophilia are treatable with medication that thins the blood to prevent excessive clotting.

References

1. "Excessive Blood Clotting," National Heart, Lung, and Blood Institute (NHLBI). June 11, 2014.

2. "Hypercoagulation," FamilyDoctor.org. March 2014.

3. Raffin, Leslie. "Thrombophilia in Children: Who to Test, How, When, and Why?" National Center for Biotechnology Information (NCBI). January 1, 2008.

4. "What Is Excessive Blood Clotting (Hypercoagulation)?" American Heart Association, November 30, 2015.

Section 16.6

von Willebrand Disease

This section includes text excerpted from "Von Willebrand
Disease (VWD)," Centers for Disease Control and
Prevention (CDC), August 6, 2019.

What Is von Willebrand Disease?

Von Willebrand disease (VWD) is a blood disorder in which the
blood does not clot properly. Blood contains many proteins that help
the body stop bleeding. One of these proteins is called "von Willebrand factor" (VWF). People with VWD either have a low level of
VWF in their blood or the VWF protein does not work the way it
should.

Normally, when a child is injured and starts to bleed, the VWF in
the blood attaches to small blood cells called "platelets." This helps the
platelets stick together, like glue, to form a clot at the site of injury
and stop the bleeding. When a child has VWD, because the VWF does
not work the way it should, the clot might take longer to form or not
form the way it should, and bleeding might take longer to stop. This
can lead to heavy, hard-to-stop bleeding. Although rare, the bleeding
can be severe enough to damage joints or internal organs, or even be
life-threatening.

Who Is Affected by von Willebrand Disease?

Von Willebrand disease is the most common bleeding disorder,
found in up to one percent of the United States population. This means
that 3.2 million (or about 1 in every 100) people in the United States
have the disease.

Types of von Willebrand Disease
Type 1

This is the most common and mildest form of VWD, in which
a child has lower than normal levels of VWF. Children with Type
1 VWD also might have low levels of factor VIII, another type of
blood-clotting protein. This should not be confused with hemophilia,
in which there are low levels or a complete lack of factor VIII but
normal levels of VWF.

Type 2

With this type of VWD, although the body makes normal amounts of the VWF, the factor does not work the way it should. Type 2 is further broken down into four subtypes; 2A, 2B, 2M, and 2N, depending on the specific problem with the child's VWF. Because the treatment is different for each type, it is important that a parent should know which subtype their child has.

Type 3

This is the most severe form of VWD, in which a child has very little or no VWF and low levels of factor VIII. This is the rarest type of VWD.

Causes of von Willebrand Disease

Most people who have VWD are born with it. It almost always is inherited, or passed down, from a parent to a child. VWD can be passed down from either the mother or the father, or both, to the child.

While rare, it is possible for a person to get VWD without a family history of the disease. This happens when a "spontaneous mutation" occurs. That means there has been a change in the person's gene. Whether the child received the affected gene from a parent or as a result of a mutation, once the child has it, the child can later pass it along to her or his children. Rarely, a person who is not born with VWD can acquire it or have it first occur later in life. This can happen when a person's own immune system destroys her or his VWF, often as a result of the use of a medication or as a result of another disease. If VWD is acquired, meaning it was not inherited from a parent, it cannot be passed along to any children.

Signs and Symptoms of von Willebrand Disease

The major signs of VWD are:

Frequent or Hard-to-Stop Nosebleeds

Children with VWD might have nosebleeds that:

- Start without injury (spontaneous)
- Occur often, usually 5 times or more in a year
- Last more than 10 minutes
- Need packing or cautery to stop the bleeding

Easy Bruising

Children with VWD might experience easy bruising that:

- Occurs with very little or no trauma or injury
- Occurs often (one to four times per month)
- Is larger than the size of a quarter
- Is not flat and has a raised lump

Longer than Normal Bleeding after Injury, Surgery, or Dental Work

Children with VWD might have longer than normal bleeding after injury or a surgery, for example:

- After a cut to the skin, the bleeding lasts more than five minutes
- Heavy or longer bleeding occurs after surgery. Bleeding sometimes stops but starts up again hours or days later.

Children with VWD might have longer than normal bleeding during or after dental work, for example:

- Heavy bleeding occurs during or after dental surgery
- The surgery site oozes blood longer than three hours after the surgery
- The surgery site needs packing or cautery to stop the bleeding

The amount of bleeding depends on the type and severity of VWD. Other common bleeding events include:

- Blood in the stool (feces) from bleeding into the stomach or intestines
- Blood in the urine from bleeding into the kidneys or bladder
- Bleeding into joints or internal organs in severe cases (Type 3)

Diagnosis of von Willebrand Disease

To find out if a child has VWD, the doctor will ask questions about personal and family histories of bleeding. The doctor also will check for unusual bruising or other signs of recent bleeding and order some blood tests that will measure how the blood clots. The tests will provide information about the amount of clotting proteins present in the blood and if the clotting proteins are working properly. Because certain medications can cause bleeding, even among children without a bleeding disorder, the doctor will ask about recent or routine medications taken that could cause bleeding or make bleeding symptoms worse.

Treatments of von Willebrand Disease

The type of treatment prescribed for VWD depends on the type and severity of the disease. For minor bleeds, treatment might not be needed.

The most commonly used types of treatment include:

- **Desmopressin acetate injection.** This medicine (DDAVP®) is injected into a vein to treat milder forms of VWD (mainly type 1). It works by making the body release more VWF into the blood. It helps increase the level of factor VIII in the blood as well.

- **Desmopressin acetate nasal spray.** This high-strength nasal spray (Stimate®) is used to treat milder forms of VWD. It works by making the body release more VWF into the blood.

- **Factor replacement therapy.** Recombinant VWF (such as Vonvendi®) and medicines rich in VWF and factor VIII (for example, Humate P®, Wilate®, Alphanate®, or Koate DVI®) are used to treat more severe forms of VWD or milder forms of VWD (for those who do not respond well to the nasal spray). These medicines are injected into a vein in the arm to replace the missing factor in the blood.

- **Antifibrinolytic drugs.** These drugs (for example, Amicar®, Lysteda®) are either injected or taken orally to help slow or prevent the breakdown of blood clots.

Chapter 17

Cancer in Children

Chapter Contents

Section 17.1

Childhood Acute Lymphoblastic Leukemia

This section contains text excerpted from the following
sources: Text in this section begins with excerpts from "Childhood
Leukemia," MedlinePlus, National Institutes of Health (NIH),
May 20, 2016. Reviewed September 2019; Text beginning with
the heading "What Is Childhood Acute Lymphoblastic Leukemia?"
is excerpted from "Childhood Acute Lymphoblastic Leukemia
Treatment (PDQ®)—Patient Version," National Cancer
Institute (NCI), July 23, 2019.

Leukemia is a cancer of the white blood cells (WBCs). It is the most
common type of childhood cancer. Your blood cells form in your bone
marrow. WBCs help your body fight infection. In leukemia, the bone
marrow produces abnormal WBCs. These cells crowd out the healthy
blood cells, making it hard for blood to do its work.

Leukemia can develop quickly or slowly. Acute leukemia is a
fast-growing type while chronic leukemia grows slowly. Children with
leukemia usually have one of the acute types.

Symptoms of leukemia include:

- Infections

- Fever

- Loss of appetite

- Tiredness

- Easy bruising or bleeding

- Swollen lymph nodes

- Night sweats

- Shortness of breath

- Pain in the bones or joints

What Is Childhood Acute Lymphoblastic Leukemia?

Childhood acute lymphoblastic leukemia (also called "ALL" or
"acute lymphocytic leukemia") is a cancer of the blood and bone
marrow. This type of cancer usually gets worse quickly if it is not
treated.

How Leukemia Affect Blood Cells and Platelets

In a healthy child, the bone marrow makes blood stem cells (immature cells) that become mature blood cells over time. A blood stem cell may become a myeloid stem cell or a lymphoid stem cell.

A myeloid stem cell becomes one of three types of mature blood cells:

- Red blood cells (RBCs) that carry oxygen and other substances to all tissues of the body

- Platelets that form blood clots to stop bleeding

- WBCs that fight infection and disease

A lymphoid stem cell becomes a lymphoblast cell and then one of three types of lymphocytes (WBCs):

- B lymphocytes that make antibodies to help fight infection.

- T lymphocytes that help B lymphocytes make the antibodies that help fight infection.

- Natural killer cells that attack cancer cells and viruses.

In a child with ALL, too many stem cells become lymphoblasts, B lymphocytes, or T lymphocytes. The cells do not work like normal lymphocytes and are not able to fight infection very well. These cells are cancer (leukemia) cells. Also, as the number of leukemia cells increases in the blood and bone marrow, there is less room for healthy WBCs, RBCs, and platelets. This may lead to infection, anemia, and easy bleeding.

Risks of Childhood Acute Lymphoblastic Leukemia

Anything that increases your risk of getting a disease is called a "risk factor." Having a risk factor does not mean that you will get cancer; not having risk factors does not mean that you will not get cancer. Talk with your child's doctor if you think your child may be at risk.

Possible risk factors for ALL include the following:

- Being exposed to x-rays before birth

- Being exposed to radiation

- Past treatment with chemotherapy

- Having certain genetic conditions, such as:

  - Down syndrome

- Neurofibromatosis type 1 (NF1)
- Bloom syndrome
- Fanconi anemia (FA)
- Ataxia-telangiectasia (A-T)
- Li-Fraumeni syndrome
- Constitutional mismatch repair deficiency (CMMRD) (mutations in certain genes that stop deoxyribonucleic acid (DNA) from repairing itself, which leads to the growth of cancers at an early age)
- Having certain changes in the chromosomes or genes

Signs of Childhood Acute Lymphoblastic Leukemia

These and other signs and symptoms may be caused by childhood ALL or by other conditions. Check with your child's doctor if your child has any of the following:

- Fever
- Easy bruising or bleeding
- Petechiae (flat, pinpoint, dark-red spots under the skin caused by bleeding)
- Bone or joint pain
- Painless lumps in the neck, underarm, stomach, or groin
- Pain or feeling of fullness below the ribs
- Weakness, feeling tired, or looking pale
- Loss of appetite

Diagnosis of Childhood Acute Lymphoblastic Leukemia

The following tests and procedures may be used to diagnose childhood ALL and find out if leukemia cells have spread to other parts of the body such as the brain or testicles:

- **Physical exam and history:** An exam of the body to check general signs of health, including checking for signs of disease, such as lumps or anything else that seems unusual. A history of the patient's health habits and past illnesses and treatments will also be taken.

- **Complete blood count (CBC) with differential:** A procedure in which a sample of blood is drawn and checked for the following:

  - The number of RBCs and platelets

  - The number and type of WBCs

  - The amount of hemoglobin (the protein that carries oxygen) in the RBCs

  - The portion of the sample made up of RBCs

- **Blood chemistry studies:** A procedure in which a blood sample is checked to measure the amounts of certain substances released into the blood by organs and tissues in the body. An unusual (higher or lower than normal) amount of a substance can be a sign of disease.

- **Bone marrow aspiration and biopsy:** The removal of bone marrow and a small piece of bone by inserting a hollow needle into the hipbone or breastbone. A pathologist views the bone marrow and bone under a microscope to look for signs of cancer.

Factors Affecting Prognosis and Treatment Options of Childhood Acute Lymphoblastic Leukemia

The prognosis (chance of recovery) depends on:

- How quickly and how low the leukemia cell count drops after the first month of treatment

- Age at the time of diagnosis, sex, race, and ethnic background

- The number of WBCs in the blood at the time of diagnosis

- Whether the leukemia cells began from B lymphocytes or T lymphocytes

- Whether there are certain changes in the chromosomes or genes of the lymphocytes with cancer

- Whether the child has Down syndrome

- Whether leukemia cells are found in the cerebrospinal fluid

- The child's weight at the time of diagnosis and during treatment

Treatment options depend on:

- Whether the leukemia cells began from B lymphocytes or T lymphocytes

- Whether the child has a standard-risk, high-risk, or very high-risk ALL

- The age of the child at the time of diagnosis

- Whether there are certain changes in the chromosomes of lymphocytes, such as the Philadelphia chromosome

- Whether the child was treated with steroids before the start of induction therapy

- How quickly and how low the leukemia cell count drops during treatment

For leukemia that relapses (comes back) after treatment, the prognosis and treatment options depend partly on the following:

- How long it is between the time of diagnosis and when leukemia comes back

- Whether leukemia comes back in the bone marrow or in other parts of the body

Section 17.2

Childhood Acute Myeloid Leukemia

This section includes text excerpted from "Childhood Acute Myeloid Leukemia/Other Myeloid Malignancies Treatment (PDQ®)—Patient Version," National Cancer Institute (NCI), July 23, 2019.

What Is Childhood Acute Myeloid Leukemia?

Childhood acute myeloid leukemia (AML) is a cancer of the blood and bone marrow. AML is also called "acute myelogenous leukemia," "acute myeloblastic leukemia," "acute granulocytic leukemia," and "acute nonlymphocytic leukemia." Cancers that are acute usually get worse quickly if they are not treated. Chronic cancer usually get worse slowly.

How Leukemia and Other Diseases of the Blood and Bone Marrow Affect Blood Cells and Platelets

Normally, the bone marrow makes blood stem cells (immature cells) that become mature blood cells over time. A blood stem cell may become a myeloid stem cell or a lymphoid stem cell. A lymphoid stem cell becomes a white blood cell (WBC).

A myeloid stem cell becomes one of three types of mature blood cells:

- Red blood cells (RBCs) that carry oxygen and other substances to all tissues of the body

- WBCs that fight infection and disease

- Platelets that form blood clots to stop bleeding

In AML, the myeloid stem cells usually become a type of immature WBC called "myeloblasts" (or myeloid blasts). The myeloblasts, or leukemia cells, in AML are abnormal and do not become healthy WBCs. The leukemia cells can build up in the blood and bone marrow so there is less room for healthy WBCs, RBCs, and platelets. When this happens, infection, anemia, or easy bleeding may occur.

The leukemia cells can spread outside the blood to other parts of the body, including the central nervous system (CNS) (brain and spinal cord), skin, and gums. Sometimes leukemia cells form a solid tumor called a "granulocytic sarcoma" or "chloroma."

Types of Myeloid Diseases
Transient Abnormal Myelopoiesis

Transient abnormal myelopoiesis (TAM) is a disorder of the bone marrow that can develop in newborns who have Down syndrome. It usually goes away on its own within the first three months of life. Infants who have TAM have an increased chance of developing AML before the age of three years. TAM is also called "transient myeloproliferative disorder" (TMD) or "transient leukemia" (TL).

Acute Promyelocytic Leukemia

Acute promyelocytic leukemia (APL) is a subtype of AML. In APL, some genes on chromosome 15 switch places with some genes on chromosome 17 and an abnormal gene called *"promyelocytic leukemia/ retinoic acid receptor alpha" (PML-RARA)* is made. The *PML-RARA* gene sends a message that stops promyelocytes (a type of WBC) from maturing. The promyelocytes (leukemia cells) can build up in the blood and bone marrow so there is less room for healthy WBCs, RBCs, and platelets. Problems with severe bleeding and blood clots may also occur. This is a serious health problem that needs treatment as soon as possible.

Juvenile Myelomonocytic Leukemia

Juvenile myelomonocytic leukemia (JMML) is a rare childhood cancer that is most common in children around the age of two years and is more common in boys. In JMML, too many myeloid blood stem cells become myelocytes and monocytes (two types of WBCs). Some of these myeloid blood stem cells never become mature WBCs. These immature cells, called "blasts," are unable to do their usual work. Over time, the myelocytes, monocytes, and blasts crowd out the RBCs and platelets in the bone marrow. When this happens, infection, anemia, or easy bleeding may occur.

Chronic Myelogenous Leukemia

Chronic myelogenous leukemia (CML) often begins in an early myeloid blood cell when a certain gene change occurs. A section of genes, that includes the *Abelson murine leukemia* (ABL) gene, on chromosome 9 changes place with a section of genes on chromosome 22, which has the *breakpoint cluster region (BCR)* gene. This makes a very short chromosome 22 (called the "Philadelphia chromosome") and a very long chromosome 9. An abnormal *BCR-ABL* gene is formed on chromosome 22. The *BCR-ABL* gene tells the blood cells to make too much of a protein called "tyrosine kinase." Tyrosine kinase causes too many WBCs (leukemia cells) to be made in the bone marrow. The leukemia cells can build up in the blood and bone marrow so there is less room for healthy WBCs, RBCs, and platelets. When this happens, infection, anemia, or easy bleeding may occur. CML is rare in children.

Myelodysplastic Syndromes

Myelodysplastic syndromes (MDS) occur less often in children than in adults. In MDS, the bone marrow makes too few RBCs, WBCs, and platelets. These blood cells may not mature and enter the blood. The type of MDS depends on the type of blood cell that is affected.

The treatment for MDS depends on how low the numbers of RBCs, WBCs, or platelets are. Over time, MDS may become AML.

Acute Myeloid Leukemia or Myelodysplastic Syndromes after Treatment

Cancer treatment with certain chemotherapy drugs and/or radiation therapy may cause therapy-related AML (t-AML) or therapy-related MDS (t-MDS). The risk of these therapy-related myeloid diseases depends on the total dose of the chemotherapy drugs used and the radiation dose and treatment field. Some patients also have an inherited risk for t-AML and t-MDS. These therapy-related diseases usually occur within seven years after treatment but are rare in children.

Risks of Childhood Acute Myeloid Leukemia

Anything that increases your risk of getting a disease is called a "risk factor." Having a risk factor does not mean that you will get cancer; not having risk factors does not mean that you will not get cancer. Talk with your child's doctor if you think your child may be at risk. These and other factors may increase the risk of childhood AML, APL, JMML, CML, and MDS:

- Having a brother or sister, especially a twin, with leukemia
- Being Hispanic
- Being exposed to cigarette smoke or alcohol before birth
- Having a personal history of aplastic anemia.
- Having a personal or family history of MDS
- Having a family history of AML
- Past treatment with chemotherapy or radiation therapy
- Being exposed to ionizing radiation or chemicals such as benzene
- Having certain syndromes or inherited disorders, such as:
  - Down syndrome
  - Aplastic anemia
  - Fanconi anemia
  - Neurofibromatosis type 1
  - Noonan syndrome

- Shwachman-Diamond syndrome (SDS)
- Li-Fraumeni syndrome (LFS)

Signs and Symptoms of Childhood Acute Myeloid Leukemia

These and other signs and symptoms may be caused by childhood AML, APL, JMML, CML, or MDS or by other conditions. Check with a doctor if your child has any of the following:

- Fever with or without an infection
- Night sweats
- Shortness of breath
- Weakness or feeling tired
- Easy bruising or bleeding
- Petechiae (flat, pinpoint spots under the skin caused by bleeding)
- Pain in the bones or joints
- Pain or feeling of fullness below the ribs
- Painless lumps in the neck, underarm, stomach, groin, or other parts of the body. In childhood AML, these lumps, called "leukemia cutis," maybe blue or purple.
- Painless lumps that are sometimes around the eyes. These lumps, called "chloromas," are sometimes seen in childhood AML and may be blue-green.
- An eczema-like skin rash

The signs and symptoms of TAM may include the following:

- Swelling all over the body
- Shortness of breath
- Trouble breathing
- Weakness or feeling tired
- Bleeding a lot, even from a small cut
- Petechiae (flat, pinpoint spots under the skin caused by bleeding)

- Pain below the ribs

- Skin rash

- Jaundice (yellowing of the skin and whites of the eyes)

- Headache, trouble seeing, and confusion

- Sometimes TAM does not cause any symptoms at all and is diagnosed after a routine blood test

Diagnosis of Childhood Acute Myeloid Leukemia

The following tests and procedures may be used:

- **Physical exam and history:** An exam of the body to check general signs of health, including checking for signs of disease, such as lumps or anything else that seems unusual. A history of the patient's health habits and past illnesses and treatments will also be taken.

- **Complete blood count (CBC) with differential:** A procedure in which a sample of blood is drawn and checked for the following:

  - The number of RBCs and platelets

  - The number and type of WBCs

  - The amount of hemoglobin (the protein that carries oxygen) in the RBCs

  - The portion of the blood sample made up of RBCs

- **Blood chemistry studies:** A procedure in which a blood sample is checked to measure the amounts of certain substances released into the blood by organs and tissues in the body. An unusual (higher or lower than normal) amount of a substance can be a sign of disease.

- **Chest x-ray:** An x-ray of the organs and bones inside the chest. An x-ray is a type of energy beam that can go through the body and onto film, making a picture of areas inside the body.

- **Biopsy:** The removal of cells or tissues so they can be viewed under a microscope by a pathologist to check for signs of cancer. Biopsies that may be done include the following:

- **Bone marrow aspiration and biopsy:** The removal of bone marrow, blood, and a small piece of bone by inserting a hollow needle into the hipbone or breastbone.

- **Tumor biopsy:** A biopsy of a chloroma may be done.

- **Lymph node biopsy:** The removal of all or part of a lymph node.

- **Immunophenotyping:** A laboratory test that uses antibodies to identify cancer cells based on the types of antigens or markers on the surface of the cells. This test is used to help diagnose specific types of leukemia.

- **Cytogenetic analysis:** A laboratory test in which the chromosomes of cells in a sample of blood or bone marrow are counted and checked for any changes, such as broken, missing, rearranged, or extra chromosomes. Changes in certain chromosomes may be a sign of cancer. Cytogenetic analysis is used to help diagnose cancer, plan treatment, or find out how well treatment is working.

Section 17.3

Lymphoma

This section contains text excerpted from the following sources: Text in this section begins with excerpts from "Childhood Hodgkin Lymphoma Treatment (PDQ®)—Health Professional Version," National Cancer Institute (NCI), May 29, 2019; Text beginning with the heading "What Is Childhood Non-Hodgkin Lymphoma?" is excerpted from "Childhood Non-Hodgkin Lymphoma Treatment (PDQ®)—Patient Version," National Cancer Institute (NCI), July 29, 2019.

Childhood Hodgkin lymphoma (HL) is one of the few pediatric malignancies that share aspects of its biology and natural history with adult cancer. Approximately 90 to 95 percent of children with Hodgkin lymphoma can be cured, prompting increased attention to devising therapy that lessens long-term morbidity for these patients.

What Is Childhood Non-Hodgkin Lymphoma?

Childhood non-Hodgkin lymphoma is a type of cancer that forms in the lymph system, which is part of the body's immune system. It helps protect the body from infection and disease.

The lymph system is made up of the following:

- **Lymph:** Colorless, watery fluid that travels through the lymph vessels and carries T and B lymphocytes. Lymphocytes are a type of white blood cell (WBC).

- **Lymph vessels:** A network of thin tubes that collect lymph from different parts of the body and return it to the bloodstream.

- **Lymph nodes:** Small, bean-shaped structures that filter lymph and store WBCs that help fight infection and disease. Lymph nodes are found along with a network of lymph vessels throughout the body. Groups of lymph nodes are found in the neck, underarm, mediastinum, abdomen, pelvis, and groin.

- **Spleen:** An organ that makes lymphocytes, stores red blood cells (RBCs) and lymphocytes, filters the blood, and destroys old blood cells. The spleen is on the left side of the abdomen near the stomach.

- **Thymus:** An organ in which T lymphocytes mature and multiply. The thymus is in the chest behind the breastbone.

- **Tonsils:** Two small masses of lymph tissue at the back of the throat. There is one tonsil on each side of the throat.

- **Bone marrow:** The soft, spongy tissue in the center of certain bones, such as the hip bone and breastbone. WBCs, RBCs, and platelets are made in the bone marrow.

Non-Hodgkin lymphoma can begin in B lymphocytes, T lymphocytes, or natural killer cells. Lymphocytes can also be found in the blood and collect in the lymph nodes, spleen, and thymus.

Lymph tissue is also found in other parts of the body, such as the stomach, thyroid gland, brain, and skin.

Types of Lymphoma

Lymphomas are divided into two general types: Hodgkin lymphoma and non-Hodgkin lymphoma. The type of lymphoma is determined by how the cells look under a microscope.

There are three major types of childhood non-Hodgkin lymphoma.

Mature B-Cell Non-Hodgkin Lymphoma

Mature B-cell non-Hodgkin lymphomas include:

- **Burkitt and Burkitt-like lymphoma/leukemia:** Burkitt lymphoma and Burkitt leukemia are different forms of the same disease. Burkitt lymphoma/leukemia is an aggressive (fast-growing) disorder of B lymphocytes that is most common in children and young adults. It may form in the abdomen, Waldeyer ring, testicles, bone, bone marrow, skin, or central nervous system (CNS). Burkitt leukemia may start in the lymph nodes as Burkitt lymphoma and then spread to the blood and bone marrow, or it may start in the blood and bone marrow without forming in the lymph nodes first.

  Both Burkitt leukemia and Burkitt lymphoma have been linked to infection with the Epstein-Barr virus (EBV), although EBV infection is more likely to occur in patients in Africa than in the United States. Burkitt and Burkitt-like lymphoma/leukemia are diagnosed when a sample of tissue is checked and a certain change to the *MYC* gene is found.

- **Diffuse large B-cell lymphoma:** Diffuse large B-cell lymphoma is the most common type of non-Hodgkin lymphoma. It is a type of B-cell non-Hodgkin lymphoma that grows quickly in the lymph nodes. The spleen, liver, bone marrow, or other organs are also often affected. Diffuse large B-cell lymphoma occurs more often in adolescents than in children.

- **Primary mediastinal B-cell lymphoma:** A type of lymphoma that develops from B cells in the mediastinum (the area behind the breastbone). It may spread to nearby organs including the lungs and the sac around the heart. It may also spread to lymph nodes and distant organs including the kidneys. In children and adolescents, primary mediastinal B-cell lymphoma occurs more often in older adolescents.

Lymphoblastic Lymphoma

Lymphoblastic lymphoma is a type of lymphoma that mainly affects T-cell lymphocytes. It usually forms in the mediastinum (the area behind the breastbone). This causes trouble breathing, wheezing, trouble swallowing, or swelling of the head and neck. It may spread to lymph nodes, bone, bone marrow, skin, the CNS, abdominal organs, and other areas. Lymphoblastic lymphoma is a lot like acute lympho-blastic leukemia (ALL).

Anaplastic Large Cell Lymphoma

Anaplastic large cell lymphoma is a type of lymphoma that mainly affects T-cell lymphocytes. It usually forms in the lymph nodes, skin, or bone, and sometimes forms in the gastrointestinal tract (GI), lung, tissue that covers the lungs, and muscle. Patients with anaplastic large cell lymphoma have a receptor, called "CD30," on the surface of their T cells. In many children, anaplastic large cell lymphoma is marked by changes in the *ALK* gene that makes a protein called "anaplastic lymphoma kinase" (ALK). A pathologist checks for these cell and gene changes to help diagnose anaplastic large cell lymphoma.

Some Types of Non-Hodgkin Lymphoma Are Rare in Children

Some types of childhood non-Hodgkin lymphoma are less common. These include:

- **Pediatric-type follicular lymphoma (PFL):** In children, follicular lymphoma occurs mainly in males. It is more likely to be found in one area and does not spread to other places in the body. It usually forms in the tonsils and lymph nodes in the neck, but may also form in the testicles, kidney, gastrointestinal tract, and salivary gland.

- **Marginal zone lymphoma:** Marginal zone lymphoma is a type of lymphoma that tends to grow and spread slowly and is usually found at an early stage. It may be found in the lymph nodes or in areas outside the lymph nodes. Marginal zone lymphoma found outside the lymph nodes in children is called "mucosa-associated lymphoid tissue" (MALT) lymphoma. MALT may be linked to *Helicobacter pylori* (*H. Pylori*) infection of the gastrointestinal tract and *Chlamydophila psittaci* infection of the conjunctival membrane which lines the eye.

- **Primary CNS lymphoma:** Primary CNS lymphoma is extremely rare in children.

- **Peripheral T-cell lymphoma:** Peripheral T-cell lymphoma is an aggressive (fast-growing) non-Hodgkin lymphoma that begins in mature T lymphocytes. The T lymphocytes mature in the thymus gland and travel to other parts of the lymph system, such as the lymph nodes, bone marrow, and spleen.

• **Cutaneous T-cell lymphoma:** Cutaneous T-cell lymphoma begins in the skin and can cause the skin to thicken or form a tumor. It is very rare in children, but is more common in adolescents and young adults. There are different types of cutaneous T-cell lymphoma, such as cutaneous anaplastic large cell lymphoma, subcutaneous panniculitis-like T-cell lymphoma, gamma-delta T-cell lymphoma, and mycosis fungoides. Mycosis fungoides rarely occurs in children and adolescents.

Risks of Childhood Non-Hodgkin Lymphoma

Anything that increases your risk of getting a disease is called a "risk factor." Having a risk factor does not mean that you will get cancer; not having risk factors does not mean that you will not get cancer. Talk with your child's doctor if you think your child may be at risk.

Possible risk factors for childhood non-Hodgkin lymphoma include the following:

• Past treatment for cancer

• Being infected with the EBV or human immunodeficiency virus (HIV)

• Having a weakened immune system after a transplant or from medicines given after a transplant

• Having certain inherited diseases (such as deoxyribonucleic acid (DNA) repair defect syndromes which include ataxia-telangiectasia, Nijmegen breakage syndrome, and constitutional mismatch repair deficiency (CMMRD))

If lymphoma or lymphoproliferative disease is linked to a weakened immune system from certain inherited diseases, HIV infection, a transplant or medicines given after a transplant, the condition is called "lymphoproliferative disease" associated with immunodeficiency. The different types of lymphoproliferative disease associated with immunodeficiency include:

• Lymphoproliferative disease associated with primary immunodeficiency

- HIV-associated non-Hodgkin lymphoma
- Post-transplant lymphoproliferative disease

Signs of Childhood Non-Hodgkin Lymphoma

These and other signs may be caused by childhood non-Hodgkin lymphoma or by other conditions. Check with a doctor if your child has any of the following:

- Trouble breathing
- Wheezing
- Coughing
- High-pitched breathing sounds
- Swelling of the head, neck, upper body, or arms
- Trouble swallowing
- Painless swelling of the lymph nodes in the neck, underarm, stomach, or groin
- Painless lump or swelling in a testicle
- Fever for no known reason
- Weight loss for no known reason
- Night sweats

Diagnosis of Childhood Non-Hodgkin Lymphoma

The following tests and procedures may be used:

- **Physical exam and history:** An exam of the body to check general signs of health, including checking for signs of disease, such as lumps or anything else that seems unusual. A history of the patient's health habits and past illnesses and treatments will also be taken.

- **Blood chemistry studies:** A procedure in which a blood sample is checked to measure the amounts of certain substances released into the blood by organs and tissues in the body, including electrolytes, lactate dehydrogenase (LDH), uric acid, blood urea nitrogen (BUN), creatinine, and liver function values. An unusual (higher or lower than normal) amount of a substance can be a sign of disease.

- **Liver function tests:** A procedure in which a blood sample is checked to measure the amounts of certain substances released into the blood by the liver. A higher than normal amount of a substance can be a sign of cancer.

- **Computerized tomography (CT) scan:** A procedure that makes a series of detailed pictures of areas inside the body, taken from different angles. The pictures are made by a computer linked to an x-ray machine. A dye may be injected into a vein or swallowed to help the organs or tissues show up more clearly. This procedure is also called "computed tomography," "computerized tomography," or "computerized axial tomography."

- **Positron emission tomography (PET) scan:** A procedure to find malignant tumor cells in the body. A small amount of radioactive glucose (sugar) is injected into a vein. The PET scanner rotates around the body and makes a picture of where glucose is being used in the body. Malignant tumor cells show up brighter in the picture because they are more active and take up more glucose than normal cells do. Sometimes a PET scan and a CT scan are done at the same time. If there is any cancer, this increases the chance that it will be found.

- **Magnetic resonance imaging (MRI):** A procedure that uses a magnet, radio waves, and a computer to make a series of detailed pictures of areas inside the body. This procedure is also called "nuclear magnetic resonance imaging" (NMRI).

- **Lumbar puncture:** A procedure used to collect cerebrospinal fluid (CSF) from the spinal column. This is done by placing a needle between two bones in the spine and into the CSF around the spinal cord and removing a sample of the fluid. The sample of CSF is checked under a microscope for signs that the cancer has spread to the brain and spinal cord. This procedure is also called an "LP" or "spinal tap."

- **Chest x-ray:** An x-ray of the organs and bones inside the chest. An x-ray is a type of energy beam that can go through the body and onto film, making a picture of areas inside the body.

- **Ultrasound exam:** A procedure in which high-energy sound waves (ultrasound) are bounced off internal tissues or organs and make echoes. The echoes form a picture of body tissues called a "sonogram."

Section 17.4

Neuroblastoma

This section includes text excerpted from "Neuroblastoma Treatment (PDQ®)—Patient Version," National Cancer Institute (NCI), March 28, 2019.

What Is Neuroblastoma?

Neuroblastoma often begins in the nerve tissue of the adrenal glands. There are two adrenal glands, one on top of each kidney in the back of the upper abdomen. The adrenal glands make important hormones that help control heart rate, blood pressure, blood sugar, and the way the body reacts to stress. Neuroblastoma may also begin in nerve tissue in the neck, chest, abdomen or pelvis.

Neuroblastoma most often begins in infancy and may be diagnosed in the first month of life. It is found when the tumor begins to grow and cause signs or symptoms. Sometimes it forms before birth and is found during a fetal ultrasound.

By the time neuroblastoma is diagnosed, the cancer has usually metastasized (spread). Neuroblastoma spreads most often to the lymph nodes, bones, bone marrow, and liver. In infants, it also spreads to the skin.

Gene Mutation and Neuroblastoma

Gene mutations that increase the risk of neuroblastoma are sometimes inherited (passed from the parent to the child). In children with a gene mutation, neuroblastoma usually occurs at a younger age and more than one tumor may form in the adrenal glands.

Children with certain gene mutations and/or hereditary (inherited) syndromes should be checked for signs of neuroblastoma until they are aged 10 years. The following tests and procedures may be used:

- **Abdominal ultrasound:** A procedure in which high-energy sound waves (ultrasound) are bounced off the abdomen and make echoes. The echoes form a picture of the abdomen called a "sonogram."

- **Urine catecholamine studies:** A procedure in which a urine sample is checked to measure the amount of certain substances, vanillylmandelic acid (VMA) and homovanillic acid (HVA), that

341

are made when catecholamines break down and are released into the urine. A higher than normal amount of VMA or HVA can be a sign of neuroblastoma.

- **Chest x-ray:** An x-ray of the organs and bones inside the chest. An x-ray is a type of energy beam that can go through the body and onto film, making a picture of areas inside the body.

Signs and Symptoms of Neuroblastoma

The most common signs and symptoms of neuroblastoma are caused by the tumor pressing on nearby tissues as it grows or by cancer spreading to the bone. These and other signs and symptoms may be caused by neuroblastoma or by other conditions.

Check with your child's doctor if your child has any of the following:

- Lump in the abdomen, neck, or chest
- Bulging eyes
- Dark circles around the eyes ("black eyes")
- Bone pain
- Swollen stomach and trouble breathing (in infants)
- Painless, bluish lumps under the skin (in infants)
- Weakness or paralysis (loss of ability to move a body part)

Less common signs and symptoms of neuroblastoma include the following:

- Fever
- Shortness of breath
- Feeling tired
- Easy bruising or bleeding
- Petechiae (flat, pinpoint spots under the skin caused by bleeding)
- High blood pressure
- Severe watery diarrhea
- Horner syndrome (droopy eyelids, smaller pupil, and less sweating on one side of the face)

- Jerky muscle movements

- Uncontrolled eye movements

Diagnosis of Neuroblastoma

The following tests and procedures may be used:

- **Physical exam and history:** An exam of the body to check general signs of health, including checking for signs of disease, such as lumps or anything else that seems unusual. A history of the patient's health habits and past illnesses and treatments will also be taken.

- **Neurological exam:** A series of questions and tests to check the brain, spinal cord, and nerve function. The exam checks a person's mental status, coordination, and ability to walk normally, and how well the muscles, senses, and reflexes work. This may also be called a "neuro exam" or a "neurologic exam."

- **Urine catecholamine studies:** A procedure in which a urine sample is checked to measure the amount of certain substances, vanillylmandelic acid (VMA) and homovanillic acid (HVA), that are made when catecholamines break down and are released into the urine. A higher than normal amount of VMA or HVA can be a sign of neuroblastoma.

- **Blood chemistry studies:** A procedure in which a blood sample is checked to measure the amounts of certain substances released into the blood by organs and tissues in the body. An unusual (higher or lower than normal) amount of a substance can be a sign of disease.

- **X-ray:** An x-ray is a type of energy beam that can go through the body and onto film, making a picture of areas inside the body.

- **Computerized Tomography (CT) scan:** A procedure that makes a series of detailed pictures of areas inside the body, taken from different angles. The pictures are made by a computer linked to an x-ray machine. A dye may be injected into a vein or swallowed to help the organs or tissues show up more clearly. This procedure is also called "computed tomography," "computerized tomography," or "computerized axial tomography."

- **Magnetic resonance imaging (MRI) with gadolinium:** A procedure that uses a magnet, radio waves, and a computer to make a series of detailed pictures of areas inside the body. A substance called "gadolinium" is injected into a vein. The gadolinium collects around the cancer cells so they show up brighter in the picture. This procedure is also called "nuclear magnetic resonance imaging" (NMRI).

- **Metaiodobenzylguanidine (MIBG) scan:** A procedure used to find neuroendocrine tumors, such as neuroblastoma. A very small amount of a substance called "radioactive MIBG" is injected into a vein and travels through the bloodstream. Neuroendocrine tumor cells take up the radioactive MIBG and are detected by a scanner. Scans may be taken over one to three days. An iodine solution may be given before or during the test to keep the thyroid gland from absorbing too much of the MIBG. This test is also used to find out how well the tumor is responding to treatment. MIBG is used in high doses to treat neuroblastoma.

- **Bone marrow aspiration and biopsy:** The removal of bone marrow, blood, and a small piece of bone by inserting a hollow needle into the hipbone or breastbone. A pathologist views the bone marrow, blood, and bone under a microscope to look for signs of cancer.

- **Ultrasound exam:** A procedure in which high-energy sound waves (ultrasound) are bounced off internal tissues or organs and make echoes. The echoes form a picture of body tissues called a "sonogram." The picture can be printed to be looked at later. An ultrasound exam is not done if a CT/MRI has been done.

Section 17.5

Sarcoma and Bone Tumors

This section includes text excerpted from "Childhood Soft Tissue Sarcoma Treatment (PDQ®)—Patient Version," National Cancer Institute (NCI), June 7, 2019.

What Is Childhood Soft Tissue Sarcoma?

Childhood soft tissue sarcoma is a disease in which malignant (cancer) cells form in soft tissues of the body.

Soft tissues of the body connect, support, and surround other body parts and organs. The soft tissue includes the following:

- Fat
- A mix of bone and cartilage
- Fibrous tissue
- Muscles
- Nerves
- Tendons (bands of tissue that connect muscles to bones)
- Synovial tissues (tissues around joints)
- Blood vessels
- Lymph vessels

Soft tissue sarcoma may be found anywhere in the body. In children, the tumors form most often in the arms, legs, chest, or abdomen.

Soft Tissue Sarcoma in Children and Adults

Soft tissue sarcoma in children may respond differently to treatment, and may have a better prognosis than soft tissue sarcoma in adults.

Risk of Childhood Soft Tissue Sarcoma

Anything that increases your risk of getting a disease is called a risk factor. Having a risk factor does not mean that you will get cancer; not having risk factors does not mean that you will not get cancer. Talk with your child's doctor if you think your child may be at risk.

Risk factors for childhood soft tissue sarcoma include having the following inherited disorders:

- Li-Fraumeni syndrome (LFS)

- Familial adenomatous polyposis (FAP)

- *RB1* gene changes

- *SMARCB1* (INI[1]) gene changes

- Neurofibromatosis type 1 (NF1)

- Werner syndrome

- Tuberous sclerosis

- Adenosine deaminase-deficient severe combined immunodeficiency

Other risk factors include the following:

- Past treatment with radiation therapy

- Having acquired immune deficiency syndrome (AIDS) and Epstein-Barr virus (EBV) infection at the same time

Common Sign of Childhood Soft Tissue Sarcoma

A sarcoma may appear as a painless lump under the skin, often on an arm, a leg, the chest, or the abdomen. There may be no other signs or symptoms at first. As the sarcoma gets bigger and presses on nearby organs, nerves, muscles, or blood vessels, it may cause signs or symptoms, such as pain or weakness.

Other conditions may cause the same signs and symptoms. Check with your child's doctor if your child has any of these problems.

Diagnosis of Childhood Soft Tissue Sarcoma

- **Physical exam and history:** An exam of the body to check general signs of health, including checking for signs of disease, such as lumps or anything else that seems unusual. A history of the patient's health habits and past illnesses and treatments will also be taken.

- **X-rays:** An x-ray is a type of energy beam that can go through the body onto film, making pictures of areas inside the body.

- **Magnetic resonance imaging (MRI):** A procedure that uses a magnet, radio waves, and a computer to make a series of detailed pictures of areas of the body, such as the chest, abdomen, arms, or legs. This procedure is also called "nuclear magnetic resonance imaging (NMRI)."

- **Computed tomography (CAT) scan:** A procedure that makes a series of detailed pictures of areas inside the body, such as the chest or abdomen, taken from different angles. The pictures are made by a computer linked to an x-ray machine. A dye may be injected into a vein or swallowed to help the organs or tissues show up more clearly. This procedure is also called "computed tomography," "computerized tomography," or "computerized axial tomography."

- **Ultrasound exam:** A procedure in which high-energy sound waves (ultrasound) are bounced off internal tissues or organs and make echoes. The echoes form a picture of body tissues called a "sonogram."

Treatment of Childhood Soft Tissue Sarcoma

The type of biopsy depends, in part, on the size of the mass and whether it is close to the surface of the skin or deeper in the tissue. One of the following types of biopsies is usually used:

- **Core needle biopsy:** The removal of tissue using a wide needle. Multiple tissue samples are taken. This procedure may be guided using ultrasound, CT scan, or MRI.

- **Incisional biopsy:** The removal of part of a lump or a sample of tissue.

- **Excisional biopsy:** The removal of an entire lump or area of tissue that does not look normal. A pathologist views the tissue under a microscope to look for cancer cells. An excisional biopsy may be used to completely remove smaller tumors that are near the surface of the skin. This type of biopsy is rarely used because cancer cells may remain after the biopsy. If cancer cells remain, the cancer may come back or it may spread to other parts of the body.

Types of Soft Tissue Sarcomas

The cells of each type of sarcoma look different under a microscope. The soft tissue tumors are grouped based on the type of soft tissue cell where they first formed.

347

Fat Tissue Tumors

Liposarcoma. This is a cancer of the fat cells. Liposarcoma usually forms in the fat layer just under the skin. In children and adolescents, liposarcoma is often low grade (likely to grow and spread slowly). There are several different types of liposarcoma, including:

- **Myxoid liposarcoma.** This is usually a low-grade cancer that responds well to treatment.

- **Pleomorphic liposarcoma.** This is usually a high-grade cancer that is less likely to respond well to treatment.

Bone and Cartilage Tumors

Bone and cartilage tumors are a mix of bone cells and cartilage cells. Bone and cartilage tumors include the following types:

- **Extraskeletal mesenchymal chondrosarcoma.** This type of bone and cartilage tumor often affects young adults and occurs in the head and neck.

- **Extraskeletal osteosarcoma.** This type of bone and cartilage tumor is very rare in children and adolescents. It is likely to come back after treatment and may spread to the lungs.

Prognosis of Sarcoma and Bone Tumors

The prognosis (chance of recovery) and treatment options depend on the following:

- The part of the body where the tumor first formed

- The size and grade of the tumor

- The type of soft tissue sarcoma

- How deep the tumor is under the skin

- Whether the tumor has spread to other places in the body and where it has spread

- The amount of tumor remaining after surgery to remove it

- Whether radiation therapy was used to treat the tumor

- Whether cancer has just been diagnosed or has recurred (come back)

Section 17.6

Wilms Tumor and Other Childhood Kidney Tumors

This section includes text excerpted from "Wilms Tumor and Other Childhood Kidney Tumors Treatment (PDQ®)—Patient Version (Nephroblastoma)," National Cancer Institute (NCI), May 22, 2019.

What Are Childhood Kidney Tumors?

There are two kidneys, one on each side of the backbone, above the waist. Tiny tubules in the kidneys filter and clean the blood. They take out waste products and make urine. The urine passes from each kidney through a long tube called a ureter into the bladder. The bladder holds the urine until it passes through the urethra and leaves the body.

Types of Childhood Kidney Tumors
Wilms Tumor

In Wilms tumor (WT), one or more tumors may be found in one or both kidneys. Wilms tumor may spread to the lungs, liver, bone, brain, or nearby lymph nodes. In children and adolescents younger than 15 years old, most kidney cancers are Wilms tumors.

Renal Cell Cancer

Renal cell cancer (RCC) is rare in children and adolescents younger than 15 years old. It is much more common in adolescents between 15 and 19 years old. Children and adolescents are more likely to be diagnosed with a large renal cell tumor or cancer that has spread. Renal cell cancers may spread to the lungs, liver, or lymph nodes. Renal cell cancer may also be called "renal cell carcinoma."

Rhabdoid Tumor of the Kidney

Rhabdoid tumor (RT) of the kidney is a type of kidney cancer that occurs mostly in infants and young children. It is often advanced at the time of diagnosis. Rhabdoid tumor of the kidney grows and spreads quickly, often to the lungs or brain.

Children with a certain change in the *SMARCB1* gene are checked regularly to see if a rhabdoid tumor has formed in the kidney or has spread to the brain:

- Children younger than one-year-old have an ultrasound of the abdomen every two to three months and an ultrasound of the head every month.

- Children one to four years old have an ultrasound of the abdomen and a magnetic resonance imaging (MRI) of the brain and spine every three months.

Clear Cell Sarcoma of the Kidney

Clear cell sarcoma (CCS) of the kidney is a type of kidney tumor that may spread to the lung, bone, brain, or soft tissue. It may recur (come back) up to 14 years after treatment, and it often recurs in the brain or lungs.

Congenital Mesoblastic Nephroma

Congenital mesoblastic nephroma (CMN) is a tumor of the kidney that is often diagnosed during the first year of life. It can usually be cured.

Ewing Sarcoma of the Kidney

Ewing sarcoma (previously called "neuroepithelial tumor") of the kidney is rare and usually occurs in young adults. These tumors grow and spread to other parts of the body quickly.

Primary Renal Myoepithelial Carcinoma

Primary renal myoepithelial carcinoma is a rare type of cancer that usually affects soft tissues, but sometimes forms in the internal organs (such as the kidney). This type of cancer grows and spreads quickly.

Cystic Partially Differentiated Nephroblastoma

Cystic partially differentiated nephroblastoma (CPDN) is a very rare type of Wilms tumor made up of cysts.

Multilocular Cystic Nephroma

Multilocular cystic nephroma are benign tumors made up of cysts and are most common in infants, young children, and adult women. These tumors can occur in one or both kidneys.

Children with this type of tumor also may have pleuropulmonary blastoma (PPB), so imaging tests that check the lungs for cysts or solid tumors are done. Since multilocular cystic nephroma may be an inherited condition, genetic counseling and genetic testing may be considered.

Primary Renal Synovial Sarcoma

Primary renal synovial sarcoma is a cyst-like tumor of the kidney and is most common in young adults. These tumors grow and spread quickly.

Anaplastic Sarcoma of the Kidney

Anaplastic sarcoma of the kidney is a rare tumor that is most common in children or adolescents younger than 15 years of age. Anaplastic sarcoma of the kidney often spreads to the lungs, liver, or bones. Imaging tests that check the lungs for cysts or solid tumors may be done. Since anaplastic sarcoma may be an inherited condition, genetic counseling and genetic testing may be considered.

Nephroblastomatosis Is Not Cancer but May Become Wilms Tumor

Sometimes, after the kidneys form in the fetus, abnormal groups of kidney cells remain in one or both kidneys. In nephroblastomatosis (diffuse hyperplastic perilobar nephroblastomatosis (HPLN), these abnormal groups of cells may grow in many places inside the kidney or make a thick layer around the kidney. When these groups of abnormal cells are found in a kidney after it was removed for Wilms tumor, the child has an increased risk of Wilms tumor in the other kidney. Frequent follow-up testing is important at least every three months, for at least seven years after the child is treated.

Having Certain Genetic Syndromes or Other Conditions Can Increase the Risk of Wilms Tumor

Anything that increases the risk of getting a disease is called a risk factor. Having a risk factor does not mean that you will get cancer; not having risk factors does not mean that you will not get cancer. Talk to your child's doctor if you think your child may be at risk.

Wilms tumor may be part of a genetic syndrome that affects growth or development. A genetic syndrome is a set of signs and symptoms or conditions that occur together and is caused by certain changes in the genes. Certain conditions can also increase a child's risk of developing Wilms tumor. These and other genetic syndromes and conditions have been linked to Wilms tumor:

- Wilms tumor, aniridia, abnormal genitourinary system, and mental retardation syndrome (WAGR)

- Denys-Drash syndrome (DDS) (abnormal genitourinary system)

- Frasier syndrome (abnormal genitourinary system)

- Beckwith-Wiedemann syndrome (BWS) (abnormally large growth of one side of the body or a body part, large tongue, umbilical hernia at birth, and abnormal genitourinary system)

- A family history of Wilms tumor

- Aniridia (the iris, the colored part of the eye, is missing)

- Isolated hemihyperplasia (abnormally large growth of one side of the body or a body part)

- Urinary-tract problems such as cryptorchidism or hypospadias

Screening of Wilms Tumor

Screening tests are done in children with an increased risk of Wilms tumor. These tests may help find cancer early and decrease the chance of dying from cancer.

In general, children with an increased risk of Wilms tumor should be screened for Wilms tumor every three months until they are at least eight years old. An ultrasound test of the abdomen is usually used for screening. Small Wilms tumors may be found and removed before symptoms occur.

Children with BWS or hemihyperplasia are also screened for liver and adrenal tumors that are linked to these genetic syndromes. A test to check the alpha-fetoprotein (AFP) level in the blood and an ultrasound of the abdomen are done until the child is four years old. An ultrasound of the kidneys is done between the ages of four and seven years old. A physical exam by a specialist (geneticist or pediatric oncologist) is done two times each year. In children with certain gene changes, a different schedule for an ultrasound of the abdomen may be used.

Children with aniridia and a certain gene change are screened for Wilms tumor every three months until they are eight years old. An ultrasound test of the abdomen is used for screening.

Some children develop Wilms tumor in both kidneys. These often appear when Wilms tumor is first diagnosed, but WT may also occur in the second kidney after the child is successfully treated for WT in one kidney. Children with an increased risk of a second WT in the other kidney should be screened for WT every three months for up to eight years. An ultrasound test of the abdomen may be used for screening.

Having Certain Conditions May Increase the Risk of Renal Cell Cancer

Renal cell cancer may be related to the following conditions:

- Von Hippel-Lindau disease (VHL) (an inherited condition that causes abnormal growth of blood vessels). Children with Von Hippel-Lindau disease should be checked yearly for renal cell cancer with an ultrasound of the abdomen or an MRI beginning at age 8 to 11 years.

- Tuberous sclerosis (TSC) (an inherited disease marked by noncancerous fatty cysts in the kidney)

- Familial renal cell cancer (an inherited condition that occurs when certain changes in the genes that cause kidney cancer are passed down from the parent to the child)

- Renal medullary cancer (RMC) (a rare kidney cancer that grows and spreads quickly)

- Hereditary leiomyomatosis (an inherited disorder that increases the risk of having cancer of the kidney, skin, and uterus)

Prior chemotherapy or radiation therapy for childhood cancer, such as neuroblastoma, soft tissue sarcoma, leukemia, or Wilms tumor may also increase the risk of renal cell cancer.

Wilms Tumor and Other Childhood Kidney Tumors and Genetic Counseling

Genetic counseling (a discussion with a trained professional about genetic diseases and whether genetic testing is needed) may be needed if the child has one of the following syndromes or conditions:

- A genetic syndrome or condition that increases the risk of Wilms tumor

- An inherited condition that increases the risk of renal cell cancer

- Rhabdoid tumor of the kidney

- Multilocular cystic nephroma (MLCN)

Signs of Wilms Tumor and Other Childhood Kidney Tumors

Sometimes childhood kidney tumors do not cause signs and symptoms and the parent finds a mass in the abdomen by chance or the mass is found during a well-child health check-up. These and other signs and symptoms may be caused by kidney tumors or by other conditions. Check with your child's doctor if your child has any of the following:

- A lump, swelling, or pain in the abdomen

- Blood in the urine

- High blood pressure (headache, feeling very tired, chest pain, or trouble seeing or breathing)

- Hypercalcemia (loss of appetite, nausea, and vomiting, weakness, or feeling very tired)

- Fever for no known reason

- Loss of appetite

- Weight loss for no known reason

Wilms tumor that has spread to the lungs or liver may cause the following signs and symptoms:

- Cough

- Blood in the sputum

- Trouble breathing

- Pain in the abdomen

Chapter 18

Cardiovascular Disorders in Children

Chapter Contents

Section 18.1

Congenital Heart Defects

This section includes text excerpted from "What Are
Congenital Heart Defects?" Centers for Disease Control
and Prevention (CDC), November 2, 2018.

Congenital heart defects (CHDs) are the most common type of birth
defect. As medical care and treatment have advanced, babies with
CHDs are living longer and healthier lives.

What Are Congenital Heart Defects?

Congenital heart defects are present at birth and can affect the
structure of a baby's heart and the way it works. They can affect how
blood flows through the heart and out to the rest of the body. CHDs
can vary from mild (such as a small hole in the heart) to severe (such
as missing or poorly formed parts of the heart).

About one in four babies born with a heart defect has a critical
CHD (also known as "critical congenital heart disease"). Babies with a
critical CHD need surgery or other procedures in the first year of life.

Types of Congenital Heart Defects

Listed below are examples of different types of CHDs. The types
marked with a star (*) are considered critical CHDs.

- Atrial septal defect (ASD)

- Atrioventricular septal defect (AVSD)

- Coarctation of the aorta (CoA or CoAo)*

- Double-outlet right ventricle (DORV)*

- Dextro-transposition of the great arteries (DTGA)*

- Ebstein anomaly*

- Hypoplastic left heart syndrome (HLHS)*

- Interrupted aortic arch (IAA)*

- Pulmonary atresia (PA)*

- Single ventricle*

- Tetralogy of Fallot (TOF)*

- Total anomalous pulmonary venous return (TAPVR)*
- Tricuspid atresia*
- Truncus arteriosus (TA)*
- Ventricular septal defect (VSD)

Signs and Symptoms of Congenital Heart Defects

Signs and symptoms for CHDs depend on the type and severity of the particular defect. Some defects might have few or no signs or symptoms. Others might cause a baby to have the following symptoms:

- Blue-tinted nails or lips
- Fast or troubled breathing
- Tiredness when feeding
- Sleepiness

Diagnosis of Congenital Heart Defects

Some CHDs may be diagnosed during pregnancy using a special type of ultrasound called a "fetal echocardiogram," which creates ultrasound pictures of the heart of the developing baby. However, some CHDs are not detected until after birth or later in life, during childhood or adulthood. If a healthcare provider suspects a CHD may be present, the baby can get several tests (such as an echocardiogram) to confirm the diagnosis.

Treatment of Congenital Heart Defects

Treatment for CHDs depends on the type and severity of the defect present. Some affected infants and children might need one or more surgeries to repair the heart or blood vessels. Some can be treated without surgery using a procedure called "cardiac catheterization." A long tube, called a "catheter," is threaded through the blood vessels into the heart, where a doctor can take measurements and pictures, do tests, or repair the problem. Sometimes the heart defect cannot be fully repaired, but these procedures can improve blood flow and the way the heart works. It is important to note that even if their heart defect has been repaired, many children with CHDs are not cured.

Causes of Congenital Heart Defects

The causes of CHDs among most babies are unknown. Some babies have heart defects because of changes in their individual genes or chromosomes. CHDs also are thought to be caused by a combination of genes and other factors, such as things in the environment, the mother's diet, the mother's health conditions, or the mother's medication use during pregnancy. For example, certain conditions a mother has such as pre-existing diabetes or obesity, have been linked to heart defects in the baby. Smoking during pregnancy as well as taking certain medications has also been linked to heart defects.

Living with Congenital Heart Defects

As medical care and treatments have advanced, infants with CHDs are living longer and healthier lives. Many children with CHDs are now living into adulthood. It is estimated that more than 2 million individuals in the United States are living with a CHD. Even with improved treatments, many children with CHDs are not cured, even if their heart defect has been repaired. Children with a CHD can develop other health problems over time, depending on their specific heart defect, the number of heart defects they have, and the severity of their heart defect. For example, some other health problems that might develop include irregular heartbeat (arrhythmias), increased risk of infection in the heart muscle (infective endocarditis), or weakness in the heart (cardiomyopathy).

Children with CHDs need routine checkups with a cardiologist (heart doctor) to stay as healthy as possible. They also might need further operations after initial childhood surgeries. It is important for parents of children with CHDs to visit their child's doctor on a regular basis and discuss their child's health, including their specific heart condition.

Section 18.2

Arrhythmia

This section includes text excerpted from "Arrhythmia," National
Heart, Lung, and Blood Institute (NHLBI), March 15, 2019.

What Is Arrhythmia?

An arrhythmia (also known as "dysrhythmia") is a problem with the
rate or rhythm of the heartbeat. During an arrhythmia, the heart can
beat too fast, too slowly, or with an irregular rhythm. When a heart
beats too fast, the condition is called "tachycardia." When a heart beats
too slowly, the condition is called "bradycardia."

Arrhythmia is caused by changes in heart tissue and activity or in
the electrical signals that control a person's heartbeat. These changes
can be caused by damage from disease, injury, or genetics. Often there
are no symptoms, but some people feel an irregular heartbeat. One
may feel faint or dizzy or have difficulty breathing.

The most common test used to diagnose an arrhythmia is an electrocardiogram (EKG or ECG). Your child's doctor will run other tests
as needed and may recommend medicines, placement of a device that
can correct an irregular heartbeat or surgery to repair nerves that are
overstimulating the heart. If an arrhythmia is left untreated, the heart
may not be able to pump enough blood to the body. This can damage
the heart, the brain, or other organs.

Types of Arrhythmias

Arrhythmias differ from normal heartbeats in speed or rhythm.
Arrhythmias are also grouped by where they occur—in the upper
chambers of the heart, in its lower chambers, or between the chambers. The main types of arrhythmias are bradyarrhythmias; premature, or extra, beats; supraventricular arrhythmias; and ventricular
arrhythmias.

Bradyarrhythmia

Bradyarrhythmia is a slow heart rate—also called "bradycardia."
People who are young or physically fit may normally have slow heart
rates. A doctor can determine whether a slow heart rate is appropriate
for a person.

Premature or Extra Heartbeat

A premature heartbeat happens when the signal to beat comes early. It can feel like a person's heart skipped a beat. The premature, or extra, heartbeat creates a short pause, which is followed by a stronger beat when a person's heart returns to its regular rhythm. These extra heartbeats are the most common type of arrhythmia. They are called "ectopic heartbeats" and can trigger other arrhythmias.

Supraventricular Arrhythmia

Arrhythmias that start in the heart's upper chambers called the "atrium," or at the gateway to the lower chambers are called "supraventricular arrhythmias." Supraventricular arrhythmias are known by their fast heart rates or tachycardia. Tachycardia occurs when the heart, at rest, goes above 100 beats per minute. The fast pace is sometimes paired with uneven heart rhythm. Sometimes the upper and lower chambers beat at different rates.

Types of supraventricular arrhythmias include:

- **Atrial fibrillation (AF).** This is one of the most common types of arrhythmia. The heart can race at more than 400 beats per minute.

- **Atrial flutter.** Atrial flutter can cause the upper chambers to beat 250 to 350 times per minute. The signal that tells the upper chambers to beat may be disrupted when it encounters damaged tissue, such as a scar. The signal may find an alternate path, creating a loop that causes the upper chamber to beat repeatedly. As with atrial fibrillation, some but not all of these signals travel to the lower chambers. As a result, the upper chambers and lower chambers beat at different rates.

- **Paroxysmal supraventricular tachycardia (PSVT).** In PSVT, electrical signals that begin in the upper chambers and travel to the lower chambers cause extra heartbeats. This arrhythmia begins and ends suddenly. It can happen during vigorous physical activity. It is usually not dangerous and tends to occur in young people.

Ventricular Arrhythmia

These arrhythmias start in the heart's lower chambers. They can be very dangerous and usually require medical care right away.

- **Ventricular tachycardia** is a fast, regular beating of the ventricles that may last for only a few seconds or for much longer. A few beats of ventricular tachycardia often do not cause problems. However, episodes that last for more than a few seconds can be dangerous. Ventricular tachycardia can turn into other more serious arrhythmias, such as ventricular fibrillation, or v-fib. Torsades de pointes is a type of arrhythmia that causes a unique pattern on an EKG and often leads to v-fib.

- **Ventricular fibrillation** occurs if disorganized electrical signals make the ventricles quiver instead of pumping normally. Without the ventricles pumping blood to the body, sudden cardiac arrest and death can occur within a few minutes.

Causes of Arrhythmia

Arrhythmia is caused by changes to heart tissue. It can also occur suddenly as a result of exertion or stress, imbalances in the blood, medicines, or problems with electrical signals in the heart. Typically, an arrhythmia is set off by a trigger, and the irregular heartbeat can continue if there is a problem in the heart. Sometimes the cause of an arrhythmia is unknown.

Changes to the Heart

The following conditions may cause arrhythmia:

- Changes to the heart's anatomy

- Reduced blood flow to the heart or damage to the heart's electrical system

- Restoring blood flow as part of treating a heart attack

- Stiffening of the heart tissue, known as "fibrosis," or "scarring"

Exertion or Strain

Strong emotional stress, anxiety, anger, pain, or a sudden surprise can make the heart work harder, raise blood pressure, and release stress hormones. Sometimes these reactions can lead to arrhythmias. If your child has heart disease, physical activity can trigger arrhythmia due to an excess of hormones, such as adrenaline. Sometimes vomiting or coughing can trigger arrhythmia.

Imbalances in the Blood

An excess or deficiency of electrolytes, hormones, or fluids can alter a person's heartbeat.

- An excess of thyroid hormone can cause the heart to beat faster, and thyroid deficiency can slow a person's heart rate.

- Dehydration can cause the heart to race.

- Low blood sugar, from an eating disorder or insulin doses that are too high in someone who has diabetes, can lead to slow or extra heartbeats.

- Low levels of potassium, magnesium, or calcium can trigger arrhythmia. These electrolyte disturbances can occur after a heart attack or surgery.

Medicines

Certain medicines can cause arrhythmia. These include medicines to treat high blood pressure and other conditions, including arrhythmia, depression, and psychosis. Parents need to be careful while giving certain antibiotics and over-the-counter (OTC) medicines, such as allergy and cold medicines to their children.

Problems with the Electrical Signals in the Heart

An arrhythmia can occur if the electrical signals that control the heartbeat are delayed or blocked. This can happen when the nerve cells that produce electrical signals do not work properly or when the electrical signals do not travel normally through the heart. Another part of the heart could start to produce electrical signals, disrupting a normal heartbeat.

Disorders of electrical signaling in the heart are called "conduction disorders."

Risk Factors of Arrhythmia

A person may have an increased risk of arrhythmia because of her or his age, environment, family history and genetics, habits in one's daily life, certain medical conditions, race or ethnicity, sex, or surgery.

Age

The chances of having arrhythmia grow as a person ages, in part because of changes in heart tissue and in how the heart works overtime.

Some types of arrhythmia happen more often in children and young adults, including arrhythmias due to congenital heart defects (CHDs) or inherited conduction disorders.

Environment

Some research suggests that exposure to air pollutants, especially particulates and gases, is linked to short-term risk of arrhythmia.

Family History and Genetics

A child may have an increased risk of some types of arrhythmia if her or his parent or other close relative has had an arrhythmia, too. Also, some inherited types of heart disease can raise the risk of arrhythmia. With some conduction disorders, gene mutations cause the ion channels that transmit signals through heart cells to work incorrectly or stop working.

Screening and Prevention of Arrhythmia

If your child is at increased risk of arrhythmia, your child's doctor may want to do a screening to assess the risk of a life-threatening event. Sometimes screening is required to participate in competitive sports. If your child carries a genetic risk of arrhythmia, your child's doctor may recommend regular screening to monitor your child's heart or other family members' health. The doctor may also ask about risk factors and may suggest genetic testing if your child, parent, or other family member has a known or suspected arrhythmia or other heart condition. Heart-healthy lifestyle changes and other precautions can help decrease the risk of triggering arrhythmia.

Screening Tests

Your child's doctor may recommend screening tests based on her or his risk factors, such as age or family history.

An **electrocardiogram (EKG or ECG)** is the main test for detecting arrhythmia. An EKG records the heart's electrical activity. Your child's doctor may do the test while she or he is at rest or may do a stress test, which records the heart's activity when it is working hard. Your child's doctor may also give her or him a portable monitor to wear for a day or several days if no arrhythmia was detected during testing in the clinic. If you have a child who is at risk of arrhythmia because of a genetic condition, the doctor may recommend regular testing for your child and her or his siblings.

Genetic testing is especially important if your newborn or another close relative died suddenly and had a genetic risk. Your child's doctor may also suggest genetic testing if your child has a history of fainting or has survived a near-drowning.

Imaging tests, such as cardiac magnetic resonance imaging (MRI), can help detect scarring or other problems that can increase your child's risk of arrhythmia.

Prevention Strategies

Learn about prevention strategies that your child's doctor may recommend, including:

- Avoiding triggers, such as caffeine or stimulant medicines, can cause arrhythmias or make them worse.

- Getting an implantable or wearable cardioverter defibrillator to prevent sudden cardiac arrest from arrhythmia if your child has heart disease. Defibrillators can correct arrhythmias by sending an electric shock to the heart.

- Making heart-healthy lifestyle changes, such as heart-healthy eating, being physically active, aiming for a healthy weight, and managing stress.

- Monitoring your child after surgery, if she or he is having heart surgery. The surgical team may also use medicine and maintain or supplement electrolyte levels during or after the procedure to prevent arrhythmia.

If you are the parents of a child with an inherited condition that increases the risk of arrhythmia, discuss prevention strategies with your pediatrician as part of your child's care.

- If your child is a newborn, follow safe sleep recommendations to help reduce the risk of sudden infant death syndrome (SIDS).

- Your doctor may recommend routine assessments of your child's heart activity to detect patterns or symptoms of arrhythmia that emerge over time.

Signs, Symptoms, and Complications of Arrhythmia

An arrhythmia may not cause any obvious signs or symptoms. Your child may notice something that occurs only occasionally, or her or his symptoms may become more frequent over time. Keep track of when and how often arrhythmia occurs, what your child feels, and whether these things change over time. They are all important clues your child's doctor can use. If left untreated, arrhythmia can lead to life-threatening complications, such as stroke, heart failure, or sudden cardiac arrest.

Signs and Symptoms of Arrhythmia

Your child may be able to feel a slow or irregular heartbeat or notice pauses between heartbeats. If your child has palpitations, she or he may feel like her or his heart skipped a beat or may notice it pounding or racing. These are all symptoms of arrhythmia.

More serious signs and symptoms include:

- Anxiety
- Blurred vision
- Chest pain
- Difficulty breathing
- Fainting or nearly fainting
- Foggy thinking
- Fatigue
- Sweating
- Weakness, dizziness, and light-headedness

What Else Will Your Child's Doctor Want to Know about Her or His Symptoms?

Some arrhythmias tend to happen at certain times or under certain circumstances. If you notice signs or symptoms of arrhythmia in your children, note when they happened and what they were doing. This information can help your child's doctor diagnose what is going on and find the right treatment. Here are questions to ask yourself.

- Did it happen at night?

- Did your child stand up after sitting or lying down?

- Was your child lying down?

- Was your child playing a sport or otherwise exerting herself or himself?

- Was your child swimming or diving?

Complications of Arrhythmia

Arrhythmias that are unrecognized or left untreated can cause sometimes life-threatening complications affecting the heart and brain.

- **Heart failure.** Repeat arrhythmias can lead to a rapid decline in the ability of the lower chambers to pump blood. Heart failure is especially likely to develop or to grow worse as a result of arrhythmia when a person already has heart disease.

- **Stroke.** This can occur in some people who have atrial fibrillation. With an arrhythmia, blood can pool in the atria, causing blood clots to form. If a clot breaks off and travels to the brain, it can cause a stroke.

- **Sudden cardiac arrest.** The heart may suddenly and unexpectedly stop beating as a result of ventricular fibrillation.

- **Sudden infant death syndrome (SIDS).** SIDS can be attributed to an inherited conduction disorder that causes arrhythmia.

- **Worsening arrhythmia.** Some arrhythmias trigger another type of arrhythmia or get worse over time.

Diagnosis of Arrhythmia

To diagnose an arrhythmia, your child's doctor will ask you about your child's symptoms, her or his medical history, and any signs of arrhythmia in your family. Your child's doctor may also do an EKG and a physical exam as part of the diagnosis. Additional tests may be necessary to rule out another cause or to help your child's doctor decide on treatment.

Medical History

To diagnose an arrhythmia, your child's doctor will ask about your child's eating and physical activity habits, family history, and other risk factors for arrhythmia. Your child's doctor may ask whether your child has any other signs or symptoms. This information can help the doctor determine whether your child has complications or other conditions that may be causing her or him to have an arrhythmia.

Physical Exam

During a physical exam, your child's doctor may take these steps:

- Check for swelling in your child's legs or feet, which could be a sign of an enlarged heart or heart failure
- Check your child's pulse to find out how fast her or his heart is beating
- Listen to the rate and rhythm of your child's heartbeat
- Listen to your child's heart for a heart murmur
- Look for signs of other diseases, such as thyroid disease, that could be causing the arrhythmia

Diagnostic Tests and Procedures

Your doctor may order some of the following tests to diagnose arrhythmia:

- **Blood tests** to check the level of certain substances in the blood, such as potassium and thyroid hormone, that can increase your child's risk of arrhythmia.
- **Cardiac catheterization** to see whether your child has complications from heart disease.
- **Chest x-ray** to show whether your child's heart is larger than normal.
- **Echocardiography (echo)** to provide information about the size and shape of your child's heart and how well it is working. Echocardiography may also be used to diagnose fetal arrhythmia in the womb.
- **EKG, or ECG,** to see how fast the heart is beating and whether its rhythm is steady or irregular. This is the most common test used to diagnose arrhythmias.
- **Electrophysiology study (EPS)** to look at the electrical activity of the heart. The study uses a wire to electrically

stimulate a person's heart and trigger an arrhythmia. If your child's doctor has already detected another condition that raises your child's risk, an EPS can help assess the possibility that an arrhythmia will develop. An EPS also allows your child's doctor to see whether a treatment, such as medicine, will stop the problem.

- **Holter or event monitor** to record your child's heart's electrical activity over long periods of time while your child does her or his normal activities.

- **Implantable loop recorder** to detect abnormal heart rhythms. It is placed under the skin and continuously records your child's heart's electrical activity. The recorder can transmit data to the doctor's office to help with monitoring. An implantable loop recorder helps doctors figure out why a person may be having palpitations or fainting spells, especially if these symptoms do not happen very often.

- **Sleep study** to see whether sleep apnea is causing your child's arrhythmia.

- **Stress test or exercise stress test** to detect arrhythmias that happen while the heart is working hard and beating fast. If your child cannot exercise, she or he may be given medicine to make her or his heart work hard and beat fast.

- **Tilt table testing** to help find the cause of fainting spells. Your child lies on a table that moves from a lying-down position to an upright position. The change in position may cause your child to faint. Your child's doctor watches her or his symptoms, heart rate, EKG reading, and blood pressure throughout the test.

- **Ultrasound** to diagnose a suspected fetal arrhythmia in the womb.

Treatment of Arrhythmia

Common arrhythmia treatments include heart-healthy lifestyle changes, medicines, surgically implanted devices that control the heartbeat, and other procedures that treat abnormal electrical signals in the heart.

Medicines

Your child's doctor may give medicine to your child's arrhythmia. Some medicines are used in combination with each other or together with a procedure or a pacemaker. If the dose is too high, medicines to treat arrhythmia can cause an irregular rhythm.

- **Adenosine** to slow a racing heart. Adenosine acts quickly to slow electrical signals. It can cause some chest pain, flushing, and shortness of breath, but any discomfort typically passes soon.

- **Atropine** to treat a slow heart rate. This medicine may cause difficulty swallowing.

- **Beta-blockers** to treat high blood pressure or a fast heart rate or to prevent repeat episodes of arrhythmia. Beta-blockers can cause digestive trouble, sleep problems, and can make some conduction disorders worse.

- **Blood thinners** to reduce the risk of blood clots forming. This helps prevent stroke. With blood-thinning medicines, there is a risk of bleeding.

- **Calcium channel blockers** to slow a rapid heart rate or the speed at which signals travel. Typically, they are used to control arrhythmias of the upper chambers. In some cases, calcium channel blockers can trigger ventricular fibrillation. They can also cause digestive trouble, swollen feet, or low blood pressure.

- **Digitalis, or digoxin**, to treat a fast heart rate. This medicine can cause nausea and may trigger arrhythmias.

- **Potassium channel blockers** to slow the heart rate. They work by lengthening the time it takes for heart cells to recover after firing so that they do not fire and squeeze as often. Potassium channel blockers can cause low blood pressure or another arrhythmia.

- **Sodium channel blockers** to block transmission of electrical signals, lengthen cell recovery periods, and make cells less excitable. However, these drugs can increase risk of sudden cardiac arrest in people who have heart disease.

Procedures

If medicines do not treat your child's arrhythmia, your child's doctor may recommend one of these procedures or devices.

- Cardioversion
- Catheter ablation

- Implantable cardioverter defibrillators (ICDs)

- Pacemakers

Living with Arrhythmia

If your child has been diagnosed and treated for arrhythmia, make sure their treatment plan is followed. Your ongoing care may focus on reducing the chance that your child will have another episode or a complication. Keep your regular appointments with your child's doctor. Ask about heart-healthy lifestyle changes that your child can follow to keep their arrhythmia from happening again or getting worse.

Section 18.3

Heart Murmurs

This section includes text excerpted from "Heart Murmur," National Heart, Lung, and Blood Institute (NHLBI), December 12, 2016. Reviewed September 2019.

What Is Heart Murmur?

A heart murmur is an unusual sound heard between heartbeats. Murmurs sometimes sound like a whooshing or swishing noise.

Types of Heart Murmur

Murmurs may be harmless, also called "innocent," or "abnormal."

- **Harmless murmurs** may not cause symptoms and can happen when blood flows more rapidly than normal through the heart, such as during exercise, pregnancy, or rapid growth in children.

- **Abnormal murmurs** may be a sign of a more serious heart condition, such as a congenital heart defect that is present since birth or heart valve disease. Depending on the heart problem causing the abnormal murmurs, the murmurs may be associated with other symptoms, such as shortness of breath, dizziness or fainting, bluish skin, or a chronic cough.

What the Doctor Does upon Diagnosing Heart Murmur

If a heart murmur is detected, your child's doctor will listen to the loudness, location, and timing of your child's murmur to find out whether it is harmless or a sign of a more serious condition. If your child's doctor thinks your child may have a more serious condition, she or he may refer your child to a cardiologist, or a doctor who specializes in the heart.

Treatment of Heart Murmur

A heart murmur itself does not require treatment. If it is caused by a more serious heart condition, your child's doctor may recommend treatment for that heart condition. Treatment may include medicines, cardiac catheterization, or surgery. The outlook and treatment for abnormal heart murmurs depend on the type and severity of the heart condition that is causing the murmur.

Section 18.4

Hyperlipidemia

This section includes text excerpted from "High Cholesterol in Children and Teens," MedlinePlus, National Institutes of Health (NIH), March 29, 2018.

What Is Cholesterol?

Cholesterol is a waxy, fat-like substance that is found in all the cells in the body. The liver makes cholesterol, and it is also in some foods, such as meat and dairy products. The body needs some cholesterol to work properly. But, if your child or teen has high cholesterol (too much cholesterol in the blood), she or he has a higher risk of coronary artery disease and other heart diseases.

What Causes High Cholesterol in Children and Teens

Three main factors contribute to high cholesterol in children and teens:

- An unhealthy diet, especially one that is high in fats

- A family history of high cholesterol, especially when one or both parents have high cholesterol

- Obesity

Some diseases, such as diabetes, kidney disease, and certain thyroid diseases, can also cause high cholesterol in children and teens.

What Are the Symptoms of High Cholesterol in Children and Teens

There are usually no signs or symptoms that your child or teen has high cholesterol.

How Do You Know If Your Child or Teen Has High Cholesterol?

There is a blood test to measure cholesterol levels. The test gives information about:

- **Total cholesterol**—a measure of the total amount of cholesterol in a person's blood. It includes both low-density lipoprotein (LDL) cholesterol and high-density lipoprotein (HDL) cholesterol.

- **Low-density lipoprotein (bad) cholesterol**—the main source of cholesterol buildup and blockage in the arteries

- **High-density lipoprotein (good) cholesterol**—HDL helps remove cholesterol from your arteries

- **Non-HDL**—this number is a person's total cholesterol minus HDL. A person's non-HDL includes LDL and other types of cholesterol such as very-low-density lipoprotein (VLDL).

- **Triglycerides**—another form of fat in a person's blood that can raise the risk for heart disease

For anyone aged 19 or younger, the healthy levels of cholesterol are

Table 18.1. Healthy Levels of Cholesterol

Type of Cholesterol	Healthy Level
Total Cholesterol	Less than 170mg/dL
Non-HDL	Less than 120mg/dL
LDL	Less than 100mg/dL
HDL	More than 45mg/dL

The first test should be between ages 9 to 11When and how often your child or teen should get this test depends on her or his age, risk factors, and family history. The general recommendations are:

- Children should have the test again every five years

- Some children may have this test starting at age two if there is a family history of high blood cholesterol, heart attack, or stroke

What Are the Treatments for High Cholesterol in Children and Teens?

Lifestyle changes are the primary treatment for high cholesterol in children and teens. These changes include:

- **Being more active.** This includes getting regular exercise and spending less time sitting (in front of a television, at a computer, on a phone or tablet, etc.)

- **Healthy eating.** A diet to lower cholesterol includes limiting foods that are high in saturated fat, sugar, and trans fat. It is also essential to eat plenty of fresh fruits, vegetables, and whole grains.

- **Losing weight,** if your child or teen is overweight or has obesity

If everyone in the family makes these changes, it will be easier for your child or teen to stick to them.

Sometimes these lifestyle changes are not enough to lower your child or teen's cholesterol. Your healthcare provider may consider giving your child or teen cholesterol medicines if she or he:

- Is at least 10 years old

- Has an LDL (bad) cholesterol level that is higher than 190 mg/dL, even after six months of diet and exercise changes

- Has an LDL (bad) cholesterol level that is higher than 160 mg/dL and is at high risk for heart disease

- Has an inherited type of high cholesterol

Section 18.5

Hypertension

This section includes text excerpted from "High Blood
Pressure during Childhood and Adolescence," Centers for
Disease Control and Prevention (CDC), July 18, 2018.

Too many youths have high blood pressure and other risk factors for heart disease and stroke. Using the updated 2017 American Academy of Pediatrics (AAP) *Clinical Practice Guidelines (CPG)*, a new Centers for Disease Control and Prevention (CDC) study shows that about four percent of youth aged 12 to 19 years have hypertension, and another 10 percent have elevated blood pressure (previously called "prehypertension"). Youth with obesity had the highest prevalence of hypertension.

High blood pressure in youth is linked to health problems later in life. The good news is that high blood pressure is preventable and treatable.

Study Finds Many Youth Have Hypertension

The Centers for Disease Control and Prevention analyzed data from more than 12,000 participants aged 12 to 19 years, responding to the National Health and Nutrition Examination Survey (NHANES) from 2001 to 2016. The CDC used these data to determine how the new guideline impacts hypertension trends among youth over time.

Using the criteria of the 2017 CPG, more than 1 in 7 U.S. youth aged 12 to 19 years had hypertension or elevated blood pressure from 2013 to 2016.

Key findings from the Morbidity and Mortality Weekly Report (MMWR) include:

- **Hypertension among youth has decreased, but youth are still at risk.** Between 2001 and 2016, the prevalence of hypertension declined using both the new and former guidelines. But, there are still many youths with hypertension and other cardiovascular disease risk factors, such as obesity and diabetes. Even with this downward trend, under the new guideline, more youth are classified as having hypertension than 15 years ago under the former guideline.

- **The new guideline changes the numbers and uses a lower threshold for hypertension.** Compared to the former guideline, the updated guideline reclassifies 2.6 percent of youth in the United States, or nearly 800,000 youth, as having hypertension.

  - Nearly half of the youth newly reclassified as having hypertension have obesity. Obesity in youth is defined as having a body mass index (BMI) greater than or equal to the 95th percentile.

  - Youth aged 18 to 19 years account for about half of the increase, and males account for more than two-thirds.

- **An estimated 1.3 million youth age 12 to 19 would have hypertension according to the new guidelines, which is about 4 percent of the population.** In a classroom of 30 youth, one would have hypertension, and about 3 more would have elevated blood pressure.

- **Risks for cardiovascular disease that start in childhood** are more likely to carry over into adulthood. Youth who have cardiovascular disease risk factors, such as hypertension, obesity, and diabetes, are more likely to have these risk factors as adults, putting them at greater risk for heart disease and stroke.

- **A healthy diet and exercise are important in reducing these risk factors.** Ensuring that youth are eating a healthy diet and getting enough physical activity is crucial to help prevent cardiovascular disease.

What Can Parents Do to Help Their Kid from Hypertension?

Ask your doctor to measure your child's blood pressure starting at age three. Helping children maintain a healthy weight, eat nutritious foods, and get regular physical activity can lower their blood pressure and reduce their risk for cardiovascular disease later in life. Try these tips to help youth keep a healthy weight and normal blood pressure:

Food and Drinks

- Offer nutritious, lower-calorie foods such as fruits and vegetables in place of foods high in added sugars and solid fats. Try serving more fruits and vegetables at meals and as snacks.

- Provide foods that are low in sodium (salt). Sodium raises blood pressure. Nearly 9 in 10 U.S. children eat more sodium than is recommended. Make sure drinking water is always available as a no-calorie alternative to sugary drinks, and limit juice.

Physical Activity

- Help your child get the recommended amount of physical activity each day. There are many age-appropriate activities to choose from.

Healthy Weight

- Be aware of your child's growth. Learn how obesity is measured in children.

Get Involved

- Be a role model! Eat healthy meals and snacks, and get the right amount of physical activity every day.

- Help shape a healthy school environment.

Chapter 19

Type 1 Diabetes in Children

What Is Type 1 Diabetes?

Type 1 diabetes (previously called "insulin-dependent" or "juvenile diabetes") is usually diagnosed in children, teens, and young adults, but it can develop at any age.

If you have type 1 diabetes, your pancreas is not making insulin or is making very little. Insulin is a hormone that enables blood sugar to enter the cells in your body where it can be used for energy. Without insulin, blood sugar cannot get into cells and builds up in the bloodstream. High blood sugar is damaging to the body and causes many of the symptoms and complications of diabetes.

Type 1 diabetes is less common than type 2—about 5 percent of people with diabetes have type 1. No one knows how to prevent type 1 diabetes, but it can be managed by following your doctor's recommendations for living a healthy lifestyle, controlling your blood sugar, getting regular health checkups, and getting diabetes self-management education.

For Parents of Children with Type 1 Diabetes

If your child has type 1 diabetes, you will be involved in diabetes care on a day-to-day basis, from serving healthy foods to giving insulin injections to watching for and treating hypoglycemia. You will also

---

This chapter includes text excerpted from "Type 1 Diabetes," Centers for Disease Control and Prevention (CDC), May 30, 2019.

need to stay in close contact with your child's healthcare team; they will help you understand the treatment plan and how to help your child stay healthy.

Causes of Type 1 Diabetes

Type 1 diabetes is caused by an autoimmune reaction (the body attacks itself by mistake) that destroys the cells in the pancreas that make insulin, called "beta cells." This process can go on for months or years before any symptoms appear.

Some people have certain genes (traits passed on from parent to child) that make them more likely to develop type 1 diabetes, though many would not go on to have type 1 diabetes even if they have the genes. Being exposed to a trigger in the environment, such as a virus, is also thought to play a part in developing type 1 diabetes. Diet and lifestyle habits do not cause type 1 diabetes.

Symptoms and Risk Factors of Type 1 Diabetes

It can take months or years for enough beta cells to be destroyed before symptoms of type 1 diabetes are noticed. Type 1 diabetes symptoms can develop in just a few weeks or months. Once symptoms appear, they can be severe.

Some type 1 diabetes symptoms are similar to symptoms of other health conditions. Do not guess—if you think you could have type 1 diabetes, see your doctor right away to get your blood sugar tested. Untreated diabetes can lead to very serious—even fatal—health problems.

Risk factors for type 1 diabetes are not as clear as for prediabetes and type 2 diabetes, though family history is known to play a part.

Getting Tested for Type 1 Diabetes

A simple blood test will let you know if your child has diabetes. If you have gotten your child's blood sugar tested at a health fair or pharmacy, follow-up at a clinic or doctor's office to make sure the results are accurate.

If your child's doctor thinks that she or he has type 1 diabetes, your child's blood may also be tested for autoantibodies (substances that indicate 'that body is attacking itself) that are often present with type 1 diabetes but not with type 2. You may have your child's urine tested for ketones (produced when the body burns fat for energy), which also indicate type 1 diabetes instead of type 2.

Management of Type 1 Diabetes in Children

Unlike many health conditions, diabetes is managed mostly by your child, with support from the healthcare team (including your child's primary care doctor, foot doctor, dentist, eye doctor, registered dietitian nutritionist, diabetes educator, and pharmacist), family, teachers, and other important people in their life. Managing diabetes can be challenging, but everything you do to improve your child's health is worth it!

If your child has type 1 diabetes, she or he will need to take insulin shots (or wear an insulin pump) every day to manage their blood sugar levels and get the energy their body needs. Insulin cannot be taken as a pill because the acid in the stomach would destroy it before it could get into the bloodstream. Your child's doctor will work with your child to figure out the most effective type and dosage of insulin for them.

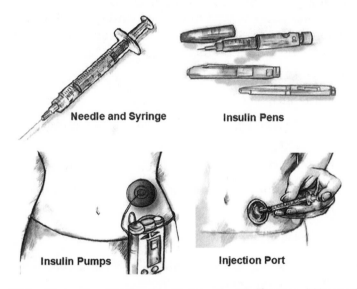

Needle and Syringe **Insulin Pens**

Insulin Pumps **Injection Port**

Figure 19.1. *Alternative Devices for Taking Insulin* (Source: "Alternative Devices for Taking Insulin," National Institute of Diabetes and Digestive and Kidney Diseases (NIDDK).)

You will also need to check your child's blood sugar regularly. Ask your child's doctor how often you should check it and what your child's target blood sugar levels should be. Keeping your child's blood sugar levels as close to the target as possible will help them to prevent or delay diabetes-related complications.

Stress is a part of life, but it can make managing diabetes harder, including controlling your child's blood sugar levels and dealing with their daily diabetes care. Regular physical activity, getting enough sleep, and relaxation exercises can help your child to cope with stress. Talk to your child's doctor and diabetes educator about these and other ways of how your child can manage stress.

Healthy lifestyle habits are really important, too:

• Making healthy food choices

• Being physically active

• Controlling your child's blood pressure

• Controlling your child's cholesterol

Make regular appointments with your child's healthcare team to be sure you are on track with your child's treatment plan and to get help with new ideas and strategies if needed.

Whether your child just got diagnosed with type 1 diabetes or have had it for some time, meeting with a diabetes educator is a great way to get support and guidance, including how to:

• Develop and stick to a healthy eating and activity plan

• Test your child's blood sugar and keep a record of the results

• Recognize the signs of high or low blood sugar and what to do about it

• Give themselves insulin by syringe, pen, or pump

• Monitor your child's feet, skin, and eyes to catch problems early

• Buy diabetes supplies and store them properly

• Manage stress and deal with daily diabetes care

Ask your child's doctor about diabetes self-management education and to recommend a diabetes educator.

Hypoglycemia

Hypoglycemia (low blood sugar) can happen quickly and needs to be treated immediately. It is most often caused by too much insulin, waiting too long for a meal or snack, not eating enough, or getting extra physical activity. Hypoglycemia symptoms are different for children to children; make sure you know their specific symptoms, which could include:

• Shakiness

• Nervousness or anxiety

- Sweating, chills, or clamminess
- Irritability or impatience
- Dizziness and difficulty concentrating
- Hunger or nausea
- Blurred vision
- Weakness or fatigue
- Anger, stubbornness, or sadness

If your child has hypoglycemia several times a week, talk to your child's doctor to see if their treatment needs to be adjusted.

Chapter 20

Ear, Nose, and Throat Disorders in Children

Chapter Contents

Section 20.1

Ear Infection

This section includes text excerpted from "Ear Infections in Children," National Institute on Deafness and Other Communication Disorders (NIDCD), May 12, 2017.

What Is an Ear Infection?

An ear infection is an inflammation of the middle ear, usually caused by bacteria, that occurs when fluid builds up behind the eardrum. Anyone can get an ear infection, but children get them more often than adults. Five out of six children will have at least one ear infection by their third birthday. In fact, ear infections are the most common reason parents bring their child to a doctor. The scientific name for an ear infection is "otitis media" (OM).

What Are the Symptoms of an Ear Infection?

There are three main types of ear infections. Each has a different combination of symptoms:

- **Acute otitis media (AOM)** is the most common ear infection. Parts of the middle ear are infected and swollen and fluid is trapped behind the eardrum. This causes pain in the ear—commonly called an "earache." Your child might also have a fever.

- **Otitis media with effusion (OME)** sometimes happens after an ear infection has run its course and fluid stays trapped behind the eardrum. A child with OME may have no symptoms, but a doctor will be able to see the fluid behind the eardrum with a special instrument.

- **Chronic otitis media with effusion (COME)** happens when fluid remains in the middle ear for a long time or returns over and over again, even though there is no infection. COME makes it harder for children to fight new infections and also can affect their hearing.

How Can You Tell If Your Child Has an Ear Infection?

Most ear infections happen to children before they have learned how to talk. If your child is not old enough to say "My ear hurts," here are a few things to look for:

- Tugging or pulling at the ear(s)

- Fussiness and crying

- Trouble sleeping

- Fever (especially in infants and younger children)

- Fluid draining from the ear

- Clumsiness or problems with balance

- Trouble hearing or responding to quiet sounds

What Causes an Ear Infection

An ear infection is usually caused by bacteria and often begins after a child has a sore throat, cold, or other upper respiratory infection. If the upper respiratory infection is bacterial, these same bacteria may spread to the middle ear; if the upper respiratory infection is caused by a virus, such as a cold, bacteria may be drawn to the microbe-friendly environment and move into the middle ear as a secondary infection. Because of the infection, fluid builds up behind the eardrum.

The ear has three major parts: the outer ear, the middle ear, and the inner ear. The outer ear also called the "pinna," includes everything we see on the outside—the curved flap of the ear leading down to the earlobe—but it also includes the ear canal, which begins at the opening to the ear and extends to the eardrum. The eardrum is a membrane that separates the outer ear from the middle ear.

The middle ear—which is where ear infections occur—is located between the eardrum and the inner ear. Within the middle ear are three tiny bones called the "malleus, incus, and stapes" that transmit sound vibrations from the eardrum to the inner ear. The bones of the middle ear are surrounded by air.

The inner ear contains the labyrinth, which helps us keep our balance. The cochlea, a part of the labyrinth, is a snail-shaped organ that converts sound vibrations from the middle ear into electrical signals. The auditory nerve carries these signals from the cochlea to the brain.

Other nearby parts of the ear also can be involved in ear infections. The eustachian tube is a small passageway that connects the upper part of the throat to the middle ear. Its job is to supply fresh air to the middle ear, drain fluid, and keep air pressure at a steady level between the nose and the ear.

Adenoids are small pads of tissue located behind the back of the nose, above the throat, and near the eustachian tubes. Adenoids are mostly made up of immune system cells. They fight off infection by trapping bacteria that enter through the mouth.

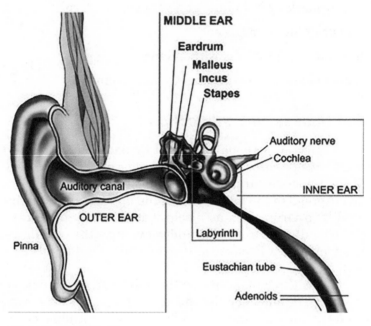

Figure 20.1. *Parts of the Ear*

Why Are Children More Likely than Adults to Get Ear Infections?

There are several reasons why children are more likely than adults to get ear infections.

Eustachian tubes are smaller and more level in children than they are in adults. This makes it difficult for fluid to drain out of the ear, even under normal conditions. If the eustachian tubes are swollen or blocked with mucus due to a cold or other respiratory illness, fluid may not be able to drain.

A child's immune system is not as effective as an adult's because it is still developing. This makes it harder for children to fight infections.

As part of the immune system, the adenoids respond to bacteria passing through the nose and mouth. Sometimes bacteria get trapped in the adenoids, causing a chronic infection that can then pass on to the eustachian tubes and the middle ear.

How Does a Doctor Diagnose a Middle Ear Infection?

The first thing a doctor will do is ask you about your child's health. Has your child had a head cold or sore throat recently? Is he having trouble sleeping? Is she pulling at her ears? If an ear infection seems likely, the simplest way for a doctor to tell is to use a lighted instrument, called an "otoscope," to look at the eardrum. A red, bulging eardrum indicates an infection.

A doctor also may use a pneumatic otoscope, which blows a puff of air into the ear canal, to check for fluid behind the eardrum. A normal eardrum will move back and forth more easily than an eardrum with fluid behind it.

Tympanometry, which uses sound tones and air pressure, is a diagnostic test a doctor might use if the diagnosis is still not clear. A tympanometer is a small, soft plug that contains a tiny microphone and speaker as well as a device that varies the air pressure in the ear. It measures how flexible the eardrum is at different pressures.

How Is an Acute Middle Ear Infection Treated?

Many doctors will prescribe an antibiotic, such as amoxicillin, to be taken over seven to 10 days. Your doctor also may recommend over-the-counter (OTC) pain relievers, such as acetaminophen or ibuprofen, or ear drops, to help with fever and pain. (Because aspirin is considered a major preventable risk factor for Reye syndrome, a child who has a fever or other flu-like symptoms should not be given aspirin unless instructed to by your doctor.)

If your doctor is not able to make a definite diagnosis of OM and your child does not have severe ear pain or a fever, your doctor might ask you to wait a day or two to see if the earache goes away. The American Academy of Pediatrics (AAP) issued guidelines in 2013 that encourage doctors to observe and closely follow these children with ear infections that cannot be definitively diagnosed, especially those between the ages of 6 months to 2 years. If there is no improvement within 48 to 72 hours from when symptoms began, the guidelines recommend doctors start antibiotic therapy. Sometimes ear pain is not caused by infection, and some ear infections may get better without antibiotics. Using antibiotics cautiously and with good reason helps prevent the development of bacteria that become resistant to antibiotics.

How Long Will It Take Your Child to Get Better?

Your child should start feeling better within a few days after visiting the doctor. If it has been several days and your child still seems sick, call your doctor. Your child might need a different antibiotic. Once the infection clears, fluid may still remain in the middle ear but usually disappears within three to six weeks.

What Happens If Your Child Keeps Getting Ear Infections?

To keep a middle ear infection from coming back, it helps to limit some of the factors that might put your child at risk, such as not being around people who smoke and not going to bed with a bottle. In spite of these precautions, some children may continue to have middle ear infections, sometimes as many as five or six a year. Your doctor may want to wait for several months to see if things get better on their own but, if the infections keep coming back and antibiotics are not helping, many doctors will recommend a surgical procedure that places a small ventilation tube in the eardrum to improve airflow and prevent fluid backup in the middle ear. The most commonly used tubes stay in place for six to nine months and require follow-up visits until they fall out.

If the placement of the tubes still does not prevent infections, a doctor may consider removing the adenoids to prevent infection from spreading to the eustachian tubes.

Can Ear Infections Be Prevented?

The best way to prevent ear infections is to reduce the risk factors associated with them. Here are some things you might want to do to lower your child's risk for ear infections.

- Vaccinate your child against the flu. Make sure your child gets influenza, or flu, vaccine every year.

- It is recommended that you vaccinate your child with the 13-valent pneumococcal conjugate vaccine (PCV13). The PCV13 protects against more types of infection-causing bacteria than the previous vaccine, the PCV7. If your child already has begun PCV7 vaccination, consult your physician about how to transition to PCV13. The Centers for Disease Control and Prevention (CDC) recommends that children under age 2 be vaccinated, starting at 2 months of age. Studies have shown that vaccinated children get far fewer ear infections than children who are not vaccinated. The vaccine is strongly recommended for children in daycare.

- Wash hands frequently. Washing hands prevents the spread of germs and can help keep your child from catching a cold or the flu.

- Avoid exposing your baby to cigarette smoke. Studies have shown that babies who are around smokers have more ear infections.

- Never put your baby down for a nap, or for the night, with a bottle.

Do not allow sick children to spend time together. As much as possible, limit your child's exposure to other children when your child or your child's playmates are sick.

Section 20.2

Enlarged Adenoids

This section includes text excerpted from "Adenoids," MedlinePlus, National Institutes of Health (NIH), January 31, 2017.

What Are Adenoids?

Adenoids are a patch of tissue that is high up in the throat, just behind the nose. They, along with the tonsils, are part of the lymphatic system. The lymphatic system clears away infection and keeps body fluids in balance. The adenoids and tonsils work by trapping germs coming in through the mouth and nose.

Adenoids usually start to shrink after about age five. By the teenage years, they are almost completely gone. By then, the body has other ways to fight germs.

What Are Enlarged Adenoids?

Enlarged adenoids are adenoids that are swollen. It is a common problem in children.

What Causes Enlarged Adenoids

Your child's adenoids can be enlarged, or swollen, for different reasons. It may just be that your child had enlarged adenoids at birth. Adenoids can also become enlarged when they are trying to fight off an infection. They might stay enlarged even after the infection is gone.

What Problems Can Enlarged Adenoids Cause?

Enlarged adenoids can make it hard to breathe through the nose. Your child might end up breathing only through the mouth. This may cause:

- A dry mouth, which can also lead to bad breath
- Cracked lips
- A runny nose

Other problems that enlarged adenoids can cause include:

- Loud breathing
- Snoring
- Restless sleep
- Sleep apnea, where you repeatedly stop breathing for a few seconds while sleeping
- Ear infections

How Can Enlarged Adenoids Be Diagnosed?

Your child's healthcare provider will take a medical history, check your child's ears, throat, and mouth, and feel your child's neck.

Since the adenoids are higher up than the throat, the healthcare provider cannot see them just by looking through your child's mouth. To check the size of your child's adenoids, your provider may use:

- A special mirror in the mouth
- A long, flexible tube with a light (an endoscope)
- An x-ray

What Are the Treatments for Enlarged Adenoids?

The treatment depends on what is causing the problem. If your child's symptoms are not too bad, she or he may not need treatment.

Your child might get the nasal spray to reduce the swelling, or antibiotics if the healthcare provider thinks that your child has a bacterial infection.

In some cases, your child may need an adenoidectomy.

What Is an Adenoidectomy and Why Might Your Child Need One?

An adenoidectomy is a surgery to remove the adenoids. Your child might need it if:

- She or he has repeated infections of the adenoids. Sometimes the infections can also cause ear infections and fluid buildup in the middle ear.

- Antibiotics cannot get rid of a bacterial infection

- The enlarged adenoids block the airways

If your child also has problems with her or his tonsils, she or he will probably have a tonsillectomy (removal of the tonsils) at the same time that the adenoids are removed.

After having the surgery, your child usually goes home the same day. She or he will probably have some throat pain, bad breath, and a runny nose. It can take several days to feel all better.

Section 20.3

Hearing Loss

This section includes text excerpted from "What Is Hearing Loss in Children?" Centers for Disease Control and Prevention (CDC), March 21, 2019.

Hearing loss can affect a child's ability to develop speech, language, and social skills. The earlier children with hearing loss start getting services, the more likely they are to reach their full potential. If you think that a child might have hearing loss, ask the child's doctor for a hearing screening as soon as possible. Do not wait!

What Is Hearing Loss?

A hearing loss can happen when any part of the ear is not working in the usual way. This includes the outer ear, middle ear, inner ear, hearing (acoustic) nerve, and auditory system.

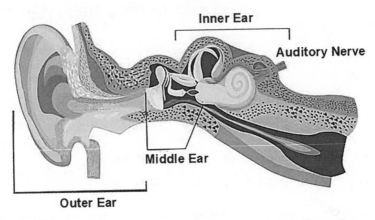

Figure 20.2. *Auditory System* (Source: "How Does Loud Noise Cause Hearing Loss?" Centers for Diseases Control and Prevention (CDC).)

Signs and Symptoms of Hearing Loss

The signs and symptoms of hearing loss are different for each child. If you think that your child might have hearing loss, ask the child's doctor for a hearing screening as soon as possible. Do not wait!

Even if a child has passed a hearing screening before, it is important to look out for the following signs.

Signs in Babies

- Does not startle at loud noises.

- Does not turn to the source of a sound after six months of age.

- Does not say single words, such as "dada" or "mama" by one year of age.

- Turns head when she or he sees you but not if you only call out her or his name. This sometimes is mistaken for not paying attention or just ignoring, but could be the result of a partial or complete hearing loss.

- Seems to hear some sounds but not others.

Signs in Children

- Speech is delayed.

- Speech is not clear.

- Does not follow directions. This sometimes is mistaken for not paying attention or just ignoring, but could be the result of a partial or complete hearing loss.

- Often says, "Huh?"

- Turns the TV volume up too high.

- Babies and children should reach milestones in how they play, learn, communicate and act. A delay in any of these milestones could be a sign of hearing loss or other developmental problems.

Screening and Diagnosis of Hearing Loss

Hearing screening can tell if a child might have hearing loss. Hearing screening is easy and is not painful. In fact, babies are often asleep while being screened. It takes a very short time—usually only a few minutes.

Babies

- All babies should be screened for hearing loss no later than one month of age. It is best if they are screened before leaving the hospital after birth.

- If a baby does not pass a hearing screening, it is very important to get a full hearing test as soon as possible, but no later than three months of age.

Older Babies and Children

- If you think a child might have hearing loss, ask the doctor for a hearing test as soon as possible.

- Children who are at risk for acquired, progressive, or delayed-onset hearing loss should have at least one hearing test by 2 to 2½ years of age. Hearing loss that gets worse over time is known as "acquired" or "progressive hearing loss." Hearing loss that develops after the baby is born is called "delayed-onset hearing loss." Find out if a child may be at risk for hearing loss.

- If a child does not pass a hearing screening, it is very important to get a full hearing test as soon as possible.

Treatments and Intervention Services

No single treatment or intervention is the answer for every person or family. Good treatment plans will include close monitoring, follow-ups and any changes needed along the way. There are many different types of communication options for children with hearing loss and for their families. Some of these options include:

- Learning other ways to communicate, such as sign language
- Technology to help with communication, such as hearing aids and cochlear implants
- Medicine and surgery to correct some types of hearing loss
- Family support services

Causes and Risk Factors of Hearing Loss

Hearing loss can happen any time during life—from before birth to adulthood.

Following are some of the things that can increase the chance that a child will have hearing loss:

- **A genetic cause.** About one out of two cases of hearing loss in babies is due to genetic causes. Some babies with a genetic cause for their hearing loss might have family members who also have a hearing loss. About one out of three babies with genetic hearing loss have a "syndrome." This means they have other conditions in addition to the hearing loss, such as Down syndrome or Usher syndrome.

- **Maternal infections during pregnancy, complications after birth, and head trauma.** One out of four cases of hearing loss in babies is due to maternal infections during pregnancy, complications after birth, and head trauma. For example, the child:

  - Was exposed to infection, such as, before birth
  - Spent five days or more in a hospital neonatal intensive care unit (NICU) or had complications while in the NICU
  - Needed a special procedure such as a blood transfusion to treat bad jaundice

- Has head, face or ears shaped or formed in a different way than usual

- Has a condition such as a neurological disorder that may be associated with hearing loss

- Had an infection around the brain and spinal cord called "meningitis"

- Received a bad injury to the head that required a hospital stay

- **Unknown causes.** For about one out of four babies born with hearing loss, the cause is unknown.

Prevention of Hearing Loss

Following are tips for parents to help prevent hearing loss in their children:

- Have a healthy pregnancy

- Make sure your child gets all the regular childhood vaccines

- Keep your child away from high noise levels, such as from very loud toys

Get Help

- If you think that your child might have hearing loss, ask the child's doctor for a hearing screening as soon as possible. Do not wait!

- If your child does not pass a hearing screening, ask the child's doctor for a full hearing test as soon as possible.

- If your child has hearing loss, talk to the child's doctor about treatment and intervention services.

Hearing loss can affect a child's ability to develop speech, language, and social skills. The earlier children with hearing loss start getting services, the more likely they are to reach their full potential. If you are a parent and you suspect your child has hearing loss, trust your instincts and speak with your child's doctor.

Section 20.4

Hoarseness

This section includes text excerpted from "Hoarseness," National
Institute on Deafness and Other Communication Disorders (NIDCD),
March 6, 2017.

What Is Hoarseness?

If your child is hoarse, your child's voice will sound breathy, raspy,
or strained, or will be softer in volume or lower in pitch. Their throat
might feel scratchy. Hoarseness is often a symptom of problems in the
vocal folds of the larynx.

How Our Voice Works

The sound of our voice is produced by the vibration of the vocal
folds, which are two bands of smooth muscle tissue that are positioned
opposite each other in the larynx. The larynx is located between the

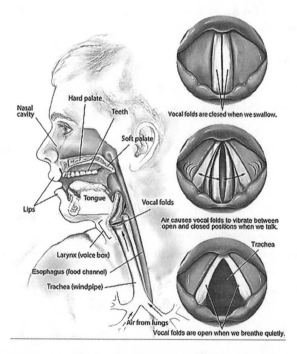

Figure 20.3. *Structures Involved in Speech and Voice Production*

base of the tongue and the top of the trachea, which is the passageway to the lungs.

When we are not speaking, the vocal folds are open so that we can breathe. When it is time to speak, however, the brain orchestrates a series of events. The vocal folds snap together while air from the lungs blows past, making them vibrate. The vibrations produce sound waves that travel through the throat, nose, and mouth, which act as resonating cavities to modulate the sound. The quality of our voice—its pitch, volume, and tone—is determined by the size and shape of the vocal folds and the resonating cavities. This is why people's voices sound so different.

Individual variations in our voices are the result of how much tension we put on our vocal folds. For example, relaxing the vocal folds makes a voice deeper; tensing them makes a voice higher.

If Your Child's Voice Is Hoarse, When Should You See Her or His Doctor Doctor?

You should see your child's doctor if her or his voice has been hoarse for more than three weeks, especially if they have not had a cold or the flu. You should also see the doctor if they are coughing up blood or if they have difficulty swallowing, feel a lump in their neck, experience pain when speaking or swallowing, have difficulty breathing, or lose their voice completely for more than a few days.

How Will Your Child's Doctor Diagnose What Is Wrong with the Child's Voice?

Your child's doctor will ask about their health history and how long they have been hoarse. Depending on their symptoms and general health, the doctor may send them to an otolaryngologist (a doctor who specializes in diseases of the ears, nose, and throat). An otolaryngologist will usually use an endoscope (a flexible, lighted tube designed for looking at the larynx) to get a better view of the vocal folds. In some cases, the doctor might recommend special tests to evaluate voice irregularities or vocal airflow.

What Are Some of the Disorders That Cause Hoarseness and How Are They Treated?

Hoarseness can have several possible causes and treatments, as described below.

Laryngitis. Laryngitis is one of the most common causes of hoarseness. It can be due to temporary swelling of the vocal folds from a cold, an upper respiratory infection, or allergies. Your child's doctor will treat laryngitis according to its cause. If it is due to a cold or upper respiratory infection, the doctor might recommend rest, fluids, and nonprescription pain relievers. Allergies might be treated similarly, with the addition of over-the-counter (OTC) allergy medicines.

Misusing or overusing your voice. Cheering at sporting events, speaking loudly in noisy situations, talking for too long without resting your child's voice, singing loudly, or speaking with a voice that is too high or too low can cause temporary hoarseness. Resting, reducing voice use, and drinking lots of water should help relieve hoarseness from misuse or overuse. If your child regularly experiences hoarseness, their doctor might suggest seeing a speech-language pathologist for voice therapy. In voice therapy, your child will be given vocal exercises and tips for avoiding hoarseness by changing the ways in which they use their voice.

Gastroesophageal reflux (GERD). GERD—commonly called "heartburn"—can cause hoarseness when stomach acid rises up the throat and irritates the tissues. Usually, hoarseness caused by GERD is worse in the morning and improves throughout the day. For some, the stomach acid rises all the way up to the throat and larynx and irritates the vocal folds. This is called "laryngopharyngeal reflux" (LPR). LPR can happen during the day or night. Some people will have no heartburn with LPR, but they may feel as if they constantly have to cough to clear their throat and they may become hoarse. GERD and LPR are treated with dietary modifications and medications that reduce stomach acid.

Vocal nodules, polyps, and cysts. Vocal nodules, polyps, and cysts are benign (noncancerous) growths within or along the vocal folds. Vocal nodules are sometimes called "singer's nodes" because they are a frequent problem among professional singers. They form in pairs on opposite sides of the vocal folds as the result of too much pressure or friction, much like the way a callus forms on the foot from a shoe that is too tight. A vocal polyp typically occurs only on one side of the vocal fold. A vocal cyst is a hard mass of tissue encased in a membrane sac inside the vocal fold. The most common treatments for nodules, polyps, and cysts are voice rest, voice therapy, and surgery to remove the tissue.

Vocal fold hemorrhage. Vocal fold hemorrhage occurs when a blood vessel on the surface of the vocal fold ruptures and the tissues fill with blood. If your child lose her or his voice suddenly during strenuous vocal use (such as yelling), they may have a vocal fold hemorrhage. Sometimes a vocal fold hemorrhage will cause hoarseness to develop quickly over a short amount of time and only affect their singing but not your speaking voice. Vocal fold hemorrhage must be treated immediately with total voice rest and a trip to the doctor.

Vocal fold paralysis. Vocal fold paralysis is a voice disorder that occurs when one or both of the vocal folds do not open or close properly. It can be caused by an injury to the head, neck or chest; lung or thyroid cancer; tumors of the skull base, neck, or chest; or infection (for example, Lyme disease). In many cases, however, the cause is unknown. Vocal fold paralysis is treated with voice therapy and, in some cases, surgery.

Neurological diseases and disorders. Neurological conditions that affect areas of the brain that control muscles in the throat or larynx can also cause hoarseness. Spasmodic dysphonia is a rare neurological disease that causes hoarseness and can also affect breathing. Treatment in these cases will depend upon the type of disease or disorder.

Other causes. Thyroid problems and injury to the larynx can cause hoarseness. Hoarseness may sometimes be a symptom of laryngeal cancer, which is why it is so important to see your child's doctor if they are hoarse for more than three weeks. Hoarseness is also the most common symptom of a disease called "recurrent respiratory papillomatosis" (RRP), or "laryngeal papillomatosis," which causes noncancerous tumors to grow in the larynx and other air passages leading from the nose and mouth into the lungs.

Section 20.5

Nosebleeds

"Nosebleeds," © 2017 Omnigraphics.
Reviewed September 2019.

A nosebleed, also known as "epistaxis," is a common condition that occurs when one of the small, delicate blood vessels inside the nose bursts open. Many children under the age of 10 are prone to nosebleeds. Although blood streaming from the nose can seem alarming, nosebleeds are usually harmless and easy to manage at home with simple first-aid techniques.

Blood vessels on the nasal septum—the tissue that separates the nostrils—are responsible for most nosebleeds. Those that occur in the front part of the nose are known as "anterior nosebleeds," and they are the most common among children and the easiest to stop. "Posterior nosebleeds," on the other hand, occur deep inside the nasal cavity. They usually affect older adults, people with high blood pressure, and people who have experienced facial injuries.

Causes of Nosebleeds

Irritation of the membranes lining the inside of the nose is the cause of most nosebleeds. Breathing cold, dry, or overheated air can cause irritation of nasal membranes, as can the accumulation of mucus from allergies, colds, sinus infections, or the flu. Medications used to dry out the sinuses, such as decongestants or antihistamines, can also cause irritation of the nasal membranes. Irritation causes crusts to form inside the nose, which can bleed when they are removed by blowing or picking the nose.

Injuries or bumps to the nose can also cause surface capillaries to burst and create nosebleeds. Children may also get nosebleeds by inserting foreign objects into their nose. In rare cases, repeated nosebleeds may be symptomatic of an underlying disorder, such as high blood pressure, hemophilia, or a tumor in the nose or sinuses.

First Aid at Home

The first step in treating a nosebleed is to remain calm and reassuring. Children often become upset at the sight or taste of blood, and it is important to let them know that everything will be fine. The next step is to stop the bleeding by applying pressure to the soft part of the nose. With the child sitting down and leaning forward slightly, use the fingers, a tissue, or a soft cloth to hold the nostrils closed for 10 minutes. Do not release the pressure to check whether the bleeding has stopped until the full time has passed. Encourage the child to spit out any blood in the mouth, as swallowing blood can cause vomiting and make the nosebleed worse. It may also be helpful to apply an icepack or cold compress to the bridge of the nose. If the bleeding has not stopped after 10 minutes, repeat the above procedures for 10 more minutes.

Once the bleeding stops, it is important to have the child pursue quiet activities for a few hours instead of running around. The child should also avoid taking hot baths or showers and drinking hot liquids for the next 24 hours to prevent dilation of blood vessels in the nose. Finally, the child should not be allowed to sniff, blow, or pick their nose for at least 24 hours following a nosebleed.

Medical Treatment

In most cases, nosebleeds can be treated successfully at home. It may be necessary to seek medical treatment, however, under the following conditions:

- The bleeding continues for more than 20 minutes
- The nosebleed accompanies a head injury
- The nose may have been fractured by a fall or blow to the face
- A foreign object may have been inserted into the nose
- The child tends to bruise easily or bleed profusely from minor wounds
- The child has recently begun taking a new medication

For a persistent nosebleed, the doctor is likely to apply a medicated cream or ointment to the inside of the nose to help stop the bleeding. The doctor may also use heat, electric current, or silver nitrate sticks to cauterize the blood vessel and stop the bleeding. Finally, the doctor may pack the child's nose with gauze, which should remain in place for 24 to 48 hours. Once the bleeding has stopped, the doctor can take steps to address any underlying causes of the nosebleed. The doctor may remove a foreign object from the nose, for instance, or reset a broken nose. If nosebleeds are related to medication, a change in prescription may be recommended.

Although it is rare, frequent, severe nosebleeds can create enough blood loss to cause anemia in children. Doctors may perform blood tests to determine whether hemoglobin levels are low. They may also check for signs of low blood pressure due to blood loss. Children who have frequent nosebleeds may also be referred to an ear, nose, and throat (ENT) specialist for further testing, such as nasal endoscopy or computerized tomography (CT) scan of the nose and sinuses.

Preventing Nosebleeds

To prevent nosebleeds caused by dry air, it may be helpful to use a vaporizer at home to add moisture. In addition, using a saline nasal spray, water-based lubricating gel, or antibiotic ointment can help prevent nasal membranes from drying out. Cutting children's fingernails can help discourage nose-picking. Finally, wearing appropriate protective headgear during sports and activities can help prevent head and facial injuries that cause nosebleeds.

References

1. Jothi, Sumana. "Nosebleed," MedlinePlus, National Institutes of Health (NIH), August 5, 2015.

2. "Nosebleeds," The Nemours Foundation/KidsHealth®, 2016.

3. "Nosebleeds," Royal Children's Hospital Melbourne, August 2015.

Section 20.6

Obstructive Sleep Apnea

This section includes text excerpted from "Obstructive
Sleep Apnea," Genetics Home Reference (GHR), National
Institutes of Health (NIH), March 2018.

What Is Obstructive Sleep Apnea?

Obstructive sleep apnea (OSA) is a condition in which individuals
experience pauses in breathing (apnea) during sleep, which are associated with partial or complete closure of the throat (upper airway).
Complete closure can lead to apnea while partial closure allows breathing but decreases the intake of oxygen (hypopnea).

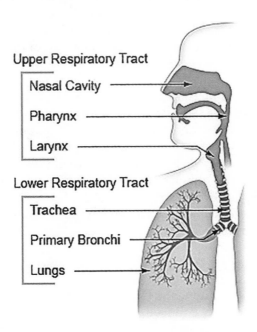

Figure 20.4. *Conducting Passages* (Source: "Conducting Passages,"
Surveillance, Epidemiology, and End Results Program (SEER), National
Cancer Institute (NCI).)

Individuals with OSA may experience interrupted sleep with frequent awakenings and loud snoring. Repeated pauses in breathing
lead to episodes of lower-than-normal oxygen levels (hypoxemia)

and the buildup of carbon dioxide (hypercapnia) in the bloodstream. Interrupted and poor-quality sleep can lead to daytime sleepiness and fatigue, impaired attention and memory, headaches, and depression.

Causes of Obstructive Sleep Apnea

The causes of OSA are often complex. This condition results from a combination of genetic, health, and lifestyle factors, many of which have not been identified. Studies suggest that variations in multiple genes, each with a small effect, combine to increase the risk of developing the condition. However, it is unclear what contribution each of these genetic changes made to disease risk. Most of the variations have been identified in single studies, and subsequent research has not verified them.

Genes thought to be associated with the development of OSA are involved in many bodily processes. These include communication between nerve cells, breathing regulation, control of inflammatory responses by the immune system, development of tissues in the head and face (craniofacial development), the sleep–wake cycle, and appetite control.

Obesity is a major risk factor for OSA. It is thought that excess fatty tissue in the head and neck constricts airways and abdominal fat may prevent the chest and lungs from fully expanding and relaxing.

Other risk factors for OSA include frequent nasal congestion, and blockages of the airways, such as by enlarged tonsils.

Obstructive sleep apnea often occurs on its own, without signs and symptoms affecting other parts of the body. However, it can also occur as part of a syndrome, such as mucopolysaccharidosis type I or polycystic ovary syndrome (PCOS).

Obstructive Sleep Apnea: Frequency

Obstructive sleep apnea is a common condition. It is estimated to affect 2 to 4 percent of children.

Section 20.7

Perforated Eardrum

"Perforated Eardrum," © 2017 Omnigraphics.
Reviewed September 2019.

A perforated eardrum—also called a "ruptured eardrum" or perforated tympanic membrane"—is a tear in the thin membrane that separates the outer ear from the middle ear. The function of this cone-shaped membrane is to transmit sound waves gathered by the outer ear to the ossicles (three small bones) in the middle ear and then to the oval window, the port to the fluid-filled inner ear. Structures in the inner ear stimulate auditory nerves, which then transmit impulses that the brain interprets as sound.

Perforated eardrums generally result in some degree of hearing loss, and in rare cases this could be permanent. Much of the time, the tear will heal on its own in a few weeks, but in more serious instances, surgery or another type of medical intervention may be necessary. And until the perforation heals or is repaired, the normally sterile middle ear is subject to infection.

Causes of Perforated Eardrum

There are numerous potential causes for a perforated eardrum, some pathological (caused by disease) and some traumatic (caused by injury). These can include:

- Middle ear infections

- Damage from foreign objects, such as cotton swabs, inserted into the ear

- Injury to the ear from a powerful slap or other impact

- Barotrauma, damage caused by a change in pressure, as with air travel or scuba diving

- Very loud noise, like as a gunshot or explosion, close to the ear

- Severe head trauma, such as a skull fracture

Symptoms of Perforated Eardrum

The primary symptom of a perforated eardrum is pain, which might initially seem like a common earache but then increases in severity. It can be extremely sharp and sudden, dull and steady, or intermittent. Other symptoms may include:

- Partial or complete hearing loss in the affected ear

- Ringing or buzzing in the ear

- Drainage from the ear, which may be pus, blood, or clear liquid

- Facial weakness

- Dizziness

- Repeated ear infections

Diagnosis of Perforated Eardrum

A physician—either a family doctor or an ear, nose, and throat specialist (ENT)—will generally begin by taking a medical history of the patient and her or his family. This will likely be followed by a series of questions about symptoms of the ailment and any medications taken by the patient. The physical examination is done with an otoscope, a specialized instrument with a light that will allow the doctor to see into the ear and determine whether or not the eardrum has been ruptured.

Other tests that may be performed include:

- **Audiology test**, which uses generated sound to assess the extent of hearing loss.

- **Tuning-fork test**, a less technical but still effective method of assessing hearing loss.

- **Tympanometry**, an examination that tests the eardrum's response to pressure changes.

- **Laboratory tests** of fluid draining from the ear, if any.

Treatment of Perforated Eardrum

Many ear infections heal on their own over the course of a few weeks, or at most a few months. In such cases, the doctor may prescribe antibiotics, either pills or ear drops, to help prevent infection, as well as pain medicine, usually over-the-counter medications like acetaminophen or ibuprofen. Warm compresses might also be recommended to relieve discomfort.

If the perforation does not begin to heal on its own, and if the hole is not too large, the ENT may apply a special patch to the eardrum.

This is done with a very thin, medicated material that both protects the wound and encourages healing of the membrane. The procedure takes only 15 to 30 minutes and can usually be done in the doctor's office using a local anesthetic.

If the eardrum does not heal on its own, and the rupture is too large for a patch, a surgical repair called a "tympanoplasty" might be required. In this procedure, the surgeon makes the repair through the ear canal itself or through an incision behind the ear. After cleaning and preparing the damaged area, the surgeon will take a small piece of tissue from elsewhere on the body and graft it onto the eardrum to seal the perforation.

Tympanoplasty is generally performed in a hospital with the patient under general anesthetic. It usually lasts up to one hour if the procedure is done through the ear canal, or up to three hours if an incision behind the ear is required.

In cases in which the ossicles—the tiny bones in the middle ear—have been damaged by injury or infection, an ossiculoplasty might need to be performed. This procedure, which is also done in a hospital under general anesthetic, involves the replacement of the damaged bones with bones from a donor or with an artificial substitute.

Complications of Perforated Eardrum

Most perforated eardrums heal well with simple treatment, and even patients with more extensive ruptures can achieve a good result with proper medical attention. However, left untreated, a punctured eardrum can lead to potentially serious complications, including:

- Fever

- Severe pain

- Dizziness

- Hearing loss, usually temporary but possibly permanent

- Middle ear infections, caused by bacteria entering through the opening

- Damage to the bones of the middle ear

- Middle ear cholesteatoma, a cyst composed of skin cells and other debris

- In rare cases, infection may spread to the brain

Prevention of Perforated Eardrum

One of the most effective ways to prevent a perforated eardrum is to keep foreign objects out of the ear. And if an object does become lodged in the ear canal, it is best to have it removed by a medical professional. Another important prevention method is to get treatment for ear infections before they become serious enough to damage the eardrum.

A few other ways to prevent ruptured eardrums include:

- Keep ears dry to help avoid infection

- If susceptible to ear infections, wear earplugs when swimming or bathing

- Protect ears while flying (yawn or chew gum to equalize pressure)

- Avoid flying with a cold or sinus infection

- Wear earplugs or earmuffs to protect against loud noises

References

1. Derrer, David T., MD. "Ruptured Eardrum: Symptoms and Treatments," WebMD, August 17, 2014.

2. "Eardrum Rupture," Healthline.com, August 25, 2016.

3. Kacker, Ashutosh, MD, BS. "Ruptured Eardrum," MedLinePlus, National Institutes of Health (NIH), May 18, 2014.

4. "Ruptured Eardrum," Mount Sinai Hospital, August 10, 2015.

5. "Ruptured Eardrum (Perforated Eardrum)," Mayo Clinic, January 4, 2014

Section 20.8

Sinusitis

This section contains text excerpted from the following sources:
Text beginning with the heading "What Is Sinusitis?" is excerpted
from "Sinus Infection (Sinusitis)," Centers for Disease Control
and Prevention (CDC), September 25, 2017; Text beginning with
the heading "Diagnosis of Sinusitis" is excerpted from "Pediatric
Treatment Recommendations," Centers for Disease Control and
Prevention (CDC), February 1, 2017.

What Is Sinusitis?

A sinus infection (sinusitis) does not typically need to be treated with antibiotics in order to get better. If your child is diagnosed with a sinus infection, the healthcare professional can decide if antibiotics are needed.

Causes of Sinusitis

Sinus infections occur when fluid is trapped or blocked in the sinuses, allowing germs to grow. Sinus infections are usually (5 to 7 out of 10 cases in children) caused by a virus. They are less commonly (3 to 5 out of 10 cases in children) caused by bacteria.

Other conditions can cause symptoms similar to a sinus infection, including:

- Allergies

- Pollutants (airborne chemicals or irritants)

- Fungal infections

Risk Factors of Sinusitis

Several conditions can increase your child's risk of getting a sinus infection:

- A previous respiratory-tract infection, such as the common cold

- Structural problems within the sinuses

- A weak immune system or taking drugs that weaken the immune system

- Nasal polyps

- Allergies
- Going to day care
- Using a pacifier
- Being exposed to secondhand smoke
- Drinking a bottle while laying down

Signs and Symptoms of Sinusitis

Common signs and symptoms of a sinus infection include:

- Headache
- Stuffy or runny nose
- Loss of the sense of smell
- Facial pain or pressure
- Postnasal drip (mucus drips down the throat from the nose)
- Sore throat
- Fever
- Coughing
- Fatigue (being tired)
- Bad breath

When your child has a sinus infection, one or more of her or his sinuses become inflamed and fluid builds up, making it hard to breathe through their nose.

When to Seek Medical Care

See a healthcare professional your child has any of the following:

- Temperature higher than 100.4°F
- Symptoms that are getting worse or lasting more than 10 days
- Multiple sinus infections in the past year
- Symptoms that are not relieved with over-the-counter (OTC) medicines

If your child is younger than three months of age and has a fever, it is important to call your healthcare professional right away.

Chronic sinusitis can be caused by nasal growths, allergies, or respiratory tract infections (viral, bacterial, or fungal).

Diagnosis of Sinusitis

Halitosis, fatigue, headache, decreased appetite, but most physical exam findings are nonspecific and do not distinguish bacterial from viral causes. A bacterial diagnosis may be established based on the presence of one of the following criteria:

- **Persistent symptoms without improvement:** Nasal discharge or daytime cough for more than 10 days.

- **Worsening symptoms:** Worsening or new-onset fever, daytime cough, or nasal discharge after initial improvement of a viral upper respiratory infection (URI).

- **Severe symptoms:** Fever more than or equal to 39°C, purulent nasal discharge for at least 3 consecutive days. Imaging tests are no longer recommended for uncomplicated cases.

Management of Sinusitis

If a bacterial infection is established:

- Watchful waiting for up to three days may be offered for children with acute bacterial sinusitis with persistent symptoms. Antibiotic therapy should be prescribed for children with acute bacterial sinusitis with severe or worsening disease.

- Amoxicillin or amoxicillin/clavulanate remain first-line therapy.

- Recommendations for treatment of children with a history of type I hypersensitivity to penicillin vary.

- In children who are vomiting or who cannot tolerate oral medication, a single dose of ceftriaxone can be used and then can be switched to oral antibiotics if improving.

Section 20.9

Stridor

"Stridor," © 2017 Omnigraphics.
Reviewed September 2019.

Stridor is a harsh, high-pitched whistling or wheezing sound that occurs while breathing. It is typically the result of a partial blockage of airflow through the throat, windpipe, or voice box. Children are particularly at risk of developing stridor because their airways are narrower and softer than those of adults.

Stridor has many possible causes, several of which are easily treated or naturally outgrown. In some cases, however, stridor can be symptomatic of a serious or potentially life-threatening disorder. Stridor and other symptoms of airway blockage should thus be considered reasons to seek immediate medical attention.

Causes of Stridor

Stridor can be caused by a variety of health conditions. Some of the most common causes include the following:

- Food or other objects obstructing the airway

- Anaphylaxis from a severe allergic reaction

- Inflammation of the throat or windpipe caused by viral or bacterial infections, such as croup, bronchitis, tonsillitis, or epiglottitis

- Irritation from phlegm or laryngitis

- Trauma to the airway from neck fractures, neck surgery, prolonged use of a breathing tube, or inhalation of smoke or harmful chemicals

- Trauma to the throat from swallowing harmful substances

- Cancer, tumors, or abscesses in the throat, windpipe, or vocal cords

- Paralysis of the vocal cords

- Congenital conditions such as subglottic stenosis (a narrow voice box), subglottic hemangioma (a mass of blood vessels obstructing the airway), or vascular rings (an artery or vein compressing the windpipe)

Among infants, the cause of up to 75 percent of inspiratory stridor cases is laryngomalacia, a condition in which soft tissues obstruct the airway. Laryngomalacia typically manifests shortly after birth, peaks around the age of six months, and gradually disappears around the age of two as the child's airway hardens. Stridor symptoms caused by laryngomalacia, such as squeaking or rattling sounds while breathing, are usually most noticeable when babies lie on their backs. Other common indicators of laryngomalacia in infants include difficulty breathing, hoarse crying, trouble nursing, and poor weight gain.

Diagnosis and Treatment of Stridor

It is important to note that unexplained stridor can be a sign of an emergency. If a child has difficulty breathing, and especially if there is a blue tint in the child's lips, skin, or nails, caregivers should seek medical attention immediately. In such cases, the doctor will take action to reopen the child's airway to allow them to breathe properly. The doctor may perform the Heimlich maneuver if a foreign object is blocking the airway, or may administer medication if the patient is experiencing anaphylaxis. In some cases, a breathing tube may be needed to support respiration until the patient is stabilized.

In many cases, however, stridor is caused by a medical condition that can be diagnosed and treated effectively. For non-emergency situations, the doctor will conduct a physical examination and take a complete medical history to find the underlying cause of the stridor. For instance, the doctor is likely to ask about when the breathing problem started, and the exact nature of the abnormal sounds. To determine whether an infection may be involved, the doctor may inquire about recent illnesses and the presence of other symptoms, such as a runny nose, cough, or sore throat. The doctor will also observe and listen to the child's breathing and look for additional symptoms, such as swelling in the face or neck or a bluish tint to the skin.

The process of diagnosing the underlying cause of stridor may also involve medical tests, including the following:

- X-rays or computerized tomography (CT) scans of the neck and chest to look for blockages

- A bronchoscopy or laryngoscopy to examine the airway and voice box

- An arterial blood gas analysis to see whether breathing problems are affecting the amount of oxygen in the bloodstream

- A sputum culture to check for bacterial or viral infections in the lungs

Treatment of stridor depends on the diagnosis of the underlying cause, as well as the severity of the condition and the child's overall health. Some cases only require monitoring until the symptoms go away on their own. In other cases, medications may be prescribed to treat infections or reduce inflammation in the airway. Referral to an ear, nose, and throat specialist may be indicated in some situations, while severe cases of stridor may require surgery to correct.

References

1. Kaneshiro, Neil K. "Stridor," MedlinePlus, National Institutes of Health (NIH), 2016.

2. Leung, Alexander K. C., and Helen Cho. "Diagnosis of Stridor in Children," American Family Physician (AFP), November 15, 1999.

3. Phillips, Natalie. "What Causes Stridor?" Healthline, 2016.

Section 20.10

Swimmer's Ear: Otitis Externa

This section includes text excerpted from "Hygiene-Related Diseases," Centers for Disease Control and Prevention (CDC), August 2, 2016. Reviewed September 2019.

Swimmer's ear is a common problem that can cause pain and discomfort for children and swimmers of all ages. In the United States, swimmer's ear results in an estimated 2.4 million healthcare visits every year and nearly half a billion dollars in healthcare costs.

What Are the Symptoms of Swimmer's Ear?

Symptoms of swimmer's ear usually appear within a few days of swimming and include:

- Itchiness inside the ear

- Redness and swelling of the ear

- Pain when the infected ear is tugged or when pressure is placed on the ear

- Pus draining from the infected ear

Although all age groups are affected by swimmer's ear, it is more common in children and can be extremely painful.

How Is Swimmer's Ear Spread at Recreational Water Venues?

Swimmer's ear can occur when water stays in the ear canal for long periods of time, providing the perfect environment for germs to grow and infect the skin. Germs found in pools and other recreational water venues are one of the most common causes of swimmer's ear.

Swimmer's ear cannot be spread from one person to another.

If you think your child has swimmer's ear, consult the healthcare provider. Swimmer's ear can be treated with antibiotic ear drops.

Is There a Difference between a Childhood Middle Ear Infection and Swimmer's Ear?

Yes. Swimmer's ear is not the same as the common childhood middle ear infection. If you can wiggle the outer ear without pain or discomfort then your ear condition is probably not swimmer's ear.

How You Can Protect Your Child from Getting Swimmer's Ear

To reduce the risk of swimmer's ear in your child:

- Do keep their ears as dry as possible:
  - Make them use a bathing cap, earplugs, or custom-fitted swim molds when swimming

- Do dry their ears thoroughly after swimming or showering:
  - Use a towel to dry your ears well
  - Tilt their head to hold each ear facing down to allow water to escape the ear canal

- Pull their earlobe in different directions while their ear is faced down to help water drain out

- If they still have water left in their ears, consider using a hairdryer to move air within the ear canal

  - Put the dryer on the lowest heat and speed or fan setting

  - Hold the dryer several inches from their ear

- Do not put objects in their ear canal (including cotton-tip swabs, pencils, paperclips, or fingers)

- Do not try to remove ear wax. Ear wax helps protect the ear canal from infection

  - If you think that their ear canal is blocked by earwax, consult the healthcare provider

- Consult with a healthcare provider about using ear drops after swimming. Drops should not be used by those with ear tubes, damaged eardrums, outer ear infections, or ear drainage (pus or liquid coming from the ear).

- Consult a healthcare provider if your child has ear pain, discomfort, or drainage from their ears

- Ask your pool or hot tub operator if disinfectant and potential of hydrogen (pH) levels are checked at least twice per day—hot tubs and pools with proper disinfectant and pH levels are less likely to spread germs

- Use pool test strips to check the pool or hot tub yourself for adequate disinfectant (chlorine or bromine) levels

Section 20.11

Tonsillitis

This section includes text excerpted from "Tonsillitis," MedlinePlus, National Institutes of Health (NIH), April 11, 2017.

What Are Tonsils?

Tonsils are lumps of tissue at the back of the throat. There are two of them, one on each side. Along with the adenoids, tonsils are part of the lymphatic system. The lymphatic system clears away infection and keeps body fluids in balance. Tonsils and adenoids work by trapping the germs coming in through the mouth and nose.

What Is Tonsillitis?

Tonsillitis is an inflammation (swelling) of the tonsils. Sometimes along with tonsillitis, the adenoids are also swollen.

What Causes Tonsillitis

The cause of tonsillitis is usually a viral infection. Bacterial infections such as strep throat can also cause tonsillitis.

Who Is at Risk for Tonsillitis?

Tonsillitis is most common in children over age 2. Almost every child in the United States gets it at least once. Tonsillitis caused by bacteria is more common in kids ages 5 to 15. Tonsillitis caused by a virus is more common in younger children.

Is Tonsillitis Contagious?

Although tonsillitis is not contagious, the viruses and bacteria that cause it are contagious. Frequent handwashing can help prevent spreading or catching the infections.

What Are the Symptoms of Tonsillitis?

The symptoms of tonsillitis include:

- A sore throat, which may be severe

- Red, swollen tonsils

- Trouble swallowing

- A white or yellow coating on the tonsils

- Swollen glands in the neck

- Fever

- Bad breath

When Should You Get Medical Help for Your Child?

You should call your healthcare provider if your child:

- Has a sore throat for more than two days

- Has trouble or pain when swallowing

- Feels very sick or very weak

You should get emergency care right away if your child:

- Has trouble breathing

- Starts drooling

- Has a lot of trouble swallowing

How Is Tonsillitis Diagnosed?

To diagnose tonsillitis, your child's healthcare provider will first ask you about your child's symptoms and medical history. The provider will look at your child's throat and neck, checking for things, such as redness or white spots on the tonsils and swollen lymph nodes.

Your child will probably also have one or more tests to check for strep throat, since it can cause tonsillitis and it requires treatment. It could be a rapid strep test, a throat culture, or both. For both tests, the provider uses a cotton swab to collect a sample of fluids from your child's tonsils and the back of the throat. With the rapid strep test, testing is done in the office, and you get the results within minutes. The throat culture is done in a lab, and it usually takes a few days to get the results. The throat culture is a more reliable test. So, sometimes if the rapid strep test is negative (meaning that it does not show any strep bacteria), the provider will also do a throat culture just to make sure that your child does not have strep.

What Are the Treatments for Tonsillitis?

Treatment for tonsillitis depends on the cause. If the cause is a virus, there is no medicine to treat it. If the cause is a bacterial infection, such as strep throat, your child will need to take antibiotics. It is important for your child to finish the antibiotics even if she or he feels better. If treatment stops too soon, some bacteria may survive and reinfect your child.

No matter what is causing the tonsillitis, there are some things you can do to help your child feel better. Make sure that your child:

- Gets a lot of rest

- Drinks plenty of fluids

- Tries eating soft foods if it hurts to swallow

- Tries eating warm liquids or cold foods, such as popsicles to soothe the throat

- Is not around cigarette smoke or do anything else that could irritate the throat

- Sleeps in a room with a humidifier

- Gargles with saltwater

- Sucks on a lozenge (but do not give them to children under four; they can choke on them)

- Takes an over-the-counter (OTC) pain reliever such as acetaminophen. Children and teenagers should not take aspirin.

In some cases, your child may need a tonsillectomy.

What Is a Tonsillectomy and Why Might Your Child Need One?

A tonsillectomy is surgery to remove the tonsils. Your child might need it if she or he:

- Keeps getting tonsillitis

- Has bacterial tonsillitis that does not get better with antibiotics

- Has tonsils are too big, and are causing trouble breathing or swallowing

Your child usually gets the surgery and goes home later that day. Very young children and people who have complications may need to stay in the hospital overnight. It can take a week or two before your child completely recovers from the surgery.

Chapter 21

Endocrine and Growth Disorders in Children

Chapter Contents

Section 21.1

Adrenal Gland Disorders

This section includes text excerpted from "Adrenal Insufficiency and
Addison Disease," National Institute of Diabetes and Digestive and
Kidney Diseases (NIDDK), October 19, 2019.

What Is Adrenal Insufficiency?

Adrenal insufficiency is a disorder that occurs when the adrenal
glands do not make enough of certain hormones. The adrenal glands
are located just above the kidneys. Adrenal insufficiency can be primary, secondary, or tertiary. Primary adrenal insufficiency is often
called "Addison disease."

Adrenal insufficiency can affect your child's body's ability to
respond to stress and maintain other essential life functions. With
treatment, most children with adrenal insufficiency can have a normal, active life.

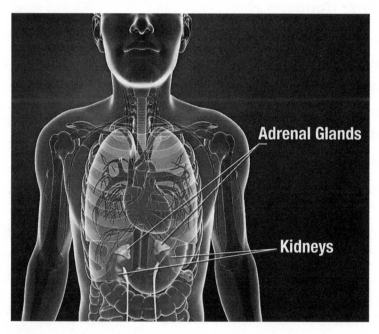

Figure 21.1. *Adrenal Gland*

*The adrenal glands, two small glands on top of the kidneys, make hormones that are
essential for life.*

Addison Disease

Addison disease occurs when the adrenal glands are damaged and cannot make enough of the hormone cortisol and sometimes the hormone aldosterone.

Secondary Adrenal Insufficiency

Secondary adrenal insufficiency starts in the pituitary—a pea-sized gland at the base of the brain. The pituitary makes adrenocorticotropin (ACTH), a hormone that tells the adrenal glands to make cortisol. If the pituitary does not make enough ACTH, the adrenal glands do not make enough cortisol. Over time, the adrenal glands can shrink and stop working.

Tertiary Adrenal Insufficiency

Tertiary adrenal insufficiency starts in the hypothalamus, a small area of the brain near the pituitary. The hypothalamus makes corticotropin-releasing hormone (CRH), a hormone that tells the pituitary to make ACTH. When the hypothalamus does not make enough CRH,

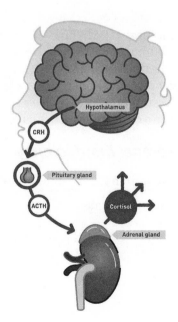

Figure 21.2. *Cortisol Creation*

CRH tells the pituitary to make ACTH, which in turn tells the adrenals to make cortisol.

the pituitary gland does not make enough ACTH. In turn, the adrenal glands do not make enough cortisol.

What Do Adrenal Hormones Do?

The adrenal glands make two main types of hormones: cortisol and aldosterone.

Cortisol

Cortisol is sometimes called the "stress hormone" because it helps the body respond to stress. Cortisol also helps:

- Control blood pressure
- Control blood glucose, also called "blood sugar"
- Reduce inflammation
- Control metabolism

Cortisol belongs to a class of hormones called "glucocorticoids."

Aldosterone

Aldosterone helps maintain the balance of the minerals sodium and potassium in blood. Sodium and potassium work together to control the salt and water balance in the body and help keep blood pressure stable. Both help to maintain normal nerve and muscle function. Potassium also helps heartbeat to stay regular.

Aldosterone belongs to a class of hormones called "mineralocorticoids."

Symptoms of Adrenal Insufficiency

The most common symptoms of adrenal insufficiency are:

- Chronic, or long-lasting, fatigue
- Muscle weakness
- Loss of appetite
- Weight loss
- Abdominal pain

Other symptoms of adrenal insufficiency can include:

- Nausea

- Vomiting

- Diarrhea

- Low blood pressure that drops further when standing up, causing dizziness or fainting

- Irritability and depression

- Joint pain

- Craving salty foods

- Hypoglycemia, or low blood glucose

- Irregular or no menstrual periods

Children with Addison disease may also have darkening of their skin. This darkening is most visible on scars; skin folds; pressure points, such as the elbows, knees, knuckles, and toes; lips; and mucous membranes, such as the lining of the cheek.

Because symptoms of adrenal insufficiency come on slowly over time, they may be overlooked or confused with other illnesses. Sometimes symptoms appear for the first time during an adrenal crisis. If your child always feel tired, weak, or are losing weight, ask the healthcare professional if your child might have adrenal insufficiency. Early treatment can help avoid an adrenal crisis.

Causes of Adrenal Insufficiency

Different types of adrenal insufficiency have different causes. The most common cause of adrenal insufficiency overall is suddenly stopping corticosteroids after taking them for a long time.

Addison Disease

Damage to the adrenal glands in Addison disease is usually caused by autoimmune disease—when your child's immune system attacks her or his body's own cells and organs. In developed countries, the autoimmune disease causes 8 or 9 of every 10 cases of Addison disease.

Certain infections can also cause Addison disease. Tuberculosis (TB) can damage the adrenal glands and used to be the most common cause of Addison disease. As treatment improved over the years, TB became a much less common cause. Children with human immunodeficiency virus (HIV), acquired immunodeficiency syndrome (AIDS), whose weakened immune systems cannot fight off infections that could cause Addison disease, are also at risk.

Less common causes of Addison disease are:

- Cancer cells in the adrenal glands.

- Surgical removal of the adrenal glands to treat other conditions.

- Bleeding into the adrenal glands.

- Genetic disorders that affect the way the adrenal glands develop or function.

- Certain medicines, such as antifungal medicines or etomidate, a type of general anesthesia.

Secondary Adrenal Insufficiency

Anything that affects the pituitary's ability to make ACTH can cause secondary adrenal insufficiency. The pituitary makes many different hormones, so ACTH may not be the only hormone that is lacking.

Causes of secondary adrenal insufficiency include:

- Autoimmune disease

- Pituitary tumors or infection

- Bleeding in the pituitary

- Genetic diseases that affect the way the pituitary gland develops or functions

- Surgical removal of the pituitary to treat other conditions

- Traumatic brain injury (TBI)

Tertiary Adrenal Insufficiency

The most common cause of tertiary adrenal insufficiency is suddenly stopping corticosteroids after taking them for a long time. Prescription doses of corticosteroids can cause higher levels of cortisol in your child's blood than her or his body normally makes. High levels in your child's blood for a long time cause the hypothalamus to make less CRH. Less CRH means less ACTH, which in turn causes the adrenal glands to stop making cortisol.

Once your child stop taking corticosteroids, their adrenal glands may be slow to start working again. To give them time to start making cortisol again, the doctor will gradually reduce their dose over a period of weeks or even months. Even so, their adrenal glands might not begin to work normally for many months. Your child's doctor should watch carefully for symptoms of adrenal insufficiency.

Tertiary adrenal insufficiency can also occur after Cushing syndrome is cured. Cushing syndrome is a hormonal disorder caused by high levels of cortisol in the blood for a long time. Sometimes Cushing syndrome is caused by tumors, usually noncancerous, in the pituitary or adrenal glands that make too much ACTH or cortisol. Once the tumors are surgically removed, the source of excess ACTH or cortisol is suddenly gone. Your child's adrenal glands may be slow to start working again.

Diagnosis of Adrenal Insufficiency

Your doctor will review your symptoms and run tests to confirm that your cortisol levels are low.

Review of Symptoms

In its early stages, adrenal insufficiency can be hard to diagnose since symptoms come on slowly. Your healthcare professional may suspect it after reviewing your medical history and symptoms. The next step is blood testing to see if your cortisol levels are too low and to help find the cause.

Blood Tests
Adrenocorticotropic Hormone Stimulation Test

The ACTH stimulation test is the test used most often to diagnose adrenal insufficiency. In this test, a healthcare professional will give you an intravenous (IV) injection of human-made ACTH, which is just like the ACTH your body makes. Your healthcare professional will take samples of your blood before and 30 minutes or 60 minutes after the injection. The cortisol levels in your blood samples are measured in a lab.

The normal response after an ACTH injection is a rise in blood cortisol levels. Children with Addison disease and most of those who have had secondary adrenal insufficiency for a long time have little or no increase in cortisol levels. The adrenal glands may be too damaged to respond to ACTH.

The ACTH test may not be accurate in children who have had secondary adrenal insufficiency for a shorter time because their adrenal glands have not yet shrunk and can still respond to ACTH.

Insulin Tolerance Test

If the results of the ACTH stimulation test are not clear or your doctor suspects a problem in the pituitary, you may have an insulin tolerance test (ITT). A healthcare professional will give you an IV injection of the hormone insulin, which lowers your levels of blood glucose. The dose is high enough to cause hypoglycemia, which occurs when your blood glucose level drops too low.

Hypoglycemia causes physical stress, which normally triggers the pituitary to make more ACTH. A healthcare professional will draw your blood at the beginning of the test and again every half hour during the next two hours. If your cortisol levels are low, your pituitary is not making enough ACTH, so your adrenal glands do not make enough cortisol. The ITT is the most reliable test to diagnose secondary adrenal insufficiency.

Very low blood glucose levels can be dangerous, so a healthcare professional must be present at all times during this test to make sure blood glucose levels do not drop too low. The ITT is not safe for children with heart disease, a history of seizures, and other serious illnesses.

Corticotropin-Releasing Hormone Stimulation Test

The CRH stimulation test is another option to help identify secondary insufficiency if the results of the ACTH test are not clear. This test can also tell secondary from tertiary adrenal insufficiency.

A healthcare professional will give you an IV injection of CRH and take samples of your blood before and 30, 60, 90, and 120 minutes after the injection to measure ACTH levels. If the pituitary is damaged, it will not make ACTH in response to CRH injection. This result shows secondary adrenal insufficiency. A slow rise in ACTH levels suggests tertiary adrenal insufficiency.

Tests to Diagnose Adrenal Insufficiency

Once doctors diagnosis and identify the type of adrenal insufficiency, they may use blood and imaging tests to find the exact cause.

Addison Disease
Antibody Blood Tests

A blood test can find antibodies that are present in autoimmune Addison disease. Antibodies are proteins made by your immune system to protect your body from bacteria or viruses. In autoimmune Addison disease, the antibodies mistakenly attack the adrenal glands. Most, but not all, children with autoimmune Addison disease have these antibodies. If the test shows antibodies, you don't need further testing.

Computed Tomography Scan

Computed tomography (CT) scans use a combination of x-rays and computer technology to create images of your organs and other internal structures. A CT scan of the abdomen can find changes in your adrenal glands. In autoimmune Addison disease, the glands are small or normal size and do not have other visible abnormalities.

Enlarged adrenal glands or a buildup of calcium in the glands can occur when Addison disease is caused by infection, bleeding in the adrenal glands, or cancer cells in the glands. However, these changes do not always occur in Addison disease caused by TB.

Tests for Tuberculosis

Tests to find tuberculosis (TB) include a chest x-ray, a urine test to look for the bacteria that causes TB, and a TB skin test. In the skin test, a healthcare professional injects a tiny amount of inactive TB bacteria under the skin of your forearm. If you develop a hard, raised bump or swelling on your arm, you have the TB bacteria in your body, even if you do not have active TB.

Secondary and Tertiary Adrenal Insufficiency
Magnetic Resonance Imaging

Magnetic resonance imaging (MRI) machines use radio waves and magnets to create detailed pictures of your internal organs and soft tissues without using x-rays. An MRI can look for changes in your pituitary and hypothalamus, such as large, noncancerous pituitary tumors.

Treatment of Adrenal Insufficiency

Your doctor will prescribe hormone medicines to replace the hormones that your adrenal glands are not making. You will need higher doses during times of physical stress.

Hormone Replacement

Cortisol is replaced with a corticosteroid, most often hydrocortisone, which you take two or three times a day by mouth. Less often, doctors prescribe prednisone or dexamethasone.

If your child's adrenal glands are not making aldosterone, you will take a medicine called "fludrocortisone," which helps balance the amount of sodium and fluids in your body. Children with secondary adrenal insufficiency usually make enough aldosterone, so they do not need to take this medicine.

Your doctor will adjust the dose of each medicine to meet your body's needs.

Treatment for adrenal crisis includes immediate IV injections of corticosteroids and large amounts of IV saline, a salt solution, with dextrose added. Dextrose is a type of sugar.

Treatment in Special Situations
Surgery

If you are having any type of surgery that uses general anesthesia, you may have treatment with IV corticosteroids and saline. IV treatment begins before surgery and continues until you are fully awake after surgery and can take medicine by mouth. Your doctor will adjust the "stress" dose as you recover until you are back to your presurgery dose.

A healthcare professional holds the opening of an IV drip bag, which hangs from an IV pole.

If you are having surgery that uses general anesthesia, you will need treatment with IV corticosteroids and saline.

Illness

Talk with your doctor about how to adjust your dose of corticosteroids during an illness. You will need to increase your dose if you have a high fever. Once you recover, your doctor will adjust your dose back to your regular, preillness level. You will need immediate medical attention if you have a severe infection or diarrhea, or are vomiting and cannot keep your corticosteroid pills down. Without treatment, in an emergency room if necessary, these conditions can lead to an adrenal crisis.

Injury or Other Serious Condition

If you have a severe injury, you may need a higher, "stress" dose of corticosteroids right after the injury and while you recover. The same is true if you have a serious health condition such as suddenly passing out or being in a coma. Often, you must get these stress doses intravenously. Once you recover, your doctor will adjust your dose back to regular, preinjury level.

Eating, Diet, and Nutrition

Some children with Addison disease who have low aldosterone can benefit from a high-sodium diet. A healthcare professional or a dietitian can recommend the best sodium sources and how much sodium you should have each day.

Section 21.2

Constitutional Growth Delay

"Constitutional Growth Delay," © 2017 Omnigraphics.
Reviewed September 2019.

Causes of Constitutional Growth Delay

Experts believe that constitutional growth delay has a genetic component, since between 60 percent and 90 percent of children affected by the condition have a family member who was also affected. Heredity may account for delays in the release of hormones that are responsible for initiating the changes associated with puberty, such as the maturation of the ovaries and testicles.

In children with constitutional growth delay, the pattern of development of secondary sexual characteristics is normal, but the age at which it begins is much later than average. The absence or disruption of this normal pattern may indicate hormonal deficiencies that warrant further investigation. Growth that is delayed or slower than expected can also result from other medical conditions, such as chronic diseases or infections, endocrine disorders, autoimmune disorders, inflammatory bowel disease, or poor nutrition. Some of the syndromes that can mimic constitutional growth delay include Turner syndrome, Noonan syndrome, Kallmann syndrome, and Russell-Silver syndrome. These conditions must be ruled out in order to form a diagnosis of constitutional growth delay.

Diagnosis of Constitutional Growth Delay

In diagnosing constitutional growth delay, a doctor will begin by taking a complete medical history of the child. The doctor is likely to inquire about the child's growth pattern over time, eating habits or feeding schedule, and any medications or supplements they might take. The doctor is also likely to ask about any other symptoms that might be present, especially delays in social interactions or other skill development. Finally, the doctor will likely inquire about the child's biological parents, including their height, weight, and age upon reaching puberty.

Next, the doctor will perform a physical examination that includes measurements of the child's height, weight, and head circumference. The doctor may order additional laboratory tests as well, including blood tests, urine tests, and stool samples to rule out infections, diseases, and nutritional deficiencies. In addition, an x-ray will typically be conducted on the child's left hand and wrist to determine the child's "bone age," or degree of skeletal maturation. The growth plates in long bones in the forearm remain open until the growth spurt that accompanies puberty. Afterward, the bones begin to fuse, meaning that further growth will be limited. The extent of skeletal maturation provides valuable clues about whether a child's growth is merely delayed or is being limited by some other biological factor.

Social and Psychological Effects of Constitutional Growth Delay

Once other causes of growth delay have been ruled out, the main priority is helping the child cope with the social and psychological challenges that often accompany the condition. Children with constitutional growth delay are likely to be quite short for their age and appear much younger than their friends. As their peers reach puberty and show signs of sexual maturation, they may feel self-conscious, left out, and anxious about their future sexual function and fertility.

Since adolescence is fraught with social changes, concerns surrounding delayed growth can create a serious emotional or psychological disturbance for some teenagers. Some may respond by behaving immaturely, or acting the age they appear rather than their chronological age. Others may respond to teasing or bullying with aggressive, antisocial behavior. Under most circumstances, constitutional growth delay does not require treatment. Doctors merely provide reassurance that children with the condition are developing normally, will experience the onset of puberty soon, and will eventually reach an appropriate adult height. But children who have trouble coping with the condition may need therapeutic help to accelerate the timing of puberty and growth.

Treatment of Constitutional Growth Delay

While medical treatment is not necessary for most cases of constitutional growth delay, it may be indicated for patients who experience psychological distress due to their slow patterns of growth and development. Short courses of therapy with growth hormones or sex hormones can accelerate growth and advance the onset of puberty. Although hormone therapy does not increase adult height, it does help speed up the process so that teenagers feel less different than their peers.

One potential benefit of medical treatment for constitutional growth delay is that it may help protect adult bone mass. Because of the activity of sex hormones and growth hormones, puberty is the peak period for bone mineralization. In fact, more than half of all bone calcium accumulates between the ages of 11 and 14 for girls, and 14 and 17 for boys. As a result, delays in the circulation of these hormones may increase the risk of osteopenia, or reduced bone mass, in adulthood. Hormone therapy thus has the potential to increase adult bone mass in children with constitutional growth delay.

References

1. Alter, Craig, and Sue Smith. "Constitutional Delay of Growth," MAGIC Foundation, n.d.

2. Clark, Pamela A. "Constitutional Growth Delay Clinical Presentation," Medscape, July 28, 2016.

3. "Delayed Growth," Agency for Healthcare Research and Quality (AHRQ), U.S. Department of Health and Human Services (HHS),

4. Stanhope, Richard. "Constitutional Delay of Growth and Puberty," Child Growth Foundation (CGF), September 2000.

Section 21.3

Growth Hormone Deficiency

This section includes text excerpted from "Isolated Growth Hormone Deficiency," Genetics Home Reference (GHR), National Institutes of Health (NIH), February 2012. Reviewed September 2019.

What Is Growth Hormone Deficiency?

Isolated growth hormone deficiency (GHD) is a condition caused by a severe shortage or absence of growth hormone. Growth hormone is a protein that is necessary for the normal growth of the body's bones and tissues. Because they do not have enough of this hormone, children with isolated growth hormone deficiency commonly experience a failure to grow at the expected rate and have unusually short stature. This condition is usually apparent by early childhood.

What Are the Types of Growth Hormone Deficiency?

There are four types of isolated growth hormone deficiency differentiated by the severity of the condition, the gene involved, and the inheritance pattern.

Isolated growth hormone deficiency type IA is caused by an absence of growth hormone and is the most severe of all the types. In children with type IA, growth failure is evident in infancy as affected babies are shorter than normal at birth.

Children with isolated growth hormone deficiency type IB produce very low levels of growth hormone. As a result, type IB is characterized by short stature, but this growth failure is typically not as severe as in type IA. Growth failure in children with type IB is usually apparent in early to mid-childhood.

Individuals with isolated growth hormone deficiency type II have very low levels of growth hormone and short stature that varies in severity. Growth failure in these individuals is usually evident in early to mid-childhood. It is estimated that nearly half of the individuals with type II have underdevelopment of the pituitary gland (pituitary hypoplasia). The pituitary gland is located at the base of the brain and produces many hormones, including growth hormone.

Isolated growth hormone deficiency type III is similar to type II in that affected individuals have very low levels of growth hormone and short stature that varies in severity. Growth failure in type III is usually evident in early to mid-childhood. Children with type III may also have a weakened immune system and are prone to frequent infections. They produce very few B cells, which are specialized white blood cells (WBCs) that help protect the body against infection (agammaglobulinemia).

Frequency of Growth Hormone Deficiency

The incidence of isolated growth hormone deficiency is estimated to be 1 in 4,000 to 10,000 individuals worldwide.

Section 21.4

Idiopathic Short Stature

"Idiopathic Short Stature," © 2017 Omnigraphics.
Reviewed September 2019.

"Idiopathic short stature" (ISS) is the term used to describe a child who is considerably shorter than others of the same age, sex, and genetic background when there is no known medical cause for the condition. ("Idiopathic" refers to a condition that arises spontaneously with no discernible origin.) Although ISS is not itself considered a disease, children who fit the definition need to be evaluated by a growth specialist in order to rule out the numerous diseases and disorders that can cause short stature before a diagnosis of ISS can be made.

When to See a Growth Specialist

Accurate height measurement is an ongoing process that should be charted by a pediatrician or family doctor throughout a child's growth years. The American Academy of Pediatrics (AAP) recommends measuring height and weight at birth, at age 2 to 4 days, periodically from 1 to 24 months, and then yearly until age 21. In this way, growth can be monitored and compared to established standards, and if there is significant deviation further evaluation and testing can be initiated.

If parents suspect that their child is small for her or his age, or if the child appears to have stopped growing, the regular physician should be consulted first for an opinion. The doctor will compare the child's height and rate of growth to demographic standards, perform a physical examination, and perhaps order some preliminary tests, such as blood work. If appropriate, the physician may then refer the child to a specialist, such as a pediatric endocrinologist.

Diagnosis of Idiopathic Short Stature

One of the first things a specialist will do is confirm that the child is actually of short stature, beginning with measurements of height, weight, and arm and leg lengths. Technically, that would mean that she or he is two standard deviations (SD) or more below average for someone of the same age, race, ethnic background, and geographical origin. The doctor will also take a thorough family history, both to learn about the height of close relatives and to ask about genetic disorders that might affect growth.

If short stature is confirmed, the next step is to determine whether it is idiopathic or the result of a medical condition. Beginning with a physical examination, the doctor would then likely order a series of tests that might include:

- Complete blood count (CBC), an indicator of overall health

- Other blood work to check kidney, liver, and immune system function

- Thyroid function tests, blood tests that ensure the thyroid gland is working properly

- Growth hormone stimulation, which tests the function of the pituitary gland

- Insulin growth factor 1 test to identify growth hormone deficiency

- Bone tests, including x-rays and scans, such as a magnetic resonance imaging (MRI)

Because short stature can be the result of such a wide variety of diseases or genetic disorders, diagnosing the underlying pathology, if any, can be a lengthy process. Eliminating possible causes can take weeks, or even months, depending on the condition and the individual child.

Causes of Idiopathic Short Stature

Since growth rate and height are the result of so many factors, ranging from genetic traits to nutrition to disease, the causes of short stature are numerous and varied. Some possible causes include:

- Growth hormone deficiency
- Thyroid disorders, such as Cushing disease and hypothyroidism
- Juvenile rheumatoid arthritis
- Celiac disease
- Kidney disorders
- Genetic conditions, such as Turner syndrome and Down syndrome
- Sickle cell anemia
- Gastrointestinal disease
- Rickets
- Malnutrition

If no specific medical cause of short stature can be determined, then it may be diagnosed as ISS. In that case, assuming all relevant tests have been completed and the conditions is not judged to be dangerous, the physician may recommend regular follow-up examinations, testing, and measurement to monitor the child's condition and growth patterns.

Treatment of Idiopathic Short Stature

If testing reveals an underlying medical cause of short stature, then treatment will be based on that disease or disorder. For example, hypothyroidism is normally treated with thyroid hormone replacement pills; juvenile rheumatoid arthritis could be treated with nonsteroidal anti-inflammatory drugs, such as ibuprofen or naproxen; and celiac disease would be addressed with a gluten-free diet.

Children for whom testing reveals growth hormone deficiency are commonly treated with growth hormone (GH) injections. These can be given at home, usually once per day, and have proven effective, particularly when treatment is begun at least five years before the onset of puberty.

In 2003, the use of GH was approved by the U.S. Food and Drug Administration (FDA) for the treatment of children with ISS, if a doctor predicts that they will attain a very short final height (under 4 feet 11 inches for a girl, and under 5 feet 4 inches for a boy). Again, the treatments, when started well before puberty, have been shown to aid growth and increase final height. But the use of GH to treat ISS is not without controversy.

For one thing, children with ISS, by definition, have normal GH levels, and some healthcare professionals are not comfortable administering medicine that tests indicate is not required. Others feel it unwise to administer hormone treatments—or any medication—when the condition is not physically harmful and the underlying cause is unknown. Another point of contention is that response to GH is highly variable, with some children experiencing only a moderate increase in height.

In addition, GH treatments can be very expensive and, if low hormone levels have not been supported by tests, some insurance plans will not cover the cost. And although GH is generally considered a safe treatment, its benefits must be weighed against the possible side effects, which can include allergic reactions, headaches, blurred vision, nervousness, and, in rare cases, chest pain, abdominal pain, rash, nausea, and vomiting.

Resources

1. "Childhood Growth and Height Issues," Children's Hospital of Philadelphia, n.d.

2. "Controversies in the Definition and Treatment of Idiopathic Short Stature (ISS)," National Center for Biotechnology Information (NCBI), February 1, 2009.

3. Geffner, Mitchell, MD. "Idiopathic Short Stature," MAGIC Foundation, n.d

4. Lee, Kimberly G., MD, MSc, IBCLC. "Short Stature," University of Maryland Medical Center (UMMC), December 12, 2014.

5. Rogol, Alan D., MD, PhD. "Causes of Short Stature," UpToDate.com, August 16, 2016.

6. Rosenbloom, Arlan L., MD. " Idiopathic Short Stature: Conundrums of Definition and Treatment," National Center for Biotechnology Information (NCBI), March 12, 2009.

7. Sinha, Sunil, MD. "Short Stature," Medscape, June 17, 2016.

Section 21.5

Klinefelter Syndrome

This section includes text excerpted from "Klinefelter Syndrome (KS): Condition Information," *Eunice Kennedy Shriver* National Institute of Child Health and Human Development (NICHD), December 1, 2016, Reviewed September 2019.

What Is Klinefelter Syndrome?

The term "Klinefelter syndrome" (KS), describes a set of features that can occur in a male who is born with an extra X chromosome in his cells. It is named after Dr. Henry Klinefelter, who identified the condition in the 1940s.

Usually, every cell in a male's body, except sperm and red blood cells, contains 46 chromosomes. The 45th and 46th chromosomes—the X and Y chromosomes—are sometimes called "sex chromosomes" because they determine a person's sex. Normally, males have one X and one Y chromosome, making them XY. Males with KS have an extra X chromosome, making them XXY.

KS is sometimes called "47,XXY" (47 refers to total chromosomes) or the "XXY condition." Those with KS are sometimes called "XXY males."

Some males with KS may have both XY cells and XXY cells in their bodies. This is called "mosaic." Mosaic males may have fewer symptoms of KS depending on the number of XY cells they have in their bodies and where these cells are located. For example, males who have normal XY cells in their testes may be fertile.

In very rare cases, males might have two or more extra X chromosomes in their cells, for instance, XXXY or XXXXY, or an extra Y, such as XXYY. This is called "poly-X Klinefelter syndrome," and it causes more severe symptoms.

What Causes Klinefelter Syndrome

The extra chromosome results from a random error that occurs when a sperm or egg is formed; this error causes an extra X cell to be included each time the cell divides to form new cells. In very rare cases, more than one extra X or an extra Y is included.

What Are Common Symptoms of Klinefelter Syndrome?

Because XXY males do not really appear different from other males and because they may not have any or have mild symptoms, XXY males often do not know they have KS.

In other cases, males with KS may have mild or severe symptoms. Whether or not a male with KS has visible symptoms depends on many factors, including how much testosterone his body makes, if he is mosaic (with both XY and XXY cells), and his age when the condition is diagnosed and treated.

KS symptoms fall into these main categories:

• Physical symptoms

• Language and learning symptoms

• Social and behavioral symptoms

• Symptoms of poly-X KS

Physical Symptoms

Many physical symptoms of KS result from low testosterone levels in the body. The degree of symptoms differs based on the amount of testosterone needed for a specific age or developmental stage and the amount of testosterone the body makes or has available.

During the first few years of life, when the need for testosterone is low, most XXY males do not show any obvious differences from typical male infants and young boys. Some may have slightly weaker muscles, meaning they might sit up, crawl, and walk slightly later than average. For example, on average, baby boys with KS do not start walking until age of 18 months.

After age 5 years, when compared to typically developing boys, boys with KS may be slightly:

• Taller

• Fatter around the belly

• Clumsier

• Slower in developing motor skills, coordination, speed, and muscle strength

Puberty for boys with KS usually starts normally. But because their bodies make less testosterone than nonKS boys, their pubertal development may be disrupted or slow.

Language and Learning Symptoms

Most males with KS have normal intelligence quotients (IQs) and successfully complete education at all levels. (IQ is a frequently used intelligence measure, but does not include emotional, creative, or other types of intelligence.) Between 25 percent and 85 percent of all males with KS have some kind of learning or language-related problem, which makes it more likely that they will need some extra help in school. Without this help or intervention, KS males might fall behind their classmates as schoolwork becomes harder.

Social and Behavioral Symptoms

Many of the social and behavioral symptoms in KS may result from the language and learning difficulties. For instance, boys with KS who have language difficulties might hold back socially and could use help building social relationships.

Boys with KS, compared to typically developing boys, tend to be:

- Quieter
- Less assertive or self-confident
- More anxious or restless
- Less physically active
- More helpful and eager to please
- More obedient or more ready to follow directions

In the teenage years, boys with KS may feel their differences more strongly. As a result, these teen boys are at higher risk of depression, substance abuse, and behavioral disorders. Some teens might withdraw, feel sad, or act out their frustration and anger.

As adults, most men with KS have lives similar to those of men without KS. They successfully complete high school, college, and other levels of education. They have successful and meaningful careers and professions. They have friends and families.

Contrary to research findings published several decades ago, males with KS are no more likely to have serious psychiatric disorders or to get into trouble with the law.

Symptoms of Poly-X KS

Males with poly-X KS have more than one extra X chromosome, so their symptoms might be more pronounced than in males with KS. In childhood, they may also have seizures, crossed eyes, constipation, and recurrent ear infections. Poly-KS males might also show slight differences in other physical features.

What Are the Treatments for Symptoms in Klinefelter Syndrome?

It is important to remember that because symptoms can be mild, many males with KS are never diagnosed or treated.

The earlier in life that KS symptoms are recognized and treated, the more likely it is that the symptoms can be reduced or eliminated. It is especially helpful to begin treatment by early puberty. Puberty is a time of rapid physical and psychological change, and treatment can successfully limit symptoms. However, treatment can bring benefits at any age.

The type of treatment needed depends on the type of symptoms being treated.

How Do Healthcare Providers Diagnose Klinefelter Syndrome?

The only way to confirm the presence of an extra chromosome is by a karyotype test. A healthcare provider will take a small blood or skin sample and send it to a laboratory, where a technician inspects the cells under a microscope to find the extra chromosome. A karyotype test shows the same results at any time in a person's life.

Tests for chromosome disorders, including KS, may be done before birth. To obtain tissue or liquid for this test, a pregnant woman undergoes chorionic villus sampling or amniocentesis. These types of prenatal testing carry a small risk for miscarriage and are not routinely conducted unless the woman has a family history of chromosomal disorders, has other medical problems, or is above 35 years of age.

Section 21.6

Precocious and Delayed Puberty

This section contains text excerpted from the following sources: Text in this section begins with excerpts from "Puberty and Precocious Puberty," *Eunice Kennedy Shriver* National Institute of Child Health and Human Development (NICHD), December 1, 2016. Reviewed September 2019; Text beginning with the heading "What Causes Normal Puberty, Precocious Puberty, and Delayed Puberty" is excerpted from "Puberty and Precocious Puberty: Condition Information," *Eunice Kennedy Shriver* National Institute of Child Health and Human Development (NICHD), December 1, 2016. Reviewed September 2019.

The onset of puberty, the time in life when a person becomes sexually mature, typically occurs between ages 8 and 13 for girls, and ages 9 and 14 for boys. Precocious puberty is puberty that begins abnormally early, and delayed puberty is puberty that begins abnormally late.

What Causes Normal Puberty, Precocious Puberty, and Delayed Puberty
Normal Puberty

Puberty is the body's natural process of sexual maturation. Puberty's trigger lies in a small part of the brain called the "hypothalamus," a gland that secretes a gonadotropin-releasing hormone (GnRH). GnRH stimulates the pituitary gland, a pea-sized organ connected to the bottom of the hypothalamus, to emit two hormones: luteinizing hormone (LH) and follicle-stimulating hormone (FSH). These two hormones signal the female and male sex organs (ovaries and testes, respectively) to begin releasing the appropriate sex hormones, including estrogens and testosterone, which launch the other signs of puberty in the body.

Precocious Puberty

In the majority of cases of precocious puberty, no underlying cause can be identified. When a cause cannot be identified, the condition is called "idiopathic precocious puberty."

Sometimes the cause is an abnormality involving the brain. In other children, the signs of puberty occur because of a problem, such as a tumor or genetic abnormality in the ovaries, testes, or adrenal glands, causing the overproduction of sex hormones.

Precocious puberty can be divided into two categories, depending on where in the body the abnormality occurs—*central precocious puberty* and *peripheral precocious puberty.*

Central Precocious Puberty

This type of early puberty, also known as "gonadotropin-dependent precocious puberty," occurs when the abnormality is located in the brain. The brain signals the pituitary gland to begin puberty at an early age. Central precocious puberty (CPP) is the most common form of precocious puberty and affects many more girls than boys.

The causes of central precocious puberty include:

- Brain tumors

- Prior radiation to the brain

- Prior infection of the brain

- Other brain abnormalities

Peripheral Precocious Puberty

This form of early puberty is also called "gonadotropin-independent precocious puberty." In peripheral precocious puberty, the abnormality is not in the brain but in the testicles, ovaries, or adrenal glands, causing overproduction of sex hormones, such as testosterone and estrogens.

Peripheral precocious puberty (PPP) may be caused by:

- Tumors of the ovary, testis, or adrenal gland

- In boys, tumors that secrete a hormone called "hCG, or human chorionic gonadotropin."

- Certain rare genetic syndromes, such as McCune-Albright syndrome (MAS) or familial male precocious puberty (FMPP)

- Severe hypothyroidism, in which the thyroid gland secretes abnormally low levels of hormones

- Disorders of the adrenal gland, such as congenital adrenal hyperplasia

- Exposure of the child to medicines or creams that contain estrogens or androgens

Delayed Puberty

Many children with delayed puberty will eventually go through otherwise normal puberty, just at a late age. Sometimes, this delay occurs because the child is just maturing more slowly than average, a condition called "constitutional delay of puberty." This condition often runs in families.

Puberty can be delayed in children who have not gotten proper nutrition due to long-term illnesses. Also, some young girls who undergo intense physical training for a sport, such as running or gymnastics, start puberty later than normal.

In other cases, the delay in puberty is not just due to slow maturation but occurs because the child has a long-term medical condition known as "hypogonadism," in which the sex glands (the testes in men and the ovaries in women) produce few or no hormones. Hypogonadism can be divided into two categories: secondary hypogonadism and primary hypogonadism.

- *Secondary hypogonadism* (central hypogonadism or hypogonadotropic hypogonadism, is caused by a problem with the pituitary gland or hypothalamus (part of the brain). In secondary hypogonadism, the hypothalamus and the pituitary gland fail to signal the gonads to properly release sex hormones. Causes of secondary hypogonadism include:

- Kallmann syndrome, a genetic problem that also diminishes the sense of smell

- Isolated hypogonadotropic hypogonadism, a genetic condition that only affects sexual development but not the sense of smell

- Prior radiation, trauma, surgery, or other injuries to the brain or pituitary

- Tumors of the brain or pituitary

- In *primary hypogonadism,* the problem lies in the ovaries or testes, which fail to make sex hormones normally. Some causes include:

- Genetic disorders, especially Turner syndrome (in women) and Klinefelter syndrome (in men)

- Certain autoimmune disorders

- Developmental disorders

445

- Radiation or chemotherapy
- Infection
- Surgery

How Do Healthcare Providers Diagnose Precocious Puberty and Delayed Puberty?

To identify whether a child is entering puberty, a pediatrician (a physician specializing in the treatment of children) will carefully examine the following:

- In girls, the growth of pubic hair and breasts
- In boys, the increase in size of the testicles and penis and the growth of pubic hair

The pediatrician will compare what she or he finds against the Tanner scale, a five-point scale that gauges the extent of puberty development in children.

Precocious Puberty

After giving a child a complete physical examination and analyzing her or his medical history, a healthcare provider may perform tests to diagnose precocious puberty, including:

- A blood test to check the level of hormones, such as the gonadotropins (luteinizing hormone (LH) and follicle-stimulating hormone (FSH)), estradiol, testosterone, dehydroepiandrosterone sulfate (DHEAS), and thyroid hormones
- A gonadotropin-releasing hormone agonist (GnRHa) stimulation test, which can tell whether a child's precocious puberty is gonadotropin-dependent or gonadotropin-independent
- Measuring blood 17-hydroxyprogesterone to test for congenital adrenal hyperplasia
- A "bone age" x-ray to determine if bones are growing at a normal rate

The healthcare provider may also use imaging techniques to rule out a tumor or other organ abnormality as a cause. These imaging methods may include:

- Ultrasound (sonography) to examine the gonads. An ultrasound painlessly creates an image on a computer screen of blood vessels and tissues, allowing a healthcare provider to monitor organs and blood flow in real-time.

- A magnetic resonance imaging (MRI) scan of the brain and pituitary gland using an instrument that produces detailed images of organs and bodily structures

Delayed Puberty

To diagnose hypogonadotropic hypogonadism, a healthcare provider may prescribe these tests:

- Blood tests to measure hormone levels

- Blood tests to measure if the pituitary gland can correctly respond to GnRH

- An MRI of the brain and pituitary gland

What Are Common Treatments for Problems of Puberty?

Precocious Puberty

There are a number of reasons to treat precocious puberty.

Treatment for precocious puberty can help stop puberty until the child is closer to the normal time for sexual development. One reason to consider treating precocious puberty is that rapid growth and bone maturation, caused by precocious puberty, can prevent a child from reaching her or his full height potential. Children grow rapidly in height during puberty and reach their final adult height after puberty. Children who go through puberty too early may not reach their full adult height potential because their growth stops too soon.

Another reason to consider treating precocious puberty is that a young child may not be psychologically ready for the physical and hormonal changes that occur in puberty.

However, not all children with precocious puberty require treatment, particularly if the onset of puberty is only slightly early. The goal of treatment is to prevent the production of sex hormones to prevent the early halt of growth, short stature in adulthood, emotional effects, social problems, and problems with libido (especially in boys).

If precocious puberty is caused by a specific medical problem, treating the underlying problem can often stop the progression of precocious puberty. In addition, precocious puberty can often be stopped by medical treatment to block the hormones that cause puberty. For example, medications called "gonadotropin-releasing hormone agonists" (GnRHa) are used to treat central precocious puberty. These medications, some of which are injected, suppress the production of luteinizing hormone (LH) and follicle-stimulating hormone (FSH).

Delayed Puberty

With delayed puberty or hypogonadism, treatment varies with the origin of the problem but may involve:

- In males, testosterone injections, skin patches, or gel

- In females, estrogen and/or progesterone given as pills or skin patches

Section 21.7

Turner Syndrome

This section includes text excerpted from "Turner Syndrome: Condition Information," *Eunice Kennedy Shriver* National Institute of Child Health and Human Development (NICHD), December 1, 2016. Reviewed September 2019.

Turner syndrome is a disorder caused by a partially or completely missing X chromosome. This condition affects only females.

Most people have 46 chromosomes in each cell—23 from their mother and 23 from their father. The 23rd pair of chromosomes is called the "sex chromosomes"—X and Y—because they determine whether a person is male or female. Females have two X chromosomes (XX) in most of their cells, and males have one X chromosome and one Y chromosome (XY) in most of their cells. A female with all of her chromosomes is referred to as 46, XX. A male is 46, XY.

Turner syndrome most often occurs when a female has one normal X chromosome, but the other X chromosome is missing (45, X). Other forms of Turner syndrome result when one of the two chromosomes is partially missing or altered in some way.

What Are the Symptoms of Turner Syndrome?

Turner syndrome causes a variety of symptoms in girls and women. For some children, symptoms are mild, but for others, Turner syndrome can cause serious health problems. In general, women with Turner syndrome have female sex characteristics, but these characteristics are underdeveloped compared to the typical female. Turner syndrome can affect:

- **Appearance.** Features of Turner syndrome may include a short neck with a webbed appearance, low hairline at the back of the neck, low-set ears, hands and feet that are swollen or puffy at birth, and soft nails that turn upward.

- **Stature.** Girls with Turner syndrome grow more slowly than other children. Without treatment, they tend to have short stature (around four feet, eight inches) as adults.

- **Puberty.** Most girls with Turner syndrome do not start puberty naturally.

- **Cardiovascular.** Turner syndrome can cause problems with the heart or major blood vessels. In addition, some women and girls with Turner syndrome have high blood pressure.

- **Kidney.** Kidney function is usually normal in Turner syndrome, but some of the children with this condition have kidneys that look abnormal.

- **Diabetes.** Children with Turner syndrome are at higher risk for type 2 diabetes.

- **Thyroid.** Many children with Turner syndrome have thyroid problems. The most common one is hypothyroidism or an underactive thyroid gland.

- **Cognitive.** Children with Turner syndrome have normal intelligence. Some, however, have problems learning mathematics and can have trouble with visual-spatial coordination (such as determining the relative positions of objects in space).

What Causes Turner Syndrome

Turner syndrome occurs when part or all of an X chromosome is missing from most or all of the cells in a girl's body. A girl normally receives one X chromosome from each parent. The error that leads to the missing chromosome appears to happen during the formation of the egg or sperm.

Most commonly, a girl with Turner syndrome has only one X chromosome. Occasionally, she may have a partial second X chromosome. Because she is missing part or all of a chromosome, certain genes are missing. The loss of these genes leads to the symptoms of Turner syndrome.

Sometimes, girls with Turner syndrome have some cells that are missing one X chromosome (45, X) and some that are normal. This is because not every cell in the body is exactly the same, so some cells might have the chromosome, while others might not. This condition is called "mosaicism." If the second sex chromosome is lost from most of a girl's cells, then it is likely that she will have symptoms of Turner syndrome. If the chromosome is missing from only some of her cells, she may have no symptoms or only mild symptoms.

How Do Healthcare Providers Diagnose Turner Syndrome?

Healthcare providers use a combination of physical symptoms and the results of a genetic blood test, called a "karyotype," to determine the chromosomal characteristics of the cells in a female's body. The test will show if one of the X chromosomes is partially or completely missing.

Turner syndrome also can be diagnosed during pregnancy by testing the cells in the amniotic fluid. Newborns may be diagnosed after heart problems are detected or after certain physical features, such as swollen hands and feet or webbed skin on the neck, are noticed. Other characteristics, such as widely spaced nipples or low-set ears, also may lead to a suspicion of Turner syndrome. Some girls may be diagnosed as teenagers because of a slow growth rate or a lack of puberty-related changes. Still, others may be diagnosed as adults when they have difficulty becoming pregnant.

What Are Common Treatments for Turner Syndrome?

Although there is no cure for Turner syndrome, some treatments can help minimize its symptoms. These include:

- **Human growth hormone.** If given in early childhood, hormone injections can often increase adult height by a few inches.

- **Estrogen replacement therapy (ERT).** ERT can help start the secondary sexual development that normally begins at puberty (around age 12). This includes breast development and the development of wider hips. Healthcare providers may prescribe a combination of estrogen and progesterone to girls who have not started menstruating by age 15. ERT also provides protection against bone loss.

Regular health checks and access to a wide variety of specialists are important to care for the various health problems that can result from Turner syndrome. These include ear infections, high blood pressure, and thyroid problems.

Chapter 22

Gastrointestinal Disorders in Children

Chapter Contents

Section 22.1

Functional Abdominal Pain

"Functional Abdominal Pain," © 2017 Omnigraphics.
Reviewed September 2019.

Functional abdominal pain (FAP) in children refers to chronic stomachaches that have no apparent underlying physical cause. The pain may be intermittent or constant and is usually experienced in the area surrounding the navel. According to the medical definition, functional abdominal pain occurs at least once per week over a period of two months or more. Even if the child undergoes extensive medical examination and testing, no abnormality, infection, or blockage will be found to explain the condition. FAP is relatively common, affecting between 10 and 15 percent of school-aged children—most of whom are otherwise healthy—and accounting for one-fourth of all visits to gastroenterologists by children and adolescents.

Although the exact mechanism is not well understood, doctors believe that FAP is caused by increased nerve sensitivity in the digestive organs. This sensitivity may be triggered by psychological stress, constipation, or some sort of infection in the digestive system. As a result, the nerves and muscles that help move food through the stomach and intestines overreact to normal functions, such as gas or bloating, that usually only cause mild discomfort. Instead, children with FAP experience recurrent episodes of significant pain that may interfere with their participation in school, sports, and family activities. While the pain is real, the lack of an identifiable cause can be frustrating or frightening for children and parents.

Causes and Risk Factors of Functional Abdominal Pain

Occasional, mild abdominal pain is common in children and does not usually require medical attention. It may be caused by such issues as constipation, gas, food allergy, lactose intolerance, food poisoning, colic, or a viral, bacterial, or parasitic infestation of the digestive tract. Chronic abdominal pain also has many possible causes, including appendicitis, acid reflux, ulcers, gallstones, hernia, intestinal obstruction, urinary-tract infection, and cancer. These conditions warrant medical examination and treatment.

If a child experiences frequent, recurring abdominal pain—but medical examination and testing rules out other possible causes—then the likely cause is functional abdominal pain. The triggers for FAP vary depending on the individual and may be difficult to identify. In many cases the condition appears to be related to traumatic experiences or emotional disturbances. FAP also tends to affect children with underlying anxiety or depression, as these conditions are often associated with an increased or exaggerated pain response. Many children with FAP have previously contracted a gastrointestinal infection. The condition may also have a genetic component, as many children with FAP have a family member who also experienced recurrent abdominal pain in childhood.

Symptoms of Functional Abdominal Pain

The main symptom of FAP is recurrent pain that centers around the navel, although the characteristics of the pain may vary. FAP includes different types or categories, each of which has its own distinct symptoms:

- **Functional dyspepsia (FD)** includes upper abdominal pain along with nausea, vomiting, and loss of appetite.

- **Irritable bowel syndrome (IBS)** includes abdominal pain along with changes in bowel movements, such as constipation or diarrhea, or abdominal pain that is relieved by bowel movements.

- **Abdominal migraine** includes recurring attacks of stomach pain along with nausea, vomiting, and pallor that last between 2 and 72 hours.

Diagnosis of Functional Abdominal Pain

The first step in diagnosis involves taking a medical history. The doctor is likely to inquire about the location and severity of the child's abdominal pain, how often it occurs, and how long each episode lasts. The doctor may also ask the patient to keep a food log to identify any relationships between foods and beverages and abdominal pain. Finally, the doctor is likely to inquire about the patient's overall health, including sleep, exercise, and psychological stress.

The next step in diagnosis involves physical examination and testing to rule out underlying health conditions that could be contributing to the abdominal pain. The initial screening tests are likely to include blood, urine, and stool samples. If any concerning symptoms are present—such as weight loss, poor growth, fever, joint pains, unusual rashes, or blood in the vomit or stool—then further testing may be indicated. Additional tests that may be performed include an ultrasound or computerized tomography (CT) scan of the abdomen or an endoscopy of the digestive tract. If all of these tests fail to turn up evidence of abnormalities, infections, blockages, or other disorders, then the diagnosis for an otherwise healthy child is likely to be FAP.

Treatment of Functional Abdominal Pain

One of the challenges in treating FAP is that no specific cause of the symptoms can be found. It is important to note that FAP symptoms are nonetheless real and not simply a product of the child's imagination or an example of attention-seeking behavior. Although no single cure is available, many patients find relief from some combination of the following treatment options:

- Identifying sources of emotional or psychological stress and assisting the child in developing coping skills and relaxation techniques

- Undergoing psychological treatments, such as cognitive-behavioral therapy

- Implementing dietary changes, such as avoiding greasy and spicy foods, cabbage, beans, caffeine, fruit juices, carbonated beverages, and anything sweetened with sorbitol

- Taking medications, such as tricyclic antidepressants, anti-spasmodic medications, laxatives, or acid reducers

Nearly half of all children with FAP experience improvement in symptoms within a few months, either on their own or with some form of treatment. Studies have shown that parental acceptance of the reality of the condition, along with family support for the emotional needs of the child, is key to recovery. The outlook is not as positive for children whose FAP is related to family dysfunction, sexual abuse, or stressful life events. Up to 30 percent of children with FAP may continue to experience chronic abdominal pain in adulthood, and evidence also suggests that FAP in childhood may increase the risk of emotional and psychiatric disorders later in life.

References

1. "Functional Abdominal Pain," GI Kids, 2016.

2. Khan, Seema. "Functional Abdominal Pain in Children," American College of Gastroenterology (ACG), December 2012.

3. Tidy, Colin. "Recurrent Abdominal Pain in Children," Patient. info, July 27, 2016.

Section 22.2

Appendicitis

This section includes text excerpted from "Appendicitis," National Institute of Diabetes and Digestive and Kidney Diseases (NIDDK), November 2014. Reviewed September 2019.

Definition and Facts of Appendicitis
What Is Appendicitis?

Appendicitis is an inflammation of appendix.

How Common Is Appendicitis?

In the United States, appendicitis is the most common cause of acute abdominal pain requiring surgery. Over five percent of the population develops appendicitis at some point.

Who Is More Likely to Develop Appendicitis?

Appendicitis most commonly occurs in the teens and twenties but may occur at any age.

What Are the Complications of Appendicitis?

If appendicitis is not treated, it may lead to complications. The complications of a ruptured appendix are:

- Peritonitis, which can be a dangerous condition. Peritonitis happens if your appendix bursts and the infection spreads in your abdomen. If you have peritonitis, you may be very ill and have:

- Fever

- Nausea

- Severe tenderness in your abdomen

- Vomiting

- An abscess of the appendix called an "appendiceal abscess."

Symptoms and Causes of Appendicitis
What Are the Symptoms of Appendicitis?

The most common symptom of appendicitis is a pain in your abdomen.

If you have appendicitis, you will most often have pain in your abdomen that:

- Begins near your belly button and then moves lower and to your right

- Gets worse in a matter of hours

- Gets worse when you move around, take deep breaths, cough, or sneeze

- Is severe and often described as different from any pain you have felt before

- Occurs suddenly and may even wake you up if you are sleeping

- Occurs before other symptoms

Other symptoms of appendicitis may include:

- Loss of appetite

- Nausea

- Vomiting

- Constipation or diarrhea

- An inability to pass gas

- A low-grade fever

- Swelling in your abdomen

- The feeling that having a bowel movement will relieve discomfort

Symptoms can be different for each person and can seem like the following conditions that also cause pain in the abdomen:

- Abdominal adhesions

- Constipation

- Inflammatory bowel disease (IBD), which includes Crohn disease and ulcerative colitis, long-lasting disorders that cause irritation and ulcers in the gastrointestinal (GI) tract

- Intestinal obstruction

- Pelvic inflammatory disease (PID)

What Causes Appendicitis

Appendicitis can have more than one cause, and in many cases, the cause is not clear. Possible causes include:

- Blockage of the opening inside the appendix

- Enlarged tissue in the wall of your appendix, caused by an infection in the GI tract or elsewhere in your body

- Inflammatory bowel disease

- Stool, parasites, or growths that can clog your appendiceal lumen

- Trauma to your abdomen

When Should I Seek a Doctor's Help?

Appendicitis is a medical emergency that requires immediate care. See a healthcare professional or go to the emergency room right away if you think you or a child has appendicitis. A doctor can help treat the appendicitis and reduce symptoms and the chance of complications.

Diagnosis of Appendicitis
How Do Doctors Diagnose Appendicitis?

Most often, healthcare professionals suspect the diagnosis of appendicitis based on your symptoms, your medical history, and a physical exam. A doctor can confirm the diagnosis with an ultrasound, x-ray, or magnetic resonance imaging (MRI) exam.

Medical History

A healthcare professional will ask specific questions about your symptoms and health history to help rule out other health problems. The healthcare professional will want to know:

- When your abdominal pain began
- The exact location and severity of your pain
- When your other symptoms appeared
- Your other medical conditions, previous illnesses, and surgical procedures
- Whether you use medicines, alcohol, or illegal drugs

Physical Exam

Healthcare professionals need specific details about the pain in your abdomen to diagnose appendicitis correctly. A healthcare professional will assess your pain by touching or applying pressure to specific areas of your abdomen.

The following responses to touch or pressure may indicate that you have appendicitis:

- Rovsing sign
- Psoas sign
- Obturator sign
- Guarding
- Rebound tenderness
- Digital rectal exam
- Pelvic exam

Lab Tests

Doctors use lab tests to help confirm the diagnosis of appendicitis or find other causes of abdominal pain.

Blood tests. A healthcare professional draws your blood for a blood test at a doctor's office or a commercial facility. The healthcare professional sends the blood sample to a lab for testing. Blood tests can show a high white blood cell (WBC) count, a sign of infection. Blood tests also may show dehydration or fluid and electrolyte imbalances.

Urinalysis. Urinalysis is the testing of a urine sample. You will provide a urine sample in a special container in a doctor's office, a commercial facility, or a hospital. Healthcare professionals can test the urine in the same location or send it to a lab for testing. Doctors use urinalysis to rule out a urinary-tract infection (UTI) or a kidney stone.

Pregnancy test. For women, healthcare professionals also may order blood or urine samples to check for pregnancy.

Imaging Tests

Doctors use imaging tests to confirm the diagnosis of appendicitis or find other causes of pain in the abdomen.

Abdominal ultrasound. In an ultrasound, a healthcare professional uses a device, called a "transducer," to bounce safe, painless sound waves off of your organs to create an image of their structure. She or he can move the transducer to different angles to examine different organs.

In an abdominal ultrasound, a healthcare professional applies a gel to your abdomen and moves a handheld transducer over your skin. A healthcare professional performs this procedure in a doctor's office, an outpatient center, or a hospital, and you do not need anesthesia.

A radiologist reviews the images, which can show signs of:

- A blockage in your appendiceal lumen

- A burst appendix

- Inflammation

- Other sources of abdominal pain

Healthcare professionals use ultrasound as the first imaging test for possible appendicitis in infants, children, young adults, and pregnant women.

Magnetic resonance imaging (MRI). MRI machines use radio waves and magnets to produce detailed pictures of your body's internal organs and soft tissues without using x-rays.

A healthcare professional performs the procedure in an outpatient center or a hospital. A radiologist reviews the images. Patients do not need anesthesia, although a healthcare professional may give light sedation, taken by mouth, to children and people with a fear of small spaces. A healthcare professional may inject a special dye, called "contrast medium," into your body.

In most cases, you will lie on a table that slides into a tunnel-shaped device. The tunnel may be open-ended or closed at one end.

An MRI can show signs of:

- A blockage in your appendiceal lumen

- A burst appendix

- Inflammation

- Other sources of abdominal pain

When diagnosing appendicitis and other sources of abdominal pain, doctors can use an MRI as a safe, reliable alternative to computerized tomography (CT) scan.

Computed tomography (CT) scan. CT scans use x-rays and computer technology to create images.

A healthcare professional may give you a solution to drink and an injection of contrast medium. You will lie on a table that slides into a tunnel-shaped device that takes the x-rays. X-ray technicians perform CT scans in an outpatient center or a hospital. Radiologists review the images.

Patients do not need anesthesia, although healthcare professionals may give children a sedative to help them fall asleep for the test.

A CT scan of the abdomen can show signs of inflammation, such as:

- An enlarged or a burst appendix

- An appendiceal abscess

- A blockage in your appendiceal lumen

Women of childbearing age should have a pregnancy test before having a CT scan. The radiation from CT scans can be harmful to a developing fetus.

Treatment of Appendicitis
How Do Doctors Treat Appendicitis?

Doctors typically treat appendicitis with surgery to remove the appendix. Surgeons perform the surgery in a hospital with general anesthesia. Your doctor will recommend surgery if you have continuous abdominal pain and fever, or signs of a burst appendix and infection. Prompt surgery decreases the chance that your appendix will burst.

Healthcare professionals call the surgery to remove the appendix an appendectomy. A surgeon performs the surgery using one of the following methods:

- **Laparoscopic surgery.** During laparoscopic surgery, surgeons use several smaller incisions and special surgical tools that they feed through the incisions to remove your appendix. Laparoscopic surgery leads to fewer complications, such as hospital-related infections, and has a shorter recovery time.

- **Laparotomy.** Surgeons use laparotomy to remove the appendix through a single incision in the lower right area of your abdomen.

After surgery, most patients completely recover from appendicitis and do not need to make changes to their diet, exercise, or lifestyle. Surgeons recommend that you limit physical activity for the first 10 to 14 days after laparotomy and for the first 3 to 5 days after laparoscopic surgery.

What If the Surgeon Finds a Normal Appendix?

In some cases, a surgeon finds a normal appendix during surgery. In this case, many surgeons will remove it to eliminate the future possibility of appendicitis. Sometimes surgeons find a different problem, which they may correct during surgery.

Can Doctors Treat Appendicitis without Surgery?

Some cases of mild appendicitis may be cured with antibiotics alone. All patients suspected of having appendicitis are treated with antibiotics before surgery, and some patients may improve completely before surgery is performed.

How Do Doctors Treat Complications of a Burst Appendix?

Treating the complications of a burst appendix will depend on the type of complication. In most cases of peritonitis, the surgeon will remove your appendix immediately with surgery. The surgeon will use laparotomy to clean the inside of your abdomen to prevent infection and then remove your appendix. Without prompt treatment, peritonitis can cause death.

A surgeon may drain the pus from an appendiceal abscess during surgery or, more commonly, before surgery. To drain an abscess, the surgeon places a tube in the abscess through the abdominal wall. You leave the drainage tube in place for about two weeks while you take antibiotics to treat an infection. When the infection and inflammation are under control, about six to eight weeks later, surgeons operate to remove what remains of the burst appendix.

Section 22.3

Celiac Disease

This section includes text excerpted from "Celiac Disease," National Institute of Diabetes and Digestive and Kidney Diseases (NIDDK), June 2016. Reviewed September 2019.

Definition and Facts of Celiac Disease
What Is Celiac Disease?

Celiac disease is a digestive disorder that damages the small intestine. The disease is triggered by eating foods containing gluten. Gluten is a protein found naturally in wheat, barley, and rye, and is common in foods, such as bread, pasta, cookies, and cakes. Many prepackaged foods, lip balms and lipsticks, hair and skin products, toothpaste, vitamin and nutrient supplements, and, rarely, medicines, contain gluten.

Celiac disease can be very serious. The disease can cause long-lasting digestive problems and keep your body from getting all the nutrients it needs. Celiac disease can also affect the body outside the intestine.

Celiac disease is different from gluten sensitivity or wheat intolerance. If you have gluten sensitivity, you may have symptoms similar to those of celiac disease, such as abdominal pain and tiredness. Unlike celiac disease, gluten sensitivity does not damage the small intestine.

Celiac disease is also different from a wheat allergy. In both cases, your body's immune system reacts to wheat. However, some symptoms in wheat allergies, such as having itchy eyes or a hard time breathing, are different from celiac disease. Wheat allergies also do not cause long-term damage to the small intestine.

How Common Is Celiac Disease?

As many as one in 141 Americans have celiac disease, although most do not know it.

Who Is More Likely to Develop Celiac Disease?

Although celiac disease affects children in all parts of the world, the disease is more common in Caucasians and more often diagnosed in females. You are more likely to develop celiac disease if someone in your family has the disease. Celiac disease also is more common among people with certain other diseases, such as Down syndrome, Turner syndrome (TS), and type 1 diabetes.

What Other Health Problems Do People with Celiac Disease Have?

If you have celiac disease, you also may be at risk for

- Addison disease

- Hashimoto disease

- Primary biliary cirrhosis

- Type 1 diabetes

Symptoms and Causes of Celiac Disease
What Are the Symptoms of Celiac Disease?

Most people with celiac disease have one or more symptoms. However, some people with the disease may not have symptoms or feel sick. Sometimes health issues, such as surgery, pregnancy, childbirth, bacterial gastroenteritis, a viral infection, or severe mental stress can trigger celiac disease symptoms.

If you have celiac disease, you may have digestive problems or other symptoms. Digestive symptoms are more common in children and can include:

- Bloating, or a feeling of fullness or swelling in the abdomen

- Chronic diarrhea

- Constipation

- Gas

- Nausea

- Pale, foul-smelling, or fatty stools that float

- Stomach pain

- Vomiting

For children with celiac disease, being unable to absorb nutrients when they are so important to normal growth and development can lead to:

- Damage to the permanent teeth's enamel

- Delayed puberty

- Failure to thrive in infants

- Mood changes or feeling annoyed or impatient

- Slowed growth and short height

- Weight loss

Celiac disease also can produce a reaction in which your immune system or your body's natural defense system attacks healthy cells in your body. This reaction can spread outside your digestive tract to other areas of your body, including your:

- Bones

- Joints

- Nervous system

- Skin

- Spleen

Depending on how old you are when a doctor diagnoses your celiac disease, some symptoms, such as short height and tooth defects, will not improve.

Dermatitis Herpetiformis

Dermatitis herpetiformis is an itchy, blistering skin rash that usually appears on the elbows, knees, buttocks, back, or scalp. The rash affects about 10 percent of people with celiac disease. The rash can affect people of all ages but is most likely to appear for the first time between the ages of 30 and 40. Some people with celiac disease may have a rash and no other symptoms.

Why Are Celiac Disease Symptoms so Varied?

Symptoms of celiac disease vary from person to person. Your symptoms may depend on:

- How long you were breastfed as an infant; some studies have shown that the longer you were breastfed, the later celiac disease symptoms appear

- How much gluten you eat

- How old you were when you started eating gluten

- The amount of damage to your small intestine

- Your age—symptoms can vary between young children

- People with celiac disease who have no symptoms can still develop complications from the disease over time if they do not get treatment.

What Causes Celiac Disease

Research suggests that celiac disease only happens to individuals who have particular genes. These genes are common and are carried by about one-third of the population. Individuals also have to be eating food that contains gluten to get celiac disease. Researchers do not know exactly what triggers celiac disease in people at risk who eat gluten over a long period of time. Sometimes the disease runs in families. About 10 to 20 percent of close relatives of people with celiac disease also are affected.

Your chances of developing celiac disease increase when you have changes in your genes or variants. Certain gene variants and other factors, such as things in your environment, can lead to celiac disease.

Diagnosis of Celiac Disease
How Do Doctors Diagnose Celiac Disease?

Celiac disease can be hard to diagnose because some of the symptoms are like symptoms of other diseases, such as irritable bowel syndrome (IBS) and lactose intolerance. Your doctor may diagnose celiac disease with a medical and family history, physical exam, and tests. Tests may include blood tests, genetic tests, and biopsy.

Medical and Family History

Your doctor will ask you for information about your family's health — specifically if anyone in your family has a history of celiac disease.

Physical Exam

During a physical exam, a doctor most often:

- Checks your body for a rash or malnutrition, a condition that arises when you do not get enough vitamins, minerals, and other nutrients you need to be healthy
- Listens to sounds in your abdomen using a stethoscope
- Taps on your abdomen to check for pain and fullness or swelling

Dental Exam

For some people, a dental visit can be the first step toward discovering celiac disease. Dental enamel defects, such as white, yellow, or brown spots on the teeth, are a pretty common problem in people with celiac disease, especially children. These defects can help dentists and other healthcare professionals identify celiac disease.

What Tests Do Doctors Use to Diagnose Celiac Disease?
Blood Tests

A healthcare professional may take a blood sample from you and send the sample to a lab to test for antibodies common in celiac disease. If blood test results are negative and your doctor still suspects celiac disease, she or he may order more blood tests.

Genetic Tests

If a biopsy and other blood tests do not clearly confirm celiac disease, your doctor may order genetic blood tests to check for certain gene changes or variants. You are very unlikely to have celiac disease if these gene variants are not present. Having these variants alone is not enough to diagnose celiac disease because they also are common in people without the disease. In fact, most people with these genes will never get celiac disease.

Intestinal Biopsy

If blood tests suggest you have celiac disease, your doctor will perform a biopsy to be sure. During a biopsy, the doctor takes a small piece of tissue from your small intestine during a procedure called an "upper gastrointestinal (GI) endoscopy."

Skin Biopsy

If a doctor suspects you have dermatitis herpetiformis, she or he will perform a skin biopsy. For a skin biopsy, the doctor removes tiny pieces of skin tissue to examine with a microscope.

A doctor examines the skin tissue and checks the tissue for antibodies common in celiac disease. If the skin tissue has the antibodies, a doctor will perform blood tests to confirm celiac disease. If the skin biopsy and blood tests both suggest celiac disease, you may not need an intestinal biopsy.

Do Doctors Screen for Celiac Disease?

Screening is testing for diseases when you have no symptoms. Doctors in the United States do not routinely screen people for celiac disease. However, blood relatives of people with celiac disease and those with type 1 diabetes should talk with their doctor about their chances of getting the disease.

Many researchers recommend routine screening of all family members, such as parents and siblings, for celiac disease. However, routine genetic screening for celiac disease is not usually helpful when diagnosing the disease.

Treatment of Celiac Disease
How Do Doctors Treat Celiac Disease?
A Gluten-Free Diet

Doctors treat celiac disease with a gluten-free diet. Gluten is a protein found naturally in wheat, barley, and rye that triggers a reaction if you have celiac disease. Symptoms greatly improve for most people with celiac disease who stick to a gluten-free diet. In recent years, grocery stores and restaurants have added many more gluten-free foods and products, making it easier to stay gluten-free.

Your doctor may refer you to a dietitian who specializes in treating people with celiac disease. The dietitian will teach you how to avoid gluten while following a healthy diet. She or he will help you:

- Check food and product labels for gluten

- Design everyday meal plans

- Make healthy choices about the types of foods to eat

For most people, following a gluten-free diet will heal damage in the small intestine and prevent more damage. You may see symptoms improve within days to weeks of starting the diet. The small intestine usually heals in three to six months in children. Once the intestine heals, the villi, which were damaged by the disease, regrow and will absorb nutrients from food into the bloodstream normally.

Gluten-Free Diet and Dermatitis Herpetiformis

If you have dermatitis herpetiformis—an itchy, blistering skin rash—skin symptoms generally respond to a gluten-free diet. However, skin symptoms may return if you add gluten back into your diet. Medicines such as dapsone, taken by mouth, can control the skin symptoms. People who take dapsone need to have regular blood tests to check for side effects from the medicine.

Dapsone does not treat intestinal symptoms or damage, which is why you should stay on a gluten-free diet if you have the rash. Even when you follow a gluten-free diet, the rash may take months or even years to fully heal—and often comes back over the years.

Avoiding Medicines and Nonfood Products That May Contain Gluten

In addition to prescribing a gluten-free diet, your doctor will want you to avoid all hidden sources of gluten. If you have celiac disease, ask a pharmacist about ingredients in:

- Herbal and nutritional supplements

- Prescription and over-the-counter (OTC) medicines

- Vitamin and mineral supplements

You also could take in or transfer from your hands to your mouth other products that contain gluten without knowing it. Products that may contain gluten include:

- Children's modeling dough, such as Play-Doh

- Cosmetics

- Lipstick, lip gloss, and lip balm
- Skin and hair products
- Toothpaste and mouthwash
- Communion wafers

Medications are rare sources of gluten. Even if gluten is present in medicine, it is likely to be in such small quantities that it would not cause any symptoms.

Reading product labels can sometimes help you avoid gluten. Some product makers label their products as being gluten-free. If a product label does not list the product's ingredients, ask the maker of the product for an ingredients list.

What If Changing to a Gluten-Free Diet Is Not Working?

If you do not improve after starting a gluten-free diet, you may still be eating or using small amounts of gluten. You probably will start responding to the gluten-free diet once you find and cut out all hidden sources of gluten. Hidden sources of gluten include additives made with wheat, such as:

- Modified food starch
- Malt flavoring
- Preservatives
- Stabilizers

If you still have symptoms even after changing your diet, you may have other conditions or disorders that are more common with celiac disease, such as irritable bowel syndrome (IBS), lactose intolerance, microscopic colitis, dysfunction of the pancreas, and small intestinal bacterial overgrowth.

Section 22.4

Constipation

This section includes text excerpted from "Constipation in Children," National Institute of Diabetes and Digestive and Kidney Diseases (NIDDK), May 2018.

Definition and Facts of Constipation in Children
What Is Constipation in Children?

Constipation in children is a condition in which your child may have:

- Fewer than two bowel movements a week

- Stools that are hard, dry, or lumpy

- Stools that are difficult or painful to pass

Your child also may tell you that she or he feels that not all stool has passed.

Some children have more bowel movements than others, so what is normal for one child may be different from another child. Also, as children get older, their bowel movement patterns may change. Even an infant's bowel movements change a lot in the first few weeks and months of life.

Constipation is not a disease but may be a symptom of another medical problem. In most cases, constipation in children lasts a short time and is not dangerous.

How Common Is Constipation in Children?

Constipation is common in children of all ages. Almost 1 of every 20 visits children make to a doctor are because of constipation.

What Are the Complications of Constipation in Children?

Children who have constipation that lasts for a short time usually do not have complications. However, avoiding or delaying a bowel movement may lead to:

- Long-lasting constipation

- Painful bowel movements

- Bladder-control problems
- Fecal impaction

Complications of long-lasting constipation, especially in older children, may include:

- Hemorrhoids
- Anal fissures
- Rectal prolapse

Symptoms and Causes of Constipation in Children
What Are the Symptoms of Constipation in Children?

Symptoms of constipation in children may include your child:

- Having fewer than two bowel movements a week
- Passing stools that are hard, dry, or lumpy
- Having stools that are difficult or painful to pass
- Telling you that she or he feels that not all stool has passed
- Changing positions to avoid or delay having a bowel movement, including:
  - Standing on tiptoes and then rocking back on her or his heels
  - Clenching her or his buttocks
  - Doing unusual, dance-like movements
- Having a swollen abdomen, or bloating
- Having daytime or nighttime wetting
- Having stool in her or his underwear that looks like diarrhea

If your child avoids or delays having a bowel movement, she or he may develop a fecal impaction.

When Should My Child See a Doctor?

Your child should see a doctor if her or his symptoms last for more than two weeks or do not go away with at-home treatment.

Take your child to a doctor right away if she or he has constipation and any of the following symptoms:

- Bleeding from her or his rectum

- Blood in her or his stool
- Bloating
- Constant pain in her or his abdomen
- Vomiting
- Weight loss

What Causes Constipation in Children

Children most often get constipated from holding in their stool to avoid or delay having a bowel movement. When stool stays too long in the colon, the colon absorbs too much fluid from the stool. Then the stool becomes hard, dry, and difficult to pass.

Your child may delay or avoid a bowel movement because she or he:

- Feels stressed about potty training
- Feels embarrassed to use a public bathroom
- Does not want to interrupt playtime
- Fears having a painful or an unpleasant bowel movement

Certain Medicines

Medicines and dietary supplements that can make constipation in children worse include:

- Antacids that contain aluminum and calcium
- Anticholinergics and antispasmodics
- Anticonvulsants—used to prevent seizures
- Iron supplements
- Narcotic pain medicines
- Some medicines used to treat depression

Certain Health and Nutrition Problems

Certain health and nutrition problems can cause constipation in children:

- Not eating enough fiber
- Not drinking enough liquids or dehydration

- Hirschsprung disease

- Celiac disease

- Disorders that affect your brain and spine, such as spina bifida

- Spinal cord or brain injuries

- Conditions that affect their metabolism, such as diabetes

- Conditions that affect their hormones, such as hypothyroidism

- Problems that can block or narrow the colon or rectum, including tumors

Diagnosis of Constipation in Children
How Do Doctors Find the Cause of Constipation in Children?

Doctors use your child's medical and family history, a physical exam, or medical tests to diagnose and find the cause of constipation.

Medical and Family History

Your child's doctor is likely to ask questions about lifestyle habits and symptoms, such as:

- How often does your child have a bowel movement?

- How long has your child had symptoms?

- What do your child's stools look like?

- Do your child's stools have red streaks in them?

- Are there streaks of blood on the toilet paper when she or he wipes?

- What is your child's daily routine, including potty training, physical activity, and daycare?

- What are your child's eating habits?

- What medicines does she or he take?

You may want to track your child's bowel movements and what her or his stools look like for several days or weeks before the doctor's visit. Write down or record the information so you can share it with the doctor.

Physical Exam

During a physical exam, a doctor may:

- Check your child's blood pressure, temperature, and heart rate
- Check for dehydration
- Use a stethoscope to listen to sounds in your child's abdomen
- Check your child's abdomen for:
  - Swelling
  - Tenderness or pain
  - Masses, or lumps
- Perform a rectal exam

What Medical Tests Do Doctors Use to Find the Cause of Constipation in Children?

Doctors do not normally need medical tests to diagnose constipation in children. However, in some cases, your child's doctor may use medical tests to help find the cause of constipation.

Lab Tests

Your child's doctor may look for signs of certain diseases and conditions that may be causing your child's constipation or are related to your child's constipation. The doctor may use one or more of the following lab tests.

- Blood tests can show signs of anemia, hypothyroidism, and celiac disease.
- Stool tests can show the presence of blood and signs of infection and inflammation.
- Urine tests can show signs of conditions such as bladder infections, which could be caused by constipation.

Bowel Function Tests

If your child's constipation does not improve with nutrition changes, your child's doctor may use bowel function tests, including colorectal transit studies. These tests help a doctor see how well stool moves through your child's colon.

Imaging Tests

In some cases, your child's doctor may use imaging tests of your child's abdomen to look for problems that may be causing her or his constipation. Imaging tests include:

- Ultrasound
- X-rays
- Computed tomography (CT) scan

Other Tests

Your child's doctor may suggest a rectal biopsy. The rectal biopsy is the best test to diagnose or rule out Hirschsprung disease. A rectal biopsy is a procedure that involves taking small pieces of tissue from the rectum and examining them with a microscope. The doctor will look at the tissue for signs of medical problems.

Treatment of Constipation in Children
How Can I Treat My Child's Constipation?

You can most often treat your child's constipation at home by doing the following:

Change What Your Child Eats and Drinks

Changing what your child eats and drinks may make her or his stools softer and easier to pass. To help relieve symptoms, have her or his:

- Eat more high-fiber foods
- Drink plenty of water and other liquids if your child eats more fiber

Change Your Child's Behavior

Changing your child's bowel movement patterns and behaviors may help treat constipation.

- Ask your potty-trained child to use the toilet after meals to build a routine.
- Use a reward system when your child uses the bathroom regularly.
- Take a break from potty training until constipation stops.

How Do Doctors Treat Constipation in Children?

Your child's doctor may recommend giving your child an enema or laxative to help treat her or his constipation. Most laxatives are over-the-counter (OTC) medicines taken by mouth until your child's bowel movements are normal. Your child's doctor may recommend stopping the laxative once your child has better eating and bowel habits. You should not give a child a laxative unless told to do so by a doctor.

If your child is taking an OTC or prescription medicine or supplement that can cause constipation, your child's doctor may recommend stopping it, changing the dose, or switching to a different one. Talk with your child's doctor before stopping any medicines.

How Can I Treat My Child's Constipation Complication?

Your doctor may recommend treating your child's hemorrhoids or anal fissures by:

- Making changes in her or his diet to prevent constipation

- Using an OTC enema or laxative suggested by your child's doctor

- Have her or him take warm tub baths to soothe the area

How Do Doctors Treat the Complications of Constipation in Children?

Doctors may be able to treat complications of constipation in children during an office visit. Your child's doctor may recommend at-home treatments, too.

For a child at the age of two or older, your doctor may recommend giving mineral oil. Your child will take the mineral oil by mouth or through an enema.

Your child's doctor may be able to treat rectal prolapse during an office visit by manually pushing the rectum back through the child's anus. Helping a child prevent constipation is the best way to prevent rectal prolapse.

How Can I Prevent My Child from Becoming Constipated?

You can help prevent constipation in your child with the same things that treat constipation:

- Provide enough fiber in your child's diet
- Have your child drink plenty of water and other liquids
- Make having a bowel movement part of your child's routine

Section 22.5

Cyclic Vomiting Syndrome

This section includes text excerpted from "Cyclic Vomiting Syndrome," National Institute of Diabetes and Digestive and Kidney Diseases (NIDDK), December 2017.

Definitions and Facts of Cyclic Vomiting Syndrome
What Is Cyclic Vomiting Syndrome?

Cyclic vomiting syndrome, or CVS, is a functional gastrointestinal (GI) disorder that causes sudden, repeated attacks—called "episodes"—of severe nausea and vomiting. Episodes can last from a few hours to several days. The episodes are separated by periods without nausea or vomiting. The time between episodes can be a few weeks to several months. Episodes can happen regularly or at random. Episodes can be so severe that you may have to stay in bed for days, unable to go to school or work. You may need treatment at an emergency room or a hospital during episodes. CVS can affect you for years or decades.

Cyclic vomiting syndrome is not chronic vomiting that lasts weeks without stopping. CVS is not a condition that has a definite cause, such as chemotherapy.

How Common Is Cyclic Vomiting Syndrome?

Experts do not know how common CVS. However, experts believe that CVS may be just as common in children. Doctors diagnose about 3 out of 100,000 children with CVS every year.

Who Is More Likely to Get Cyclic Vomiting Syndrome?

You may be more likely to get CVS if you have:

- Migraines or a family history of migraines
- A history of long-term marijuana use
- A tendency to get motion sickness

What Other Health Problems Do People with Cyclic Vomiting Syndrome Have?

People with CVS may have other health problems, including:

- Migraines
- Anxiety and depression
- Gastroparesis
- Autonomic nervous system disorders
- High blood pressure
- Gastroesophageal reflux disease (GERD)
- Irritable bowel syndrome

What Are the Complications of Cyclic Vomiting Syndrome?

The severe vomiting and retching that happen during CVS may cause the following complications:

- Dehydration
- Esophagitis
- Mallory-Weiss tears
- Tooth decay or damage to tooth enamel

Symptoms and Causes of Cyclic Vomiting Syndrome
What Are the Main Symptoms of Cyclic Vomiting Syndrome?

The main symptoms of CVS are sudden, repeated attacks—called "episodes"—of severe nausea and vomiting. You may vomit several times an hour. Episodes can last from a few hours to several days. Episodes may make you feel very tired and drowsy.

Each episode of CVS tends to start at the same time of day, last the same length of time, and happen with the same symptoms and intensity as previous episodes. Episodes may begin at any time but often start during the early morning hours.

What Are Some Other Symptoms of Cyclic Vomiting Syndrome?

Other symptoms of CVS may include one or more of the following:

- Retching—trying to vomit but having nothing come out of your mouth, also called "dry vomiting"
- Pain in the abdomen
- Abnormal drowsiness
- Pale skin
- Headaches
- Lack of appetite
- Not wanting to talk
- Drooling or spitting
- Extreme thirst
- Sensitivity to light or sound
- Dizziness
- Diarrhea
- Fever

What Are the Phases of Cyclic Vomiting Syndrome?

Cyclic vomiting syndrome has four phases:

- Prodrome phase
- Vomiting phase
- Recovery phase
- Well phase

How Do the Symptoms Vary in the Phases of Cyclic Vomiting Syndrome?

The symptoms will vary as you go through the four phases of CVS:

- **Prodrome phase.** During the prodrome phase, you feel an episode coming on. Often marked by intense sweating and

481

nausea—with or without pain in your abdomen—this phase can last from a few minutes to several hours. Your skin may look unusually pale.

- **Vomiting phase.** The main symptoms of this phase are severe nausea, vomiting, and retching. At the peak of this phase, you may vomit several times an hour. You may be:

  - Quiet and able to respond to people around you

  - Unable to move and unable to respond to people around you

  - Twisting and moaning with intense pain in your abdomen
  Nausea and vomiting can last from a few hours to several days.

- **Recovery phase.** Recovery begins when you stop vomiting and retching and you feel less nauseated. You may feel better gradually or quickly. The recovery phase ends when your nausea stops and your healthy skin color, appetite, and energy return.

- **Well phase.** The well phase happens between episodes. You have no symptoms during this phase.

When Should I Seek Medical Help?

You should seek medical help if:

- The medicines your doctor recommended or prescribed for the prodrome phase do not relieve your symptoms

- Your episode is severe and lasts more than several hours

- You are not able to take in foods or liquids for several hours

You should seek medical help right away if you have any signs or symptoms of dehydration during the vomiting phase. These signs and symptoms may include:

- Extreme thirst and dry mouth

- Urinating less than usual

- Dark-colored urine

- Dry mouth

- Decreased skin turgor, meaning that when your skin is pinched and released, the skin does not flatten back to normal right away

- Sunken eyes or cheeks

- Light-headedness or fainting

If you are a parent or caregiver of an infant or child, you should seek medical care for them right away if they have any signs and symptoms of dehydration during the vomiting phase. These signs and symptoms may include:

- Thirst

- Urinating less than usual, or no wet diapers for three hours or more

- Lack of energy

- Dry mouth

- No tears when crying

- Decreased skin turgor

- Sunken eyes or cheeks

- Unusually cranky or drowsy behavior

What Causes Cyclic Vomiting Syndrome

Experts are not sure what causes CVS. However, some experts believe the following conditions may play a role:

- Problems with nerve signals between the brain and digestive tract

- Problems with the way the brain and endocrine system react to stress

- Mutations in certain genes that are associated with an increased chance of getting CVS

What May Trigger an Episode of Cyclic Vomiting?

Triggers for an episode of cyclic vomiting may include:

- Emotional stress

- Anxiety or panic attacks

- Infections, such as colds, flu, or chronic sinusitis

- Intense excitement before events, such as birthdays, holidays, vacations, and school outings, especially in children

- Lack of sleep
- Physical exhaustion
- Allergies
- Temperature extremes of hot or cold
- Drinking alcohol
- Menstrual periods
- Motion sickness
- Periods without eating (fasting)

Eating certain foods, such as chocolate, cheese, and foods with monosodium glutamate (MSG) may play a role in triggering episodes.

Diagnosis of Cyclic Vomiting Syndrome
How Do Doctors Diagnose Cyclic Vomiting Syndrome?

Doctors diagnose CVS based on family and medical history, a physical exam, a pattern of symptoms, and medical tests. Your doctor may perform medical tests to rule out other diseases and conditions that may cause nausea and vomiting.

Family and Medical History

Your doctor will ask about your family and medical history. She or he may ask for details about your history of health problems, such as migraines, irritable bowel syndrome, and gastroparesis. Your doctor may also ask about your history of mental health problems, the use of substances such as marijuana, and cigarette smoking.

Physical Exam

During a physical exam, your doctor will:
- Examine your body
- Check your abdomen for unusual sounds, tenderness, or pain
- Check your nerves, muscle strength, reflexes, and balance

Pattern or Cycle of Symptoms in Children

A doctor will often suspect CVS in a child when all of the following are present:

- At least 5 episodes over any time period, or a minimum of 3 episodes over a 6-month period
- Episodes lasting 1 hour to 10 days and happening at least 1 week apart
- Episodes similar to previous ones, tending to start at the same time of day, lasting the same length of time, and happening with the same symptoms and intensity
- Vomiting during episodes happening at least 4 times an hour for at least 1 hour
- Episodes are separated by weeks to months, usually with no symptoms between episodes
- After an appropriate medical evaluation, symptoms cannot be attributed to another medical condition

What Medical Tests Do Doctors Use to Diagnose Cyclic Vomiting Syndrome?

Doctors use lab tests, upper GI endoscopy, and imaging tests to rule out other diseases and conditions that cause nausea and vomiting. Once other diseases and conditions have been ruled out, a doctor will diagnose CVS based on the pattern or cycle of symptoms.

Lab Tests

Your doctor may use the following lab tests:

- **Blood tests** can show signs of anemia, dehydration, inflammation, infection, and liver problems.
- **Urine tests** can show signs of dehydration, infection, and kidney problems.

Blood and urine tests can also show signs of mitochondrial diseases.

Upper Gastrointestinal Endoscopy

Your doctor may perform an upper GI endoscopy to look for problems in your upper digestive tract that may be causing nausea and vomiting.

Imaging Tests

A doctor may perform one or more of the following imaging tests:

- **Ultrasound of the abdomen**

- **Gastric emptying test**, also called "gastric emptying scintigraphy." This test involves eating a bland meal, such as eggs or an egg substitute, that contains a small amount of radioactive material. An external camera scans the abdomen to show where the radioactive material is located. A radiologist can then measure how quickly the stomach empties after the meal. Healthcare professionals perform gastric emptying tests only between episodes.

- **Upper GI series**

- **Magnetic resonance imaging (MRI) scan or computed tomography (CT) scan** of the brain

Treatment of Cyclic Vomiting Syndrome
How Do Doctors Treat Cyclic Vomiting Syndrome?

How doctors treat CVS depends on the phase. Your doctor may

- Prescribe medicines

- Treat health problems that may trigger the disorder

- Recommend

  - Staying away from triggers

  - Ways to manage triggers

  - Getting plenty of sleep and rest

Prodrome Phase

Taking medicines early in this phase can sometimes help stop an episode from happening. Your doctor may recommend OTC medicines or prescribe medicines such as:

- Ondansetron (Zofran®) or promethazine (Phenergan™) for nausea

- Sumatriptan (Imitrex®) for migraines

- Lorazepam (Ativan®) for anxiety

- Ibuprofen for pain

Your doctor may recommend OTC medicines to reduce the amount of acid your stomach makes, such as:

- Famotidine (Pepcid®)

- Ranitidine (Zantac®)

- Omeprazole (Prilosec®)

- Esomeprazole (Nexium®)

Vomiting Phase

During this phase, you should stay in bed and sleep in a dark, quiet room. You may have to go to a hospital if your nausea and vomiting are severe or if you become severely dehydrated. Your doctor may recommend or prescribe the following for children:

- Medicines for:
  - Nausea
  - Migraines
  - Anxiety
  - Pain
- Medicines that reduce the amount of acid your stomach makes

If you go to a hospital, your doctor may treat you with:

- Intravenous (IV) fluids for dehydration
- Medicines for symptoms
- IV nutrition if an episode continues for several days

Recovery Phase

During the recovery phase, you may need IV fluids for a while. Your doctor may recommend that you drink plenty of water and liquids that contain glucose and electrolytes, such as:

- Broths
- Caffeine-free soft drinks
- Fruit juices
- Sports drinks
- Oral rehydration solutions, such as Pedialyte®

If you have lost your appetite, start drinking clear liquids and then move slowly to other liquids and solid foods. Your doctor may prescribe medicines to help prevent future episodes.

Well Phase

During the well phase, your doctor may prescribe medicines to help prevent episodes and how often and how severe they are, such as:

- Amitriptyline (Elavil®)

- Cyproheptadine (Periactin®)

- Propranolol (Inderal®)

- Topiramate (Topamax®)

- Zonisamide (Zonegran®)

Your doctor may also recommend coenzyme Q10, levocarnitine (L-carnitine), or riboflavin as dietary supplements to help prevent episodes.

How Can I Prevent Cyclic Vomiting Syndrome?

Knowing and managing your triggers can help prevent CVS, especially during the well phase. You should also:

- Get enough sleep and rest

- Treat infections and allergies

- Learn how to reduce or manage stress and anxiety

- Avoid foods and food additives that trigger episodes

How Do Doctors Treat the Complications of Cyclic Vomiting Syndrome?

Doctors treat the complications of CVS as follows:

- **Dehydration**—plenty of liquids with glucose and electrolytes; or IV fluids and hospitalization for severe dehydration

- **Esophagitis**—medicines to reduce the amount of acid your stomach makes

- **Mallory-Weiss tears**—medicines or medical procedures to stop bleeding if the tears do not heal on their own, which they generally do

- **Tooth decay or damage to tooth enamel**—dental fillings, fluoride toothpaste, or mouth rinses

Section 22.6

Diarrhea

This section includes text excerpted from "Chronic Diarrhea in Children," National Institute of Diabetes and Digestive and Kidney Diseases (NIDDK), February 2017.

Definition and Facts of Chronic Diarrhea
What Is Chronic Diarrhea in Children?

Chronic diarrhea is passing loose, watery stools three or more times a day for at least four weeks. Children with chronic diarrhea may have loose, watery stools continually, or their diarrhea may come and go. Chronic diarrhea can affect children of any age.

Diarrhea that lasts only a short time is called "acute diarrhea." Acute diarrhea, a common problem in children, usually lasts a few days and goes away on its own.

What Are the Complications of Chronic Diarrhea in Children?
Malabsorption

Certain diseases and conditions that cause chronic diarrhea may cause malabsorption—a condition in which a child's body cannot absorb nutrients from foods, resulting in shortages of protein, calories, and vitamins.

A child who does not absorb enough nutrients from the food she or he eats may become malnourished. Malnourishment during the years when nutrition is important to a child's normal growth and development can result in health problems.

Dehydration

Chronic diarrhea may lead to dehydration. With diarrhea, especially acute diarrhea, a child's body loses more fluid and electrolytes in loose stools than solid stools.

Symptoms and Causes of Chronic Diarrhea
What Are the Symptoms of Chronic Diarrhea in Children?

The main symptom of chronic diarrhea in children is passing loose, watery stools three or more times a day for at least four weeks.

Depending on the cause, children with chronic diarrhea may also have one or more of the following symptoms:

- Bloody stools
- Chills
- Fever
- Loss of control of bowel movements
- Nausea or vomiting
- Pain or cramping in the abdomen

Chronic diarrhea may cause malabsorption and may lead to dehydration.

What Are the Symptoms of Malabsorption and Dehydration in Children?

Malabsorption

Symptoms of malabsorption may include:

- Bloating
- Changes in appetite
- Gas
- Loose, greasy, foul-smelling bowel movements
- Weight loss or poor weight gain

Dehydration

Symptoms of dehydration may include:

- Thirst
- Urinating less than usual, or no wet diapers for three hours or more
- Lack of energy
- Dry mouth
- No tears when crying
- Decreased skin turgor, meaning that when your child's skin is pinched and released, the skin does not flatten back to normal right away
- Sunken eyes, cheeks, or soft spot in the skull

What Causes Chronic Diarrhea in Children

Common diseases and disorders that cause chronic diarrhea in children include:

Infections of the Digestive Tract

Infections from harmful viruses, bacteria, or parasites sometimes lead to chronic diarrhea. Children may become infected through contaminated water, beverages, or food; or through person-to-person contact. After infection, some children have problems digesting carbohydrates such as lactose or proteins in foods such as milk, milk products, or soy. These problems can cause prolonged diarrhea—often for up to six weeks—after an infection. Also, some bacterial and parasitic infections that cause diarrhea do not go away quickly without treatment.

Celiac Disease

Celiac disease is a digestive disorder that damages the small intestine. The disease is triggered by eating foods containing gluten. Gluten is a protein found naturally in wheat, barley, and rye. Gluten is common in foods, such as bread, pasta, cookies, and cakes. Celiac disease can cause chronic diarrhea in children of any age.

Functional Gastrointestinal Disorders

In functional GI disorders, symptoms are caused by changes in how the digestive tract works. Children with functional GI disorder have frequent symptoms, yet the digestive tract does not become damaged. Functional GI disorders are not diseases; they are groups of symptoms that occur together.

Two functional GI disorders that cause chronic diarrhea in children are toddler's diarrhea and irritable bowel syndrome (IBS).

Food Allergies and Intolerances

Food allergies, lactose intolerance, fructose intolerance, and sucrose intolerance are common causes of chronic diarrhea.

Inflammatory Bowel Disease

The two main types of inflammatory bowel disease (IBD) are Crohn disease and ulcerative colitis. These disorders can affect children at any age. However, they commonly begin in the grade school years or in adolescence.

Small Intestinal Bacterial Overgrowth

Small intestinal bacterial overgrowth is an increase in the number of bacteria or a change in the type of bacteria in your small intestine. SIBO is often related to diseases that damage the digestive system such as Crohn disease.

Diagnosis of Chronic Diarrhea
How Do Doctors Find the Cause of Chronic Diarrhea in Children?

To find the cause of a child's chronic diarrhea, doctors may use information from the child's medical and family history, a physical exam, or tests.

Medical and Family History

Your child's doctor will ask you for information about your child's symptoms, such as:

- How long your child has had diarrhea

- How much stool your child passes

- How often your child has diarrhea

- How your child's stool looks, such as color and consistency

- Whether your child has other symptoms along with diarrhea

The doctor will ask about the foods your child eats and beverages she or he drinks. The doctor may recommend keeping a diary of what your child eats and drinks and her or his bowel habits.

Your child's doctor may also ask about family medical history. Some of the conditions that cause chronic diarrhea, such as Crohn disease and ulcerative colitis, run in families.

Physical Exam

During a physical exam, a doctor typically:

- Checks blood pressure and pulse

- Checks for symptoms of dehydration and malabsorption

- Listens to sounds in your child's abdomen using a stethoscope

- Taps on your child's abdomen to check for pain or tenderness

What Tests Do Doctors Use to Find the Cause of Chronic Diarrhea in Children?

Doctors may use the following tests to help find the cause of a child's chronic diarrhea:

Stool Test

Stool tests can show the presence of blood and signs of infection, food allergies, and digestive tract problems, such as malabsorption of certain sugars, proteins, or nutrients. A healthcare professional will give you a container for catching and storing a sample of your child's stool, along with instructions on where to send or take the sample for testing. A doctor may also do a digital rectal exam to check for blood in your child's stool.

Blood Tests

A healthcare professional may take a sample of your child's blood to test for signs of certain diseases or disorders that can cause chronic diarrhea, such as infections or celiac disease.

Hydrogen Breath Tests

This test measures the amount of hydrogen in a child's breath. Normally, little hydrogen is found in your child's breath. However, bacteria break down sugars—such as lactose, fructose, and sucrose—that are not digested by the small intestine and produce high levels of hydrogen. By measuring the amount of hydrogen in your child's breath, a doctor can diagnose:

- Lactose intolerance

- Fructose intolerance

- Sucrose intolerance

- Small intestinal bacterial overgrowth (SIBO)

For a lactose intolerance test, your child will drink a beverage that contains a known amount of lactose. For a fructose intolerance test, your child will drink a beverage that contains a known amount of fructose For a sucrose intolerance test, your child will drink a beverage that contains a known amount of sucrose. For a SIBO test, your child will drink a beverage that contains a known amount of sugar. Your child will then breathe into a balloon-type container that measures hydrogen. If the hydrogen level is high, your doctor will diagnose one of these disorders.

Fasting Tests

To find out if a food allergy or intolerance is causing your child's chronic diarrhea, the doctor may recommend that your child avoid foods with lactose, carbohydrates, wheat, or other ingredients to see if a change in the diet reduces or stops diarrhea.

Endoscopy

Your doctor may use endoscopy to look inside your child's body to help find the cause of her or his chronic diarrhea. Endoscopic procedures include:

- Colonoscopy
- Flexible sigmoidoscopy
- Upper GI endoscopy

Treatment of Chronic Diarrhea
How Do Doctors Treat Chronic Diarrhea in Children?

How doctors treat chronic diarrhea in children depends on the cause. Doctors may be able to reduce or stop chronic diarrhea by treating the cause.

Infections of the Digestive Tract

Your child's doctor may prescribe antibiotics to treat bacterial infections and medicines that target parasites to treat parasitic infections. If your child has long-lasting problems digesting certain carbohydrates or proteins after an infection, a doctor may recommend changes in the foods your child eats.

Your child's doctor may prescribe antibiotics to treat your child's SIBO and may recommend changes in what your child eats.

Inflammatory Bowel Disease

A doctor may use medicines, surgery, and changes in what your child eats to treat inflammatory bowel diseases (IBD) such as Crohn disease and ulcerative colitis.

Section 22.7

Dysphagia

"Dysphagia (Difficulty Swallowing),"
© 2017 Omnigraphics. Reviewed September 2019.

Dysphagia, which literally means "difficulty swallowing," is a condition in which people have trouble passing foods or liquids from their mouth to their digestive system. The process of swallowing involves four stages. The brain controls this process through nerves that connect to the mouth, throat, esophagus, and stomach. Dysphagia can result from problems occurring in any of the four stages.

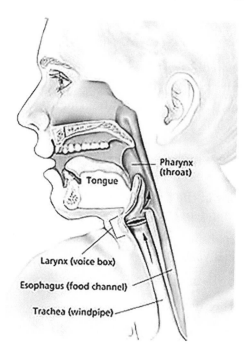

Figure 22.1. *Parts of the Mouth and Neck Involved in Swallowing* (Source: "Dysphagia," National Institute on Deafness and Other Communication Disorders (NIDCD).)

In the oral stage, food is placed in the mouth, where it is moistened by saliva, broken down by chewing, and pushed back toward the throat by the tongue. In the pharyngeal phase, food enters the throat (pharynx). The voice box (larynx) closes briefly to prevent food from entering the airway and lungs, and then the food passes down the throat and into the esophagus. In the esophageal stage, food is pushed downward through the esophagus by wave-like muscle contractions known as peristalsis. Finally, the food passes into the stomach through the lower esophageal sphincter, a band of muscle that relaxes to allow food to enter and tightens to prevent stomach contents from moving back upward into the esophagus.

Causes of Dysphagia

Swallowing difficulties have many possible causes, including the following:

- Cleft lip, cleft palate, or other problems with craniofacial development

- Dental problems

- Large tongue

- Large tonsils

- Tumors, masses, or congenital abnormalities in the throat

- Foreign objects in the esophagus

- Gastrointestinal problems that irritate or damage the esophagus, such as acid reflux

- Malformations of the digestive tract, such as esophageal atresia or tracheoesophageal fistula

- Compression of the esophagus by enlarged thyroid gland, lymph nodes, or blood vessels

- Premature birth or low birth weight

- Autism or other developmental delays

- Nervous system disorders, such as cerebral palsy

- Diseases or injuries that affect the nerves and muscles of the face and neck, such as stroke, brain injury, or muscular dystrophy

- Respiratory problems

- Tracheostomy

- Oral sensitivity or irritation of the airway from prolonged use of a ventilator

- Vocal cord paralysis

- Certain medications that decrease appetite

- Dysfunctional parent–child interaction at mealtimes

Symptoms of Dysphagia

Swallowing difficulties manifest themselves in many ways, some of which may not be obvious or may mimic other medical conditions. Some of the more common symptoms of dysphagia include the following:

- Eating very slowly

- Chewing with difficulty

- Attempting to swallow a mouthful of food several times

- Feeling as if food becomes stuck in the throat

- Trouble coordinating breathing and swallowing

- Frequent coughing, gagging, or choking during meals

- Frequent spitting up or vomiting

- Drooling

- Stuffy nose at mealtime, or food or liquid coming out of the nose

- Hoarse, raspy, or gurgling voice during or after meals

- Chest congestion after eating, or recurring respiratory infections

- Weight loss, or less than normal weight gain and growth

- Aversion to certain textures of food

- Arching the back or stiffening while feeding

- Irritability or lack of alertness while feeding

Diagnosis of Dysphagia

The medical professional that is most often involved in diagnosing swallowing difficulties is a speech-language pathologist (SLP). The SLP may consult with a team that also includes a physician or pediatrician, a dietician or nutritionist, and a physical or occupational therapist. The team will ask about the patient's medical history, including the development of the condition, symptoms experienced, and overall health. They may also evaluate the patient's posture and behavior while eating, as well as their oral movements and the strength of muscles involved in chewing and swallowing. As needed, various tests and imaging studies may be performed to further analyze the actions of the mouth, throat, and esophagus. Some of the possible tests used to diagnose dysphagia are described below.

Modified Barium Swallow Study

The patient consumes a small amount of a liquid containing barium, a metallic chemical that shows up well on x-rays. A series of x-rays are taken as the barium moves through the throat and esophagus, providing the SLP with valuable information about the source of swallowing difficulties.

Fiberoptic Endoscopic Evaluation of Swallowing

A small, flexible tube with a tiny camera on the end is inserted through the patient's nose to provide an internal view of the throat. The patient then consumes several varieties of solid and liquid foods while the SLP observes the function of the throat, vocal cords, and larynx.

Laryngoscopy

With the patient under anesthesia, the doctor uses a small tube with a light on the end to examine the patient's throat and larynx for abnormalities or narrow areas.

Gastroesophageal Endoscopy

With the patient under anesthesia, the doctor inserts a small tube with a camera on the end into the patient's mouth. The tube is gently threaded through the throat and esophagus into the stomach, and the camera captures images of the internal structures. If the doctor notices any abnormalities, the endoscope can be used to take a tissue sample.

Esophageal Manometry

A small tube containing a pressure gauge is inserted through the mouth into the esophagus, where it measures the pressure. This test is used to evaluate the effectiveness of the esophagus in moving food downward to the stomach.

Gastrointestinal Reflux Testing

Tiny probes are inserted into the patient's esophagus or stomach to measure the amount of acid present. The pH probes are used to analyze whether acid reflux may contribute to throat irritation and swallowing problems.

Treatment of Dysphagia

Based on the results of the physical examination and special tests, the medical team will recommend a course of treatment for the patient's swallowing difficulties. The treatment depends on the extent and underlying cause of the dysphagia, as well as the patient's overall health. Some of the possible forms of treatment include the following:

- Nutritional changes, including different types, tastes, textures, and temperatures of foods

- Thickening liquids to make them easier to swallow

- Medications to treat acid reflux

- Behavioral interventions

- Posture or positioning changes

- Exercises recommended by an SLP to improve chewing or sucking, strengthen muscles in the mouth, and increase tongue movement

- Referral to a dentist or craniofacial surgeon

- Surgical procedures to widen the esophagus or keep food and acid in the stomach

Prognosis of Dysphagia

Dysphagia in children can result in dehydration, poor nutrition, and a failure to gain weight or grow properly. In addition, they may develop aversion to certain foods or liquids, embarrassment in social situations involving eating, or behavioral resistance to eating. Dysphagia can also result in aspiration of food into the windpipe (trachea) and lungs. Aspiration can create a choking hazard, and it also increases the risk of respiratory infections, pneumonia, and chronic lung disease. Medical treatment can help many children with dysphagia learn to swallow more effectively so that they can eat and drink with minimal difficulty.

Some patients may not experience much improvement, however, especially those with health issues that affect the nerves and muscles.

References

1. "Difficulty Swallowing (Dysphagia)—Overview," WebMD, 2016.

2. "Dysphagia," Ann and Robert H. Lurie Children's Hospital of Chicago, 2016.

3. "Feeding and Swallowing Disorders (Dysphagia) in Children," American Speech-Language-Hearing Association (ASHA), 2016.

4. "Swallowing Problems (Dysphagia)," Stanford Children's Health, 2016.

Section 22.8

Gastroenteritis

This section includes text excerpted from "Viral Gastroenteritis (Stomach Flu)," National Institute of Diabetes and Digestive and Kidney Diseases (NIDDK), May 2018.

Definition and Facts for Viral Gastroenteritis
What Is Viral Gastroenteritis?

Viral gastroenteritis is an infection of your intestines that typically causes watery diarrhea, pain or cramping in your abdomen, nausea or vomiting, and sometimes fever.

Viral gastroenteritis is caused by viruses. Viruses invade normal cells in your body. Many viruses cause infections that can be spread from person to person.

People commonly call viral gastroenteritis "stomach flu," but the term is not medically correct. Viral gastroenteritis is an infection of the intestines, not the stomach, and it is not caused by influenza (flu) viruses. The flu vaccine does not protect against viral gastroenteritis.

Viral gastroenteritis is acute, meaning it happens suddenly and lasts a short time. Most cases of viral gastroenteritis last less than a week, and most people get better on their own without medical treatment. In some cases, viral gastroenteritis may cause severe symptoms or may lead to dehydration.

How Common Is Viral Gastroenteritis?

Viral gastroenteritis is very common. Norovirus is the most common cause of viral gastroenteritis. In the United States, norovirus causes 19 to 21 million cases of viral gastroenteritis each year. Other viruses that cause gastroenteritis are less common.

Who Is More Likely to Get Viral Gastroenteritis?

Anyone can get viral gastroenteritis. Some people are more likely to have severe symptoms, including:

- Infants and young children

- Older adults

- People with a weakened immune system

What Are the Complications of Viral Gastroenteritis?

Dehydration is the most common complication of viral gastroenteritis. When viral gastroenteritis causes you to vomit or have diarrhea, your body loses fluids and electrolytes. If you do not replace those fluids and electrolytes, you may become dehydrated. When you are dehydrated, your body does not have enough fluids and electrolytes to work properly.

Dehydration is especially dangerous in children. Without treatment, dehydration can lead to serious problems, such as organ damage, shock, coma, or even death.

Symptoms and Causes of Viral Gastroenteritis
What Are the Symptoms of Viral Gastroenteritis?

The symptoms of viral gastroenteritis include:

- Watery diarrhea

- Pain or cramping in your abdomen

- Nausea or vomiting

- Sometimes fever

What Are the Symptoms of Dehydration?

Symptoms of dehydration, if you are the parent or caretaker of an infant or young child with viral gastroenteritis, you should watch for the following signs of dehydration:

- Thirst

- Urinating less than usual, or no wet diapers for three hours or more

- Lack of energy

- Dry mouth

- No tears when crying

- Decreased skin turgor

- Sunken eyes or cheeks

What Kinds of Viruses Cause Viral Gastroenteritis?

Many different viruses can cause viral gastroenteritis. The most common causes of viral gastroenteritis include:

- **Norovirus.** Norovirus is the most common cause of viral gastroenteritis. Symptoms usually begin 12 to 48 hours after you come into contact with the virus and last 1 to 3 days.

- **Rotavirus.** Symptoms usually begin about 2 days after you come into contact with the virus and last for 3 to 8 days. Vaccines can prevent rotavirus infection.

- **Adenovirus.** Symptoms typically begin 3 to 10 days after you come into contact with the virus and last 1 to 2 weeks.

- **Astrovirus.** Symptoms typically begin 4 to 5 days after you come into contact with the virus and last 1 to 4 days.

Norovirus causes infections in people of all ages. Rotavirus, adenovirus, and astrovirus most often infect infants and young children, but they can also infect adults.

Viruses may cause viral gastroenteritis any time of the year. In the United States, norovirus, rotavirus, and astrovirus are more likely to cause infections in the winter.

Do Flu Viruses Cause Viral Gastroenteritis?

Although some people call viral gastroenteritis "stomach flu," influenza (flu) viruses do not cause viral gastroenteritis. Flu viruses cause infections of the respiratory system, while viral gastroenteritis is an infection of the intestines.

Are Viruses the Only Cause of Gastroenteritis?

No. While viruses cause viral gastroenteritis, bacteria, parasites, and chemicals may cause other kinds of gastroenteritis.

When gastroenteritis is caused by consuming foods or drinks contaminated with viruses, bacteria, parasites, or chemicals, this is called "food poisoning."

How Does Viral Gastroenteritis Spread?

Viral gastroenteritis spreads from person to person through contact with an infected person's stool or vomit.

If you have viral gastroenteritis, viruses will be present in your stool and vomit. You may spread the virus in small bits of stool or vomit, especially if you do not wash your hands thoroughly after using the bathroom and:

- Touch surfaces or objects used by other people

- Prepare or serve foods and drinks for other people

- Shake hands with or touch another person

Infected people who do not have symptoms can still spread viruses. For example, norovirus may be found in your stool before you have symptoms and up to two weeks after you recover.

Norovirus is especially contagious, meaning that it spreads easily from person to person. Norovirus can live for months on surfaces such as countertops and changing tables. When an infected person vomits, the virus may become airborne and land on surfaces or on another person.

Viral gastroenteritis may spread in households, daycare centers and schools, nursing homes, cruise ships, restaurants, and other places where people gather in groups.

If water comes into contact with stools of infected people, the water may become contaminated with a virus. The contaminated water can spread the virus to foods or drinks, and people who consume these foods or drinks may become infected. People who swim in contaminated water may also become infected.

Diagnosis of Viral Gastroenteritis
How Do Doctors Diagnose Viral Gastroenteritis?

Doctors often diagnose viral gastroenteritis based on your symptoms. If your symptoms are mild and last only a short time, you typically will not need tests.

In some cases, a medical history, a physical exam, and stool tests can help diagnose viral gastroenteritis. Your doctor may perform additional tests to check for other health problems.

Medical History

Your doctor will ask you about your symptoms, for example:

- What symptoms you have

- How long you have had symptoms

- How often you have had symptoms

Your doctor may also ask you about:

- Recent contacts with other people who are sick

- Recent travel

- Current and past medical conditions

- Prescription and over-the-counter (OTC) medicines you take

Physical Exam

During a physical exam, your doctor may:

- Check your blood pressure and pulse for signs of dehydration

- Examine you for signs of fever or dehydration

- Use a stethoscope to listen to sounds in your abdomen

- Tap on your abdomen to check for tenderness or pain

Sometimes, doctors perform a digital rectal exam. Your doctor will have you bend over a table or lie on your side while holding your knees close to your chest. After putting on a glove, the doctor will slide a lubricated finger into your anus to check for blood in your stool. Blood in your stool may be a sign of health conditions other than viral gastroenteritis that may be causing your symptoms.

Stool Tests

A healthcare professional will give you a container for catching and storing the stool. You will receive instructions on where to send or take the container for analysis. Stool tests can show signs of infection, inflammation, and digestive diseases and disorders.

Treatment of Viral Gastroenteritis
How Can I Treat Viral Gastroenteritis?

In most cases, people with viral gastroenteritis get better on their own without medical treatment. You can treat viral gastroenteritis by replacing lost fluids and electrolytes to prevent dehydration. In some cases, OTC medicines may help relieve symptoms.

Research shows that following a restricted diet does not help treat viral gastroenteritis. When you have viral gastroenteritis, you may vomit after you eat or lose your appetite for a short time. When your appetite returns, you can most often go back to eating your normal diet, even if you still have diarrhea. Find tips on what to eat when you have viral gastroenteritis.

If your child has symptoms of viral gastroenteritis, such as vomiting or diarrhea, do not hesitate to call a doctor for advice.

Replace Lost Fluids and Electrolytes

If your child has viral gastroenteritis, you should give your child an oral rehydration solution—such as Pedialyte®, Naturalyte®, Infalyte®, and CeraLyte®—as directed to replace lost fluids and electrolytes. Oral rehydration solutions are liquids that contain glucose and electrolytes. Talk with a doctor about giving these solutions to your infant. Infants should drink breast milk or formula as usual.

Over-the-Counter Medicines

Over-the-counter (OTC) medicines can be unsafe for infants and children. Talk with a doctor before giving your child an OTC medicine.

How Do Doctors Treat Viral Gastroenteritis?

Your doctor may prescribe medicine to control severe vomiting. Doctors do not prescribe antibiotics to treat viral gastroenteritis. Antibiotics do not work for viral infections.

In some cases, your doctor may recommend probiotics. Probiotics are live microbes, most often bacteria, that are like the ones you normally have in your digestive tract. Studies suggest that some probiotics may help shorten a case of diarrhea. Researchers are still studying the use of probiotics to treat viral gastroenteritis. For safety reasons, talk with your doctor before using probiotics or any other complementary or alternative medicines or practices.

Anyone with signs or symptoms of dehydration should see a doctor right away. Doctors may need to treat people with severe dehydration in a hospital.

How Can I Prevent Viral Gastroenteritis?

You can take several steps to keep from getting or spreading infections that cause viral gastroenteritis. Wash your hands thoroughly with soap and water:

- After using the bathroom

- After changing diapers

- Before and after handling, preparing, or eating food

You can clean surfaces that may have come into contact with infected stool or vomit, such as countertops and changing tables, with a mixture of 5 to 25 tablespoons of household bleach and 1 gallon of water. If clothes or linens may have come into contact with an infected person's stool or vomit, you should wash them with detergent for the longest cycle available and machine dry them. To protect yourself from infection, wear rubber gloves while handling the soiled laundry and wash your hands afterward.

If you have viral gastroenteritis, avoid handling and preparing food for others while you are sick and for 2 days after your symptoms stop. People who have viral gastroenteritis may spread the virus to any food they handle, especially if they do not thoroughly wash their hands. Contaminated water may also spread a virus to foods before they are harvested. For example, contaminated fruits, vegetables, and oysters have been linked to norovirus outbreaks. Wash fruits and vegetables before using them, and thoroughly cook oysters and other shellfish. Find tips to help keep food safe.

The flu vaccine does not protect against viral gastroenteritis. Although some people call viral gastroenteritis "stomach flu," influenza (flu) viruses do not cause viral gastroenteritis. However, rotavirus vaccines can prevent viral gastroenteritis caused by rotavirus.

Rotavirus Vaccines

Two vaccines, which infants receive by mouth, are approved to protect against rotavirus infections:

- **RotaTeq®**: Infants receive 3 doses, at ages 2 months, 4 months, and 6 months

- **Rotarix®**: Infants receive this vaccine in 2 doses, at ages 2 months and 4 months

For the rotavirus vaccine to be most effective, infants should receive the first dose by 15 weeks of age. Infants should receive all doses by 8 months of age.

If you have a baby, talk with your baby's doctor about rotavirus vaccination.

Section 22.9

Gastroesophageal Reflux

This section includes text excerpted from "Acid Reflux (GER and GERD) in Children and Teens," National Institute of Diabetes and Digestive and Kidney Diseases (NIDDK), April 2015. Reviewed September 2019.

Definition and Facts of Gastroesophageal Reflux and Gastroesophageal Reflux Disease in Children and Teens
What Is Gastroesophageal Reflux?

Gastroesophageal reflux (GER) happens when stomach contents come back up into the esophagus. Stomach acid that touches the lining of the esophagus can cause heartburn, also called "acid indigestion."

Doctors also refer to GER as:

- Acid indigestion

- Acid reflux

- Acid regurgitation

- Heartburn

- Reflux

How Common Is Gastroesophageal Reflux in Children and Teens?

Occasional GER is common in children and teens—ages 2 to 19—and does not always mean that they have gastroesophageal reflux disease (GERD).

What Is Gastroesophageal Reflux Disease?

Gastroesophageal reflux disease is a more serious and long-lasting form of GER in which acid reflux irritates the esophagus.

What Is the Difference between Gastroesophageal Reflux and Gastroesophageal Reflux Disease?

Gastroesophageal reflux that occurs more than twice a week for a few weeks could be GERD. GERD can lead to more serious health problems over time. If you think your child or teen has GERD, you should take her or him to see a doctor or a pediatrician.

How Common Is Gastroesophageal Reflux Disease in Children and Teens?

Up to 25 percent of children and teens have symptoms of GERD, although GERD is more common in adults.

What Are the Complications of Gastroesophageal Reflux Disease in Children and Teens?

Without treatment, GERD can sometimes cause serious complications over time, such as:

Esophagitis

Esophagitis may lead to ulcerations, a sore in the lining of the esophagus.

Esophageal Stricture

An esophageal stricture happens when a person's esophagus becomes too narrow. Esophageal strictures can lead to problems with swallowing.

Respiratory Problems

A child or teen with GERD might breathe stomach acid into her or his lungs. The stomach acid can then irritate her or his throat and lungs, causing respiratory problems or symptoms, such as:

- Asthma—a long-lasting lung disease that makes a child or teen extra sensitive to things that she or he is allergic to

- Chest congestion, or extra fluid in the lungs

- A dry, long-lasting cough or a sore throat

- Hoarseness—the partial loss of a child or teen's voice

- Laryngitis—the swelling of a child or teen's voice box that can lead to a short-term loss of her or his voice

- Pneumonia—an infection in one or both lungs—that keeps coming back

- Wheezing—a high-pitched whistling sound that happens while breathing

A pediatrician should monitor children and teens with GERD to prevent or treat long-term problems.

Symptoms and Causes of Gastroesophageal Reflux and Gastroesophageal Reflux Disease in Children and Teens

What Are the Symptoms of Gastroesophageal Reflux and Gastroesophageal Reflux Disease in Children and Teens?

If a child or teen has gastroesophageal reflux, she or he may taste food or stomach acid in the back of the mouth.

Symptoms of gastroesophageal reflux disease (GERD) in children and teens can vary depending on their age. The most common symptom of GERD in children 12 years and older is regular heartburn, a painful, burning feeling in the middle of the chest, behind the breastbone, and in the middle of the abdomen. In many cases, children with GERD who are younger than 12 do not have heartburn.

Other common GERD symptoms include:

- Bad breath

- Nausea

- Pain in the chest or the upper part of the abdomen
- Problems swallowing or painful swallowing
- Respiratory problems
- Vomiting
- The wearing away of teeth

What Causes Gastroesophageal Reflux and Gastroesophageal Reflux Disease in Children and Teens

Gastroesophageal reflux and gastroesophageal reflux disease happen when a child or teen's lower esophageal sphincter becomes weak or relaxes when it should not, causing stomach contents to rise up into the esophagus. The lower esophageal sphincter becomes weak or relaxes due to certain things, such as:

- Increased pressure on the abdomen from being overweight, obese, or pregnant
- Certain medicines, including:
  - Those used to treat asthma—a long-lasting disease in the lungs that makes a child or teen extra sensitive to things that she or he is allergic to
  - Antihistamines—medicines that treat allergy symptoms
  - Painkillers
  - Sedatives—medicines that help put someone to sleep
  - Antidepressants—medicines that treat depression
- Smoking, which is more likely with teens than younger children, or inhaling secondhand smoke

Other reasons a child or teen develops GERD include:

- Previous esophageal surgery
- Having a severe developmental delay or neurological condition, such as cerebral palsy

When Should I Seek a Doctor's Help?

Call a doctor right away if your child or teen:

- Vomits large amounts

- Has regular projectile, or forceful, vomiting
- Vomits fluid that is:
  - Green or yellow
  - Looks like coffee grounds
  - Contains blood
- Has problems breathing after vomiting
- Has mouth or throat pain when she or he eats
- Has problems swallowing or pain when swallowing
- Refuses food repeatedly, causing weight loss or poor growth
- Shows signs of dehydration, such as no tears when she or he cries

Diagnosis of Gastroesophageal Reflux and Gastroesophageal Reflux Disease in Children and Teens

How Do Doctors Diagnose Gastroesophageal Reflux in Children and Teens?

In most cases, a doctor diagnoses gastroesophageal reflux by reviewing a child's or teen's symptoms and medical history. If symptoms of GER do not improve with lifestyle changes and antireflux medicines, she or he may need testing.

How Do Doctors Diagnose Gastroesophageal Reflux Disease in Children and Teens?

If a child or teen's GER symptoms do not improve, if they come back frequently, or she or he has trouble swallowing, the doctor may recommend testing for gastroesophageal reflux disease (GERD).

The doctor may refer the child or teen to a pediatric gastroenterologist to diagnose and treat GERD.

What Tests Do Doctors Use to Diagnose Gastroesophageal Reflux Disease?

Several tests can help a doctor diagnose GERD. A doctor may order more than one test to make a diagnosis.

Upper Gastrointestinal Series

An upper GI series looks at the shape of the child or teen's upper GI tract.

Esophageal pH and Impedance Monitoring

The most accurate procedure to detect acid reflux is esophageal pH and impedance monitoring. Esophageal pH and impedance monitoring measure the amount of acid or liquid in a child or teen's esophagus while she or he does normal things, such as eating and sleeping.

Upper Gastrointestinal Endoscopy and Biopsy

In an upper GI endoscopy, a gastroenterologist, surgeon, or other trained healthcare professional uses an endoscope to see inside a child or teen's upper GI tract. This procedure takes place at a hospital or an outpatient center.

Treatment of Gastroesophageal Reflux and Gastroesophageal Reflux Disease in Children and Teens

How Do Doctors Treat Gastroesophageal Reflux and Gastroesophageal Reflux Disease in Children and Teens?

You can help control a child or teen's gastroesophageal reflux or gastroesophageal reflux disease (GERD) by having her or him:

- Not eat or drink items that may cause GER, such as greasy or spicy foods
- Not overeat
- Avoid smoking and secondhand smoke
- Lose weight if she or he is overweight or obese
- Avoid eating two to three hours before bedtime
- Take over-the-counter (OTC) medicines, such as Alka-Seltzer®, Maalox®, or Rolaids®

How Do Doctors Treat Gastroesophageal Reflux Disease in Children and Teens?

Depending on the severity of the child's symptoms, a doctor may recommend lifestyle changes, medicines, or surgery.

Lifestyle Changes

Helping a child or teen make lifestyle changes can reduce her or his GERD symptoms. A child or teen should:

- Lose weight, if needed.
- Eat smaller meals
- Avoid high-fat foods
- Wear loose-fitting clothing around the abdomen. Tight clothing can squeeze the stomach area and push the acid up into the esophagus.
- Stay upright for three hours after meals and avoid reclining and slouching when sitting.
- Sleep at a slight angle. Raise the head of the child or teen's bed six to eight inches by safely putting blocks under the bedposts. Just using extra pillows will not help.
- If a teen smokes, help them quit smoking and avoid secondhand smoke.

Over-the-Counter and Prescription Medicines

If a child or teen has symptoms that will not go away, you should take her or him to see a doctor. The doctor can prescribe medicine to relieve her or his symptoms. Some medicines are available OTC.

All GERD medicines work in different ways. A child or teen may need a combination of GERD medicines to control symptoms.

Antacids

Doctors often first recommend antacids to relieve GER and other mild GERD symptoms. A doctor will tell you which OTC antacids to give a child or teen, such as:

- Alka-Seltzer®
- Maalox®
- Mylanta®
- Riopan®
- Rolaids®

Antacids can have side effects, including diarrhea and constipation. Do not give your child or teen OTC antacids without first checking with her or his doctor.

Histamine H₂-Receptor Antagonists Blockers

Histamine H$_2$-receptor antagonists (H$_2$) blockers decrease acid production. They provide short-term or on-demand relief for many people with GERD symptoms. They can also help heal the esophagus, although not as well as other medicines. If a doctor recommends an H$_2$ blocker for the child or teen, you can buy them OTC or a doctor can prescribe one. Types of H$_2$ blockers include:

- Cimetidine (Tagamet HB®)

- Famotidine (Pepcid AC®)

- Nizatidine (Axid AR®)

- Ranitidine (Zantac 75®)

If a child or teen develops heartburn after eating, her or his doctor may prescribe an antacid and an H$_2$ blocker. The antacids neutralize stomach acid, and the H$_2$ blockers stop the stomach from creating acid. By the time the antacids wear off, the H$_2$ blockers are controlling the acid in the stomach.

Do not give your child or teen OTC H$_2$ blockers without first checking with her or his doctor.

Proton Pump Inhibitors

Proton pump inhibitors (PPIs) lower the amount of acid the stomach makes. PPIs are better at treating GERD symptoms than H$_2$ blockers. They can heal the esophageal lining in most people with GERD. Doctors often prescribe PPIs for long-term GERD treatment.

However, studies show that people who take PPIs for a long time or in high doses are more likely to have hip, wrist, and spinal fractures. A child or teen should take these medicines on an empty stomach so that her or his stomach acid can make them work correctly.

Several types of PPIs are available by a doctor's prescription, including:

- Esomeprazole (Nexium®)

- Lansoprazole (Prevacid®)

- Omeprazole (Prilosec®, Zegerid®)

- Pantoprazole (Protonix®)

- Rabeprazole (Aciphex®)

Talk with the child or teen's doctor about taking lower-strength omeprazole or lansoprazole, sold OTC. Do not give a child or teen OTC PPIs without first checking with her or his doctor.

Prokinetics

Prokinetics help the stomach empty faster. Prescription prokinetics include:

- Bethanechol (Urecholine®)
- Metoclopramide (Reglan®)

Both these medicines have side effects, including:

- Nausea
- Diarrhea
- Fatigue, or feeling tired
- Depression
- Anxiety
- Delayed or abnormal physical movement

Prokinetics can cause problems if a child or teen mixes them with other medicines, so tell the doctor about all the medicines she or he is taking.

Antibiotics

Antibiotics, including erythromycin, can help the stomach empty faster. Erythromycin has fewer side effects than prokinetics; however, it can cause diarrhea.

Surgery

A pediatric gastroenterologist may recommend surgery if a child or teen's GERD symptoms do not improve with lifestyle changes or medicines. A child or teen is more likely to develop complications from surgery than from medicines.

Section 22.10

Irritable Bowel Syndrome

This section includes text excerpted from "Irritable Bowel Syndrome (IBS) in Children," National Institute of Diabetes and Digestive and Kidney Diseases (NIDDK), June 2014. Reviewed September 2019.

What Is Irritable Bowel Syndrome?

Irritable bowel syndrome (IBS) is a functional gastrointestinal (GI) disorder, meaning it is a problem caused by changes in how the GI tract works. Children with functional GI disorder have frequent symptoms, but the GI tract does not become damaged. IBS is not a disease; it is a group of symptoms that occur together. The most common symptoms of IBS are abdominal pain or discomfort, often reported as cramping, along with diarrhea, constipation, or both. In the past, IBS was called "colitis," "mucous colitis," "spastic colon," "nervous colon," and "spastic bowel." The name was changed to reflect the understanding that the disorder has both physical and mental causes and is not a product of a person's imagination.

Irritable bowel syndrome is diagnosed when a child who is growing as expected has abdominal pain or discomfort once per week for at least two months without other disease or injury that could explain the pain. The pain or discomfort of IBS may occur with a change in stool frequency or consistency or may be relieved by a bowel movement.

What Is the Gastrointestinal Tract?

The GI tract is a series of hollow organs joined in a long, twisting tube from the mouth to the anus. The movement of muscles in the GI tract, along with the release of hormones and enzymes, allows for the digestion of food. Organs that make up the GI tract are the mouth, esophagus, stomach, small intestine, large intestine—which includes the appendix, cecum, colon, and rectum—and anus. The intestines are sometimes called the "bowel." The last part of the GI tract—called the "lower GI tract"—consists of the large intestine and anus.

The large intestine absorbs water and any remaining nutrients from partially digested food passed from the small intestine. The large intestine then changes waste from liquid to a solid matter called "stool." Stool passes from the colon to the rectum. The rectum is located between the last part of the colon—called the "sigmoid colon"—and the "anus." The rectum stores stool prior to a bowel movement. During a bowel movement, stool moves from the rectum to the anus, the opening through which stool leaves the body.

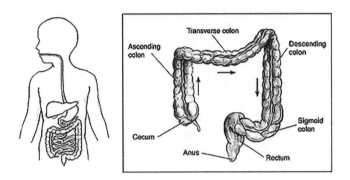

Figure 22.2. *The Lower GI Tract*

How Common Is Irritable Bowel Syndrome in Children?

Limited information is available about the number of children with IBS. Older studies have reported prevalence rates for recurrent abdominal pain in children of 10 to 20 percent. However, these studies did not differentiate IBS from functional abdominal pain, indigestion, and abdominal migraine. One study of children in North America found that 14 percent of high school students and 6 percent of middle school students have IBS. The study also found that IBS affects boys and girls equally.

What Are the Symptoms of Irritable Bowel Syndrome in Children?

The symptoms of IBS include abdominal pain or discomfort and changes in bowel habits. To meet the definition of IBS, the pain or discomfort should be associated with two of the following three symptoms:

- Start with bowel movements that occur more or less often than usual

- Start with stool that appears looser and more watery or harder and more lumpy than usual

- Improve with a bowel movement

Other symptoms of IBS may include:

- Diarrhea—having loose, watery stools three or more times a day and feeling an urgency to have a bowel movement
- Constipation—having hard, dry stools; two or fewer bowel movements in a week; or straining to have a bowel movement
- Feeling that a bowel movement is incomplete
- Passing mucus, a clear liquid made by the intestines that coats and protects tissues in the GI tract
- Abdominal bloating

Symptoms may often occur after eating a meal. To meet the definition of IBS, symptoms must occur at least once per week for at least two months.

What Causes Irritable Bowel Syndrome in Children

The causes of IBS are not well understood. Researchers believe a combination of physical and mental health problems can lead to IBS. The possible causes of IBS in children include the following:

- **Brain–gut signal problems.** Signals between the brain and nerves of the small and large intestines, also called the "gut," control how the intestines work. Problems with brain–gut signals may cause IBS symptoms, such as changes in bowel habits and pain or discomfort.

- **GI motor problems.** Normal motility, or movement, may not be present in the colon of a child who has IBS. Slow motility can lead to constipation and fast motility can lead to diarrhea. Spasms, or sudden strong muscle contractions that come and go, can cause abdominal pain. Some children with IBS also experience hyperreactivity, which is an excessive increase in contractions of the bowel in response to stress or eating.

- **Hypersensitivity.** Children with IBS have greater sensitivity to abdominal pain than children without IBS. Affected children have been found to have different rectal tone and rectal motor response after eating a meal.

- **Mental-health problems.** IBS has been linked to mental health or psychological problems such as anxiety and depression in children.

- **Bacterial gastroenteritis.** Some children who have bacterial gastroenteritis—an infection or irritation of the stomach and intestines caused by bacteria—develop IBS. Research has shown a connection between gastroenteritis and IBS in adults but not in children. But researchers believe postinfectious IBS does occur in children. Researchers do not know why gastroenteritis leads to IBS in some people and not others.

- **Small intestinal bacterial overgrowth (SIBO).** Normally, few bacteria live in the small intestine. SIBO is an increase in the number of bacteria or a change in the type of bacteria in the small intestine. These bacteria can produce excess gas and may also cause diarrhea and weight loss. Some researchers believe that SIBO may lead to IBS, and some studies have shown antibiotics to be effective in treating IBS. However, the studies were weak and more research is needed to show a link between SIBO and IBS.

- **Genetics.** Whether IBS has a genetic cause, meaning it runs in families, is unclear. Studies have shown that IBS is more common in people with family members who have a history of GI problems. However, the cause could be environmental or the result of heightened awareness of GI symptoms.

How Is Irritable Bowel Syndrome in Children Diagnosed?

To diagnose IBS, a healthcare provider will conduct a physical exam and take a complete medical history. The medical history will include questions about the child's symptoms, family members with GI disorders, recent infections, medications, and stressful events related to the onset of symptoms. IBS is diagnosed when the physical exam does not show any cause for the child's symptoms and the child meets all of the following criteria:

- Has had symptoms at least once per week for at least two months

- Is growing as expected

- Is not showing any signs that suggest another cause for the symptoms

How Is Irritable Bowel Syndrome in Children Treated?

Though there is no cure for IBS, the symptoms can be treated with a combination of the following:

- Changes in eating, diet, and nutrition
- Medications
- Probiotics
- Therapies for mental-health problems

Eating, Diet, and Nutrition

Large meals can cause cramping and diarrhea, so eating smaller meals more often, or eating smaller portions, may help IBS symptoms. Eating meals that are low in fat and high in carbohydrates, such as pasta, rice, whole-grain bread, and cereals, fruits, and vegetables may help.

Certain foods and drinks may cause IBS symptoms in some children, such as:

- Foods high in fat
- Milk products
- Drinks with caffeine
- Drinks with large amounts of artificial sweeteners, which are substances used in place of sugar
- Foods that may cause gas, such as beans and cabbage

Medications

The healthcare provider will select medications based on the child's symptoms. Caregivers should not give children any medications unless told to do so by a healthcare provider.

Probiotics

Probiotics are live microorganisms, usually bacteria, that are similar to microorganisms normally found in the GI tract. Studies have found that probiotics, specifically Bifidobacteria and certain probiotic combinations, improve symptoms of IBS when taken in large enough amounts. But more research is needed. Probiotics can be found in dietary supplements, such as capsules, tablets, and powders, and in some foods, such as yogurt. A healthcare provider can give information about the right kind and right amount of probiotics to take to improve IBS symptoms.

Therapies for Mental-Health Problems

The following therapies can help improve IBS symptoms due to mental-health problems:

- **Talk therapy.** Talking with a therapist may reduce stress and improve IBS symptoms. Two types of talk therapy used to treat IBS are cognitive-behavioral therapy (CBT) and psychodynamic, or interpersonal therapy (PIT). Cognitive-behavioral therapy focuses on the child's thoughts and actions. Psychodynamic therapy focuses on how emotions affect IBS symptoms. This type of therapy often involves relaxation and stress-management techniques.

- **Hypnotherapy.** In hypnotherapy, the therapist uses hypnosis to help the child relax into a trance-like state. This type of therapy may help the child relax the muscles in the colon.

Section 22.11

Lactose Intolerance

This section includes text excerpted from "Lactose Intolerance," National Institute of Diabetes and Digestive and Kidney Diseases (NIDDK), February 2018.

Definition and Facts of Lactose Intolerance
What Is Lactose Intolerance?

Lactose intolerance is a condition in which you have digestive symptoms—such as bloating, diarrhea, and gas—after you consume foods or drinks that contain lactose. Lactose is a sugar that is naturally found in milk and milk products, such as cheese or ice cream.

In lactose intolerance, digestive symptoms are caused by lactose malabsorption. Lactose malabsorption is a condition in which your small intestine cannot digest, or break down, all the lactose you eat or drink.

Not everyone with lactose malabsorption has digestive symptoms after they consume lactose. Only people who have symptoms are lactose intolerant.

Most people with lactose intolerance can consume some amount of lactose without having symptoms. Different people can tolerate different amounts of lactose before having symptoms.

Lactose intolerance is different from a milk allergy. A milk allergy is an immune system disorder.

How Common Is Lactose Malabsorption?

While most infants can digest lactose, many people begin to develop lactose malabsorption—a reduced ability to digest lactose—after infancy. Experts estimate that about 68 percent of the world's population has lactose malabsorption.

Lactose malabsorption is more common in some parts of the world than in others. In Africa and Asia, most people have lactose malabsorption. In some regions, such as Northern Europe, many people carry a gene that allows them to digest lactose after infancy, and lactose malabsorption is less common. In the United States, about 36 percent of people have lactose malabsorption.

While lactose malabsorption causes lactose intolerance, not all people with lactose malabsorption have lactose intolerance.

Who Is More Likely to Have Lactose Intolerance?

You are more likely to have lactose intolerance if you are from, or your family is from, a part of the world where lactose malabsorption is more common. In the United States, the following ethnic and racial groups are more likely to have lactose malabsorption:

- African Americans
- American Indians
- Asian Americans
- Hispanics/Latinos

Because these ethnic and racial groups are more likely to have lactose malabsorption, they are also more likely to have the symptoms of lactose intolerance.

Lactose intolerance is least common among people who are from, or whose families are from Europe.

What Are the Complications of Lactose Intolerance?

Lactose intolerance may affect your health if it keeps you from getting enough nutrients, such as calcium and vitamin D. Milk and milk products, which contain lactose, are some of the main sources of calcium, vitamin D, and other nutrients.

You need calcium throughout your life to grow and have healthy bones. If you do not get enough calcium, your bones may become weak and more likely to break. This condition is called "osteoporosis." If you have lactose intolerance, you can change your diet to make sure you get enough calcium while also managing your symptoms.

Symptoms and Causes of Lactose Intolerance
What Are the Symptoms of Lactose Intolerance?

If you have lactose intolerance, you may have symptoms within a few hours after you have milk or milk products, or other foods that contain lactose. Your symptoms may include:

- Bloating

- Diarrhea

- Gas

- Nausea

- Pain in your abdomen

- Stomach "growling" or rumbling sounds

- Vomiting

Your symptoms may be mild or severe, depending on how much lactose you have.

What Causes Lactose Intolerance

Lactose intolerance is caused by lactose malabsorption. If you have lactose malabsorption, your small intestine makes low levels of lactase—the enzyme that breaks down lactose—and cannot digest all the lactose you eat or drink.

The undigested lactose passes into your colon. Bacteria in your colon break down the lactose and create fluid and gas. In some people, this extra fluid and gas cause lactose intolerance symptoms.

In some cases, your genes are the reason for lactose intolerance. Genes play a role in the following conditions, and these conditions can lead to low levels of lactase in your small intestine and lactose malabsorption:

- **Lactase nonpersistence.** In people with lactase nonpersistence, the small intestine makes less lactase after infancy. Lactase levels get lower with age. Symptoms of lactose intolerance may not begin until later childhood, the teen years, or early adulthood. Lactase nonpersistence, also called "primary lactase deficiency," is the most common cause of low lactase levels.

- **Congenital lactase deficiency.** In this rare condition, the small intestine makes little or no lactase, starting at birth.

Not all causes of lactose intolerance are genetic. The following can also lead to lactose intolerance:

- **Injury to the small intestine.** Infections, diseases, or other conditions that injure your small intestine, like Crohn disease or celiac disease, may cause it to make less lactase. Treatments—such as medicines, surgery, or radiation therapy—for other conditions may also injure your small intestine. Lactose intolerance caused by injury to the small intestine is called "secondary lactose intolerance." If the cause of the injury is treated, you may be able to tolerate lactose again.

- **Premature birth.** In premature babies, or babies born too soon, the small intestine may not make enough lactase for a short time after birth. The small intestine usually makes more lactase as the baby gets older.

What Is the Difference between Lactose Intolerance and Milk Allergies?

Lactose intolerance and milk allergies are different conditions with different causes. Lactose intolerance is caused by problems digesting lactose, the natural sugar in milk. In contrast, milk allergies are caused by your immune system's response to one or more proteins in milk and milk products.

A milk allergy most often appears in the first year of life, while lactose intolerance typically appears later. Lactose intolerance can cause uncomfortable symptoms, while a serious allergic reaction to milk can be life-threatening.

Diagnosis of Lactose Intolerance
How Do Doctors Diagnose Lactose Intolerance?

To diagnose lactose intolerance, your doctor will ask about your symptoms, family and medical history, and eating habits.

Your doctor may perform a physical exam and tests to help diagnose lactose intolerance or to check for other health problems. Other conditions, such as irritable bowel syndrome (IBS), celiac disease, inflammatory bowel disease (IBD), or small bowel bacterial overgrowth (SIBO) can cause symptoms similar to those of lactose intolerance.

Your doctor may ask you to stop eating and drinking milk and milk products for a period of time to see if your symptoms go away. If your symptoms do not go away, your doctor may order additional tests.

Physical Exam

During a physical exam, your doctor may:

- Check for bloating in your abdomen

- Use a stethoscope to listen to sounds within your abdomen

- Tap on your abdomen to check for tenderness or pain

What Tests Do Doctors Use to Diagnose Lactose Intolerance?

Your doctor may order a hydrogen breath test to see how well your small intestine digests lactose.

Hydrogen Breath Test

Doctors use this test to diagnose lactose malabsorption and lactose intolerance. Normally, a small amount of hydrogen, a type of gas, is found in your breath. If you have lactose malabsorption, undigested lactose causes you to have high levels of hydrogen in your breath.

For this test, you will drink a liquid that contains a known amount of lactose. Every 30 minutes over a few hours, you will breathe into a balloon-type container that measures the amount of hydrogen in your breath. During this time, a healthcare professional will ask about your symptoms. If both your breath hydrogen levels rise and your symptoms get worse during the test, your doctor may diagnose lactose intolerance.

Treatment of Lactose Intolerance
How Can I Manage My Lactose Intolerance Symptoms?

In most cases, you can manage the symptoms of lactose intolerance by changing your diet to limit or avoid foods and drinks that contain lactose, such as milk and milk products.

Some people may only need to limit the amount of lactose they eat or drink, while others may need to avoid lactose altogether. Using lactase products can help some people manage their symptoms.

Lactase Products

Lactase products are tablets or drops that contain lactase, the enzyme that breaks down lactose. You can take lactase tablets before you eat or drink milk products. You can also add lactase drops to milk before you drink it. The lactase breaks down the lactose in foods and drinks, lowering your chances of having lactose intolerance symptoms.

Check with your doctor before using lactase products. Some people, such as young children and pregnant and breastfeeding women, may not be able to use them.

How Do Doctors Treat Lactose Intolerance?

Treatments depend on the cause of lactose intolerance. If your lactose intolerance is caused by lactase nonpersistence or congenital lactase deficiency, no treatments can increase the amount of lactase your small intestine makes. Your doctor can help you change your diet to manage your symptoms.

If your lactose intolerance is caused by an injury to your small intestine, your doctor may be able to treat the cause of the injury. You may be able to tolerate lactose after treatment.

While some premature babies are lactose intolerant, the condition usually improves without treatment as the baby gets older.

Section 22.12

Motion Sickness

This section contains text excerpted from the following sources:
Text in this section begins with excerpts from "Motion Sickness,"
Centers for Disease Control and Prevention (CDC), October
23, 2017; Text beginning with the heading "Risk for Travelers"
is excerpted from "Motion Sickness," Centers for Disease
Control and Prevention (CDC), June 24, 2019.

Motion sickness results when the movement you see is different
from what your inner ear senses. It can occur in cars, trains, airplanes,
or boats. Anyone can get motion sickness, although children and pregnant women are especially vulnerable. It can cause dizziness, nausea,
and vomiting, and although it is not a serious condition, motion sickness can make traveling very unpleasant.

Risk for Travelers

"Motion sickness" is the term attributed to physiologic responses
to travel by sea, car, train, air, and virtual reality immersion. Given
sufficient stimulus, all people with functional vestibular systems can
develop motion sickness. However, people vary in their susceptibility.
Risk factors include the following:

- **Age**—children aged 2 to 12 years are especially susceptible, but
  infants and toddlers are generally immune.

- **Sex**—women are more likely to have motion sickness, especially
  when pregnant, menstruating, or on hormones.

- **Migraines**—people who get migraine headaches are more prone
  to motion sickness, especially during a migraine.

- **Medication**—some prescriptions can worsen the nausea of
  motion sickness.

Symptoms of Motion Sickness

Travelers suffering from motion sickness commonly exhibit some
or all of the following symptoms:

- Nausea

- Vomiting/retching

- Sweating
- Cold sweats
- Excessive salivation
- Apathy
- Hyperventilation
- Increased sensitivity to odors
- Loss of appetite
- Headache
- Drowsiness
- Warm sensation
- General discomfort

Prevention of Motion Sickness

Nonpharmacologic interventions to prevent or treat motion sickness include the following:

- Being aware of and avoiding situations that tend to trigger symptoms
- Optimizing position to reduce motion or motion perception—for example, driving a vehicle instead of riding in it, sitting in the front seat of a car or bus, sitting over the wing of an aircraft, holding the head firmly against the back of the seat, and choosing a window seat on flights and trains
- Reducing sensory input—lying prone, shutting eyes, sleeping, or looking at the horizon
- Maintaining hydration by drinking water and eating small meals frequently
- Adding distractions—controlling breathing, listening to music, or using aromatherapy scents such as mint or lavender. Flavored lozenges may also help.
- Using acupressure or magnets is advocated by some to prevent or treat nausea, although scientific data on the efficacy of these interventions for preventing motion sickness are lacking.
- Gradually exposing oneself to continuous or repeated motion sickness triggers. Most people, in time, notice a reduction in motion sickness symptoms.

Treatment of Motion Sickness

Antihistamines are the most frequently used and widely available medications for motion sickness; nonsedating ones appear to be less effective. Antihistamines commonly used for motion sickness include cyclizine, dimenhydrinate, meclizine, and promethazine (oral and suppository). Other common medications used to treat motion sickness are anticholinergics, such as scopolamine (hyoscine—oral, intranasal, and transdermal), antidopaminergic drugs (such as prochlorperazine), metoclopramide, sympathomimetics, and benzodiazepines. Clinical trials have not shown that ondansetron, a drug commonly used as an antiemetic in cancer patients, is effective in the prevention of nausea associated with motion sickness.

Medications in Children

Although using antihistamines to treat motion sickness in children is considered off-label, for children aged 2 to 12 years, dimenhydrinate (Dramamine®), 1 to 1.5 mg/kg per dose, or diphenhydramine (Benadryl®), 0.5 to 1 mg/kg per dose up to 25 mg, can be given 1 hour before travel and every 6 hours during the trip. Because some children have paradoxical agitation with these medicines, a test dose should be given at home before departure. Oversedation of young children with antihistamines can be life-threatening.

Scopolamine can cause dangerous adverse effects in children and should not be used; prochlorperazine and metoclopramide should be used with caution in children.

Chapter 23

Kidney and Urologic Disorders in Children

Chapter Contents

Section 23.1

Bedwetting and Urinary Incontinence

This section includes text excerpted from "Bladder-Control Problems
and Bedwetting in Children," National Institute of Diabetes and
Digestive and Kidney Diseases (NIDDK), September 2017.

What Are Bladder-Control Problems in Children?

Children may have a bladder-control problem—also called "urinary
incontinence" (UI)—if they leak urine by accident and are past the
age of toilet training. A child may not stay dry during the day, called
"daytime wetting;" or through the night, called "bedwetting."

Children normally gain control over their bladders somewhere
between ages two and four—each in their own time. Occasional wetting is common even in four- to six-year-old children.

By age four, when most children stay dry during the day, daytime
wetting can be very upsetting and embarrassing. By ages five or six,
children might have a bedwetting problem if the bed is wet once or
twice a week over a few months.

Most bladder-control problems disappear naturally as children grow
older. When needed, a healthcare professional can check for conditions
that may lead to wetting.

Loss of urine is almost never due to laziness, a strong will, emotional problems, or poor toilet training. Parents and caregivers should
always approach this problem with understanding and patience.

Do Bladder-Control Problems Have Another Name?

Bladder-control problems are also called "urinary incontinence" or
"enuresis."

- Primary enuresis is wetting in a child who has never regularly
  stayed dry.

- Secondary enuresis is wetting that begins after at least 6
  months of staying dry.

What Are the Types of Bladder-Control Problems in Children?

Children usually have one of two main bladder-control problems:

- Daytime wetting also called "diurnal enuresis"

- Bedwetting, also called "nocturnal enuresis"

Some children may have trouble controlling their bladders both day and night.

Daytime Wetting

For infants and toddlers, wetting is a normal part of development. Children gradually learn to control their bladders as they grow older. Problems that can occur during this process and lead to daytime wetting include:

- **Holding urine too long.** Your child's bladder can overfill and leak urine.

- **Overactive bladder.** Your child's bladder squeezes without warning, causing frequent runs for the toilet and wet clothes.

- **Underactive bladder.** Your child uses the toilet only a few times a day, with little urge to do so. Children may have a weak or interrupted stream of urine.

- **Disordered urination.** Your child's bladder muscles and nerves do not work together smoothly. Certain muscles cut off urine flow too soon. Urine left in the bladder may leak.

Bedwetting

Children who wet the bed fall into two groups: those who have never been dry at night, and children who started wetting the bed again after staying dry for six months.

How Common Are Bladder-Control Problems in Children?

Bladder-control problems are common in children. About 1 in 10 children have trouble with daytime wetting at age five. Nighttime wetting is more common than daytime wetting.

Who Is More Likely to Have Bladder-Control Problems?

Daytime wetting is more common in girls than in boys.

Table 23.1. Bedwetting Numbers in Children

Age	Bedwetting Numbers
Age 5	About 1 in 6 children
Age 6	About 1 in 8 children
Age 7	1 in 10 children
Age 15	1 to 2 in 100 children

Bedwetting is more common in boys—and in all children whose parents wet the bed when they were young. Your child's chances of wetting the bed are about 1 in 3 when one parent was affected as a child. If both parents were affected, the chances that your child will wet the bed are 7 in 10.

Most children with bladder-control problems are physically and emotionally normal. Certain health conditions can make a child more likely to experience wetting, including:

- A bladder or kidney infection (urinary-tract infection)

- **Constipation**—fewer than two bowel movements a week, or bowel movements in which stool is painful or hard to pass

- **Nerve problems**, such as those seen with spina bifida, a birth defect

- **Vesicoureteral reflux**, backward flow of urine from the bladder to the kidneys

- **Diabetes**, a condition in which blood glucose, also called "blood sugar," is too high

- Problems with the structure of the urinary-tract, such as a blockage or a narrowed urethra

- **Obstructive sleep apnea (OSA)**, a condition in which breathing is interrupted during sleep, often because of inflamed or enlarged tonsils

- Attention deficit hyperactivity disorder (ADHD)

Complications of Bladder-Control Problems

Children can manage or outgrow most bladder-control problems with no lasting health effects. However, accidental wetting can cause emotional distress and poor self-esteem for a child as well as frustration for families.

Bladder-control problems can sometimes lead to bladder or kidney infections (UTIs). Bedwetting that is never treated during childhood can last into the teen years and adulthood, causing emotional distress.

Symptoms and Causes of Bladder-Control Problems and Bedwetting in Children

What Are the Signs and Symptoms of Bladder-Control Problems in Children?

Losing urine by accident is the main sign of a bladder-control problem. Your child may often have wet or stained underwear—or a wet bed.

Daytime Wetting

Signs that your child may have a condition that causes daytime wetting include:

- The urgent need to urinate, often with urine leaks

- Urinating 8 or more times a day, called "frequency"

- Infrequent urination—emptying the bladder only two to three times a day, rather than the usual four to seven times a day

- Incomplete urination—not fully emptying the bladder during bathroom visits

- Squatting, squirming, leg crossing, or heel sitting to avoid leaking urine

Bedwetting

Nighttime wetting is normal for many children—and is often not considered a health problem at all—especially when it runs in the family.

At ages five and older, signs that your child may have a nighttime bladder-control problem—whether due to slow physical development, an illness, or any cause—can include:

- Never being dry at night

- Wetting the bed two to three times a week over three months or more

- Wetting the bed again after six months of dry nights

When Should My Child See a Doctor about Bladder-Control Problems?

If you or your child are worried about accidental wetting, talk with a healthcare professional. She or he can check for medical problems and offer treatment, or reassure you that your child is developing normally.

Take your child to a healthcare professional if there are signs of a medical problem, including:

- Symptoms of bladder infection such as:
  - Pain or burning when urinating
  - Cloudy, dark, bloody, or foul-smelling urine
  - Urinating more often than usual
  - Strong urges to urinate, but passing only a small amount of urine
  - Pain in the lower belly area or back
  - Crying while urinating
  - Fever
  - Restlessness
- Your child dribbles urine or has a weak urine stream, which can be signs of a birth defect in the urinary-tract
- Your child was dry but started wetting again

Although each child is unique, providers often use a child's age to decide when to look for a bladder-control problem. In general,

- By age four, most children are dry during the day
- By ages five or six, most children are dry at night

Seek Care Right Away

If your child has symptoms of a bladder or kidney infection or has a fever without a clear cause, see a healthcare professional within 24 hours. Quick treatment is important to prevent a urinary-tract infection from causing more serious health problems.

What Causes Bladder-Control Problems in Children

Bathroom habits, such as holding urine for too long, and slow physical development cause many of bladder-control problems seen in children. Less often, a medical condition can cause wetting.

What Causes Daytime Wetting in Children

Daytime wetting in children is commonly caused by holding urine too long, constipation, or bladder systems that do not work together smoothly. Health problems can sometimes cause daytime wetting, too, such as bladder or kidney infections, structural problems in the urinary-tract, or nerve problems.

What Causes Bedwetting in Children

Nighttime wetting is often related to slow physical development, a family history of bedwetting, or making too much urine at night. In many cases, there is more than one cause. Children almost never wet the bed on purpose—and most children who wet the bed are physically and emotionally normal.

Diagnosis of Bladder-Control Problems and Bedwetting in Children

How Do Doctors Diagnose Bladder-Control Problems in Children?

To diagnose a bladder-control problem, doctors use a child's:

- Medical history
- Physical exam
- Lab tests
- Imaging tests, if needed

In addition, doctors will ask questions about:

- Symptoms
- When and how often the wetting happens
- Dry periods
- Family history of bedwetting

What Tests Do Doctors Use to Diagnose Bladder-Control Problems in Children?

Lab Tests

Healthcare professionals often test a urine sample, which is called "urinalysis," to help diagnose bladder-control problems in children.

The lab may also perform a urine culture if requested. White blood cells and bacteria in the urine can be signs of a urinary-tract infection.

Other Tests

In a few cases, healthcare professionals may order imaging tests or tests of how the urinary-tract works. These tests can show a birth defect or a blockage in the urinary-tract that may lead to wetting. Special tests can find nerve or spine problems. Testing can also help show a small bladder, weak muscles, or muscles that do not work together well.

Treatment of Bladder-Control Problems and Bedwetting in Children
How Can My Child's Doctor and I Treat a Bladder-Control Problem?

When a health condition causes the wetting—such as diabetes or a birth defect in the urinary-tract—doctors will treat the health problem, and the wetting is likely to stop.

Other common treatments for wetting include bladder training, moisture alarms, medicines, and home care. Teamwork is important among you, your child, and your child's doctor. You should reward your child for following a program, rather than for staying dry—because a child often cannot control wetting.

If your child wets both day and night, the doctor is likely to treat daytime wetting first. Children usually stay dry during the day before they gain bladder-control at night.

Daytime Wetting

Treatments for daytime wetting depend on what is causing the wetting, and will often start with changes in bladder and bowel habits. Your child's doctor will treat any constipation, so that hard stools do not press against the bladder and lead to wetting.

Bladder Training

Bladder training helps your child get to the bathroom sooner and may help reset bladder systems that do not work together smoothly. Programs can include:

• Urinating on schedule every 2 to 3 hours, called "timed voiding."

- Urinating twice during one visit, called "double voiding." This method may help the bladder empty completely in children who have an underactive or "lazy" bladder or VUR

- Relaxing the pelvic floor muscles so children can empty the bladder fully. A few sessions of biofeedback can retrain muscles that do not work together in the right order.

In extremely rare cases, doctors may suggest using a thin, flexible tube, called a "catheter," to empty the bladder. Occasional use of a catheter may help develop better bladder-control in children with a weak, underactive bladder.

Medicine

Your child's doctor may suggest medicine to limit daytime wetting or prevent a urinary-tract infection (UTI).

Oxybutynin (Ditropan®) is often the first choice of medicine to calm an overactive bladder until a child matures and outgrows the problem naturally.

If your child often has bladder infections, the doctor may prescribe an antibiotic, which is a medicine that kills the bacteria that cause infections. Your child's doctor may suggest taking a low-dose antibiotic for several months to prevent repeated bladder infections.

Home Care and Support

Changes in your child's routines and behavior may greatly improve daytime wetting, even without other treatments. Encourage your child to:

- Use the bathroom whenever the urge occurs.

- Drink more liquid, mainly water, if the doctor suggests doing so. Drinking more liquid produces more urine and more trips to the bathroom.

- Take extra time in the bathroom to relax and empty the bladder completely.

- Avoid drinks with caffeine or bubbles, citrus juices, and sports drinks. These drinks may irritate the bladder or produce extra urine.

Children need plenty of support from parents and caregivers to overcome daytime wetting, not blame or punishment. Calming your child's stresses may help—stresses about a new baby or new school, for example. A counselor or psychologist can help treat anxiety.

Bedwetting

If your child's provider suggests treatment, it is likely to start with ways to motivate your child and change her or his behavior. The next steps include moisture alarms or medicine.

For a bedwetting treatment program to work, both the parent and child must be motivated. Treatment does not always completely stop bedwetting—and there are likely to be some setbacks. However, treatment can greatly reduce how often your child wets the bed.

Motivational Therapy

For motivational therapy, you and your child agree on ways to manage bedwetting and rewards for following the program. Keep a record of your child's tasks and progress, such as a calendar with stickers. You can give rewards to your child for remembering to use the bathroom before bed, helping to change and clean wet bedding, and having a dry night.

Motivational therapy helps children gain a sense of control over bedwetting. Many children learn to stay dry with this approach, and many others have fewer wet nights. Taking back rewards, shaming, penalties, and punishments do not work; your child is not wetting the bed on purpose. If there is no change in your child's wetting after 3 to 6 months, talk with a healthcare professional about other treatments.

Moisture Alarms

Moisture alarms detect the first drops of urine in a child's underwear and sound an alarm to wake the child. A sensor clips to your child's clothes or bedding. At first, you may need to wake your child, get him or her to the bathroom, and clean up wet clothes and bedding. Eventually, your child learns to wake up when her or his bladder is full and get to the bathroom in time.

Moisture alarms work well for many children and can end bedwetting for good. Families need to use the alarm regularly for 3 to 4 months as the child learns to sense her or his signals and control the bladder. Signs of progress usually appear in the first few weeks—smaller wet spots, fewer alarms each night, and your child waking on her or his own.

Medicine

Your child's doctor may suggest medicine when other treatments have not worked well.

Desmopressin (DDAVP) is often the first choice of medicine for bedwetting. This medicine slows the amount of urine your child's body makes overnight, so the bladder does not overfill and leak. Desmopressin can work well, but bedwetting often returns when a child stops taking the medicine. You can use desmopressin for sleepovers, camp, and other short periods of time. You can also keep a child on desmopressin safely for long periods of time.

How Can I Help My Child Cope with Bladder-Control Problems?

Your patience, understanding, and encouragement are vital to help your child cope with a bladder-control problem. If you think a health problem may be causing your child's wetting, make an appointment with your child's healthcare provider.

Clothing, Bedding, and Wearable Products

For children with daytime wetting, clothes that come on and off easily may help prevent accidents. A wristwatch alarm set to vibrate can privately remind your child to visit the toilet, without help from a teacher or parent.

For children who wet the bed, the following practices can make life easier and may boost your child's confidence:

- Leave out dry pajamas and towels so your child can clean up easily.

- Layer waterproof pads and fitted sheets on the bed. Your child can quickly pull off wet bedding and put it in a hamper. Fewer signs of wetting may help your child feel less embarrassed.

- Have your child help with the clean-up and laundry the next day. However, do not make it a punishment.

- Be sure your child showers or bathes every day to wash away the smell of urine.

- Plan to stop using diapers, training pants, or disposable training pants, except when sleeping away from home. These items may discourage your child from getting out of bed to use the toilet.

Do not make a habit of waking your child during the night to use the bathroom. Researchers do not think it helps children overcome bedwetting.

Emotional Support

Let your child know that bedwetting is very common and most children outgrow it. If your child is age four or older, ask him or her for ideas on how to stop or manage the wetting. Involving your child in finding solutions may provide a sense of control.

Calming your child's stresses may help—stresses about a new baby or new school, for example. A counselor or psychologist can help treat anxiety.

Prevention of Bladder-Control Problems and Bedwetting in Children

How Can I Help My Child Prevent Bladder-Control Problems?

Often, you cannot prevent a bladder-control problem, especially bedwetting, which is a common pattern of normal child development. However, good habits may help your child have more dry days and nights, including:

- Avoid or treat constipation

- Urinate every 2 to 3 hours during the day—4 to 7 times total in a day

- Drink the right amount of liquid, with most liquids consumed between morning and about 5 p.m. Ask your child's healthcare provider how much liquid is healthy, based on age, weather, and activities.

- Avoid drinks with caffeine or bubbles, citrus juices, and sports drinks. These drinks may irritate the bladder or produce extra urine.

Section 23.2

Childhood Nephrotic Syndrome

This section includes text excerpted from "Childhood Nephrotic Syndrome," National Institute of Diabetes and Digestive and Kidney Diseases (NIDDK), September 2014. Reviewed September 2019.

What Is Childhood Nephrotic Syndrome?

Childhood nephrotic syndrome is not a disease in itself; rather, it is a group of symptoms that

- Indicate kidney damage—particularly damage to the glomeruli, the tiny units within the kidney where blood is filtered
- Result in the release of too much protein from the body into the urine

When the kidneys are damaged, the protein albumin, normally found in the blood, will leak into the urine. Proteins are large, complex molecules that perform a number of important functions in the body. The two types of childhood nephrotic syndrome are

- **Primary**—the most common type of childhood nephrotic syndrome, which begins in the kidneys and affects only the kidneys
- **Secondary**—the syndrome is caused by other diseases

A healthcare provider may refer a child with nephrotic syndrome to a nephrologist—a doctor who specializes in treating kidney disease. A child should see a pediatric nephrologist, who has special training to take care of kidney problems in children, if possible. However, in many parts of the country, pediatric nephrologists are in short supply, so the child may need to travel. If traveling is not possible, some nephrologists who treat adults can also treat children.

What Causes Childhood Nephrotic Syndrome

While idiopathic, or unknown, diseases are the most common cause of primary childhood nephrotic syndrome, researchers have linked certain diseases and some specific genetic changes that damage the kidneys with primary childhood nephrotic syndrome.

The cause of secondary childhood nephrotic syndrome is an underlying disease or infection. Called a "primary illness," it is this underlying disease or infection that causes changes in the kidney function that can result in secondary childhood nephrotic syndrome.

Congenital diseases—diseases that are present at birth—can also cause childhood nephrotic syndrome.

Which Children Are More Likely to Develop Childhood Nephrotic Syndrome?

In cases of primary childhood nephrotic syndrome for which the cause is idiopathic, researchers are unable to pinpoint which children are more likely to develop the syndrome. However, as researchers continue to study the link between genetics and childhood nephrotic syndrome, it may be possible to predict the syndrome for some children.

Children are more likely to develop secondary childhood nephrotic syndrome if they:

- Have diseases that can damage their kidneys

- Take certain medications

- Develop certain types of infections

What Are the Signs and Symptoms of Childhood Nephrotic Syndrome?

The signs and symptoms of childhood nephrotic syndrome may include:

- **Edema**—swelling, most often in the legs, feet, or ankles and less often in the hands or face

- **Albuminuria**—when a child's urine has high levels of albumin

- **Hypoalbuminemia**—when a child's blood has low levels of albumin

- **Hyperlipidemia**—when a child's blood cholesterol and fat levels are higher than normal

In addition, some children with nephrotic syndrome may have:

- Blood in their urine

- Symptoms of infection, such as fever, lethargy, irritability, or abdominal pain

- Loss of appetite

- Diarrhea

- High blood pressure

What Are the Complications of Childhood Nephrotic Syndrome?

The complications of childhood nephrotic syndrome may include:

- **Infection.** When the kidneys are damaged, a child is more likely to develop infections because the body loses proteins that normally protect against infection. Healthcare providers will prescribe medications to treat infections. Children with childhood nephrotic syndrome should receive the pneumococcal vaccine and yearly flu shots to prevent those infections. Children should also receive age-appropriate vaccinations, although a healthcare provider may delay certain live vaccines while a child is taking certain medications.

- **Blood clots.** Blood clots can block the flow of blood and oxygen through a blood vessel anywhere in the body. A child is more likely to develop clots when she or he loses proteins through the urine. The healthcare provider will treat blood clots with blood-thinning medications.

- **High blood cholesterol.** When albumin leaks into the urine, the albumin levels in the blood drop. The liver makes more albumin to make up for the low levels in the blood. At the same time, the liver makes more cholesterol. Sometimes children may need treatment with medications to lower blood cholesterol levels.

How Is Childhood Nephrotic Syndrome Diagnosed?

A healthcare provider diagnoses childhood nephrotic syndrome with:

- A medical and family history

- A physical exam

- Urine tests

- A blood test

- Ultrasound of the kidney

- Kidney biopsy

How Is Childhood Nephrotic Syndrome Treated?

Healthcare providers will decide how to treat childhood nephrotic syndrome based on the type:

- Primary childhood nephrotic syndrome: medications

- Secondary childhood nephrotic syndrome: treat the underlying illness or disease

- Congenital nephrotic syndrome: medications, surgery to remove one or both kidneys, and transplantation

How Can Childhood Nephrotic Syndrome Be Prevented?

Researchers have not found a way to prevent childhood nephrotic syndrome when the cause is idiopathic or congenital.

Eating, Diet, and Nutrition

Children who have nephrotic syndrome may need to make changes to their diet, such as:

- Limiting the amount of sodium, often from salt, they take in each day

- Reducing the amount of liquids they drink each day

- Eating a diet low in saturated fat and cholesterol to help control elevated cholesterol levels

Parents or caretakers should talk with the child's healthcare provider before making any changes to the child's diet.

Section 23.3

Hemolytic Uremic Syndrome

This section includes text excerpted from "Hemolytic Uremic Syndrome in Children," National Institute of Diabetes and Digestive and Kidney Diseases (NIDDK), June 2015. Reviewed September 2019.

What Is Hemolytic Uremic Syndrome?

Hemolytic uremic syndrome (HUS), is a kidney condition that happens when red blood cells are destroyed and block the kidneys' filtering system. Red blood cells contain hemoglobin—an iron-rich protein that gives blood its red color and carries oxygen from the lungs to all parts of the body.

When the kidneys and glomeruli—the tiny units within the kidney where blood is filtered—become clogged with the damaged red blood cells, they are unable to do their jobs. If the kidneys stop functioning, a child can develop acute kidney injury—the sudden and temporary loss of kidney function. HUS is the most common cause of acute kidney injury in children.

What Causes Hemolytic Uremic Syndrome in Children

The most common cause of HUS in children is an *Escherichia coli (E. coli)* infection of the digestive system. The digestive system is made up of the gastrointestinal (GI), tract—a series of hollow organs joined in a long, twisting tube from the mouth to the anus—and other organs that help the body break down and absorb food.

Normally, harmless strains, or types, of *E. coli* are found in the intestines and are an important part of digestion. However, if a child becomes infected with the *O157:H7* strain of E. coli, the bacteria will lodge in the digestive tract and produce toxins that can enter the bloodstream. The toxins travel through the bloodstream and can destroy the red blood cells. *E. coli O157:H7* can be found in:

- Undercooked meat, most often ground beef

- Unpasteurized, or raw, milk

- Unwashed, contaminated raw fruits and vegetables

- Contaminated juice

- Contaminated swimming pools or lakes

Less common causes, sometimes called "atypical hemolytic uremic syndrome," (aHUS) can include:

- Taking certain medications, such as chemotherapy

- Having other viral or bacterial infections

- Inheriting a certain type of hemolytic uremic syndrome that runs in families

Which Children Are More Likely to Develop Hemolytic Uremic Syndrome?

Children who are more likely to develop hemolytic uremic syndrome include those who:

- Are younger than age five and have been diagnosed with an *E. coli O157:H7* infection

- Have a weakened immune system

- Have a family history of inherited hemolytic uremic syndrome

Hemolytic uremic syndrome occurs in about two out of every 100,000 children.

What Are the Signs and Symptoms of Hemolytic Uremic Syndrome in Children?

A child with HUS may develop signs and symptoms similar to those seen with gastroenteritis—an inflammation of the lining of the stomach, small intestine, and large intestine—such as:

- Vomiting

- Bloody diarrhea

- Abdominal pain

- Fever and chills

- Headache

How Is Hemolytic Uremic Syndrome in Children Diagnosed?

A healthcare provider diagnoses hemolytic uremic syndrome with:

- A medical and family history
- A physical exam
- Urine tests
- A blood test
- A stool test
- Kidney biopsy

Medical and Family History

Taking a medical and family history is one of the first things a healthcare provider may do to help diagnose HUS.

Physical Exam

A physical exam may help diagnose HUS. During a physical exam, a healthcare provider most often:

- Examines a child's body
- Taps on specific areas of the child's body

Urine Tests

A healthcare provider may order the following urine tests to help determine if a child has kidney damage from the hemolytic uremic syndrome.

Dipstick test for albumin. A dipstick test performed on a urine sample can detect the presence of albumin in the urine, which could mean kidney damage. The child or caretaker collects a urine sample in a special container in a healthcare provider's office or a commercial facility. For the test, a nurse or technician places a strip of chemically treated paper, called a "dipstick," into the child's urine sample. Patches on the dipstick change color when albumin is present in the urine.

Urine albumin-to-creatinine ratio. A healthcare provider uses this measurement to estimate the amount of albumin passed into the urine over a 24-hour period. The child provides a urine sample during an appointment with the healthcare provider. Creatinine is a waste product that is filtered in the kidneys and passed in the urine. A high urine albumin-to-creatinine ratio indicates that the kidneys are leaking large amounts of albumin into the urine.

Blood Test

A blood test involves drawing blood at a healthcare provider's office or a commercial facility and sending the sample to a lab for analysis. A healthcare provider will test the blood sample to:

- Estimate how much blood the kidneys filter each minute, called the "estimated glomerular filtration rate" (eGFR). The test results help the healthcare provider determine the amount of kidney damage from HUS.

- Check red blood cell (RBC) and platelet levels

- Check for liver and kidney function

- Assess protein levels in the blood

Stool Test

A stool test is the analysis of a sample of stool. The healthcare provider will give the child's parent or caretaker a container for catching and storing the stool. The parent or caretaker returns the sample to the healthcare provider or a commercial facility that will send the sample to a lab for analysis. Stool tests can show the presence of *E. coli O157:H7.*

Kidney Biopsy

A biopsy is a procedure that involves taking a small piece of kidney tissue for examination with a microscope. A healthcare provider performs the biopsy in an outpatient center or a hospital. The healthcare provider will give the child light sedation and local anesthetic; however, in some cases, the child will require general anesthesia. A pathologist—a doctor who specializes in diagnosing diseases—examines the tissue in a lab. The pathologist looks for signs of kidney disease and infection. The test can help diagnose HUS.

What Are the Complications of Hemolytic Uremic Syndrome in Children?

Most children who develop hemolytic uremic syndrome and its complications recover without permanent damage to their health.

However, children with hemolytic uremic syndrome may have serious and sometimes life-threatening complications, including:

• Acute kidney injury

• High blood pressure

• Blood-clotting problems that can lead to bleeding

• Seizures

• Heart problems

• Chronic, or long-lasting, kidney disease

• Stroke

• Coma

How Is Hemolytic Uremic Syndrome in Children Treated?

A healthcare provider will treat a child with hemolytic uremic syndrome by addressing:

• Urgent symptoms and preventing complications

• Acute kidney injury

• Chronic kidney disease (CKD)

In most cases, healthcare providers do not treat children with HUS with antibiotics unless they have infections in other areas of the body. With proper management, most children recover without long-term health problems.

Treating Urgent Symptoms and Preventing Complications

A healthcare provider will treat a child's urgent symptoms and try to prevent complications by:

• Observing the child closely in the hospital

- Replacing minerals, such as potassium and salt, and fluids through an intravenous (IV) tube

- Giving the child red blood cells and platelets—cells in the blood that help with clotting—through an IV

- Giving the child IV nutrition

- Treating high blood pressure with medications

Treating Acute Kidney Injury

If necessary, a healthcare provider will treat acute kidney injury with dialysis—the process of filtering wastes and extra fluid from the body with an artificial kidney. The two forms of dialysis are hemodialysis and peritoneal dialysis. Most children with acute kidney injury need dialysis for a short time only.

Treating Chronic Kidney Disease

Some children may sustain significant kidney damage that slowly develops into CKD. Children who develop CKD must receive treatment to replace the work the kidneys do. The two types of treatment are dialysis and transplantation.

In most cases, healthcare providers treat CKD with a kidney transplant. A kidney transplant is a surgery to place a healthy kidney from someone who has just died or a living donor, most often a family member, into a person's body to take over the job of the failing kidneys. Though some children receive a kidney transplant before their kidneys fail completely, many children begin with dialysis to stay healthy until they can have a transplant.

How Can Hemolytic Uremic Syndrome in Children Be Prevented?

Parents and caregivers can help prevent childhood hemolytic uremic syndrome due to *E. coli O157:H7* by:

- Avoiding unclean swimming areas

- Avoiding unpasteurized milk, juice, and cider

- Cleaning utensils and food surfaces often

- Cooking meat to an internal temperature of at least 160°F

- Defrosting meat in the microwave or refrigerator

- Keeping children out of pools if they have had diarrhea
- Keeping raw foods separate
- Washing hands before eating
- Washing hands well after using the restroom and after changing diapers

When a child is taking medications that may cause HUS, it is important that the parent or caretaker watch for symptoms and report any changes in the child's condition to the healthcare provider as soon as possible.

Eating, Diet, and Nutrition

At the beginning of the illness, children with hemolytic uremic syndrome may need IV nutrition or supplements to help maintain fluid balance in the body. Some children may need to follow a low-salt diet to help prevent swelling and high blood pressure.

Healthcare providers will encourage children with HUS to eat when they are hungry. Most children who completely recover and do not have permanent kidney damage can return to their usual diet.

Section 23.4

Urinary-Tract Infections

This section includes text excerpted from "Bladder Infection (Urinary-Tract Infection—UTI) in Children," National Institute of Diabetes and Digestive and Kidney Diseases (NIDDK), April 2017.

What Is a Bladder Infection?

A bladder infection is an illness that is usually caused by bacteria. Bladder infections are the most common type of urinary-tract infection (UTI) in children. A UTI can develop in any part of your child's urinary-tract, including the urethra, bladder, ureters, or kidneys.

All healthy children have some bacteria on their bodies and in their bowels. Occasionally, bacteria can get into the bladder and start an infection. Children of any age can and do develop bladder infections, including infants.

Your child's body has ways to defend against infection. For example, urine normally flows from your child's kidneys, through the ureters, to the bladder. Bacteria that enter the urinary-tract are flushed out when your child urinates. This one-way flow of urine keeps bacteria from infecting the urinary-tract.

Sometimes the body's defenses fail and the bacteria cause a bladder infection. If your child has symptoms of a bladder infection or has a fever without a clear cause, see a healthcare professional within 24 hours.

Getting treatment right away for an infection in your child's urethra or bladder can prevent a kidney infection. A kidney infection can develop from an infection that moves upstream to one or both kidneys. Kidney infections are often very painful and can be dangerous and cause serious health problems, so it is best to get early treatment when your child has a bladder infection.

A healthcare professional is likely to treat your child's bladder infection with antibiotics, a type of medicine that fights bacteria. It is important for your child to take every dose on time and to finish all of the medicine.

How Common Are Bladder Infections in Children?

Bladder infections are a common reason that children visit a healthcare professional. Each year, about 3 in 100 children develop a UTI, and most of these infections are bladder infections.

- Babies under 12 months old are more likely to have a UTI than older children.

- During the first few months of life, UTIs are more common in boys than girls.

- By age one, girls are more likely to develop a UTI than boys— and girls continue to have a higher risk throughout childhood and the teen years.

Which Children Are More Likely to Develop a Bladder Infection?

Girls are much more likely to develop bladder infections than boys, except during the first year of life. Among boys younger than age one, those who have not had the foreskin of the penis removed, called a "circumcision," have a higher risk for a bladder infection. Still, most uncircumcised boys will not get a bladder infection.

In general, any condition or habit that keeps urine in your child's bladder for too long may lead to an infection.

Other factors that may make your child more likely to develop a bladder infection include:

Abnormal bladder function or habits, such as:

- **Overactive bladder**—a treatable condition that often goes away as your child grows older

  - Not emptying the bladder fully

  - Waiting too long to urinate

- **Constipation**—fewer than two bowel movements a week or hard bowel movements that are painful or difficult to pass

- **Vesicoureteral reflux (VUR)**—the backward flow of urine from the bladder toward the kidneys during urination.

- **Urinary blockage**—a problem that limits the normal flow of urine, such as a kidney stone or a ureter that is too narrow. In some cases, this can be related to a birth defect.

- Poor toilet hygiene

- Family history of UTIs

Among teen girls, those who are sexually active are more likely to get a bladder infection.

Different anatomy makes girls much more likely to develop a bladder infection than boys:

- Girls have a shorter urethra than boys, so bacteria do not have to go as far as to reach the bladder and cause an infection.

- In girls, the urethra is closer to the anus, a source of bacteria that can cause a bladder infection.

What Are the Complications of Bladder Infections in Children?

Quick treatment is likely to cure your child's bladder infection with no complications.

If an infection in the lower urinary-tract, such as a bladder infection, is not treated properly, it can lead to a kidney infection. Kidney infections that last a long time or keep coming back can cause damage to a child's kidneys that never goes away. This damage can include kidney scars, poor kidney function, high blood pressure, and problems during pregnancy. Young children have a greater risk of kidney damage from a UTI than older children and adults.

In a few cases, a kidney infection can develop suddenly and become life-threatening, particularly if bacteria get into the bloodstream, which causes a reaction called "sepsis," or "septicemia."

What Are the Symptoms of a Bladder Infection?

Do not assume that you will know when your child has a bladder infection, even if you have had one yourself. Symptoms can be very different in children than in adults, especially for infants and preschoolers. If your child is not well, contact your child's pediatrician or health clinic.

Young Children

It is not always obvious when an infant or child younger than age two has a bladder infection. Sometimes there are no symptoms. Or, your child may be too young to be able to explain what feels wrong. A urine test is the only way to know for certain whether your child has a bladder or kidney infection.

When a young child has symptoms of a UTI, they may include

- Fever, which may be the only sign

- Vomiting or diarrhea

- Irritability or fussiness

- Poor feeding or appetite; poor weight gain

Older Children

Symptoms of a bladder or kidney infection in a child ages two and older can include

- Pain or burning when urinating

- Cloudy, dark, bloody, or foul-smelling urine

- Frequent or intense urges to urinate

- Pain in the lower belly area or back

- Fever

- Wetting after a child has been toilet trained

Seek Care Right Away

If you think your child has a bladder infection, take her or him to a healthcare professional within 24 hours. A child who has a high fever and is sick for more than a day without a runny nose, earache, or other obvious cause should also be checked for a bladder infection. Quick treatment is important to prevent the infection from getting more dangerous.

What Causes Bladder Infection

Most often a bladder infection is caused by bacteria that are normally found in the bowel. The bladder has several systems to prevent infection. For example, urinating most often flushes out bacteria before it reaches the bladder. Sometimes, your child's body cannot fight the bacteria and the bacteria cause an infection. Certain health conditions can put children at risk for bladder infections.

How Do Healthcare Professionals Diagnose a Bladder Infection?

Healthcare professionals use your child's medical history, a physical exam, and tests to diagnose a bladder infection. A healthcare professional will ask about health conditions that may make your child more likely to develop a bladder infection. During a physical exam, the healthcare professional will also ask about your child's symptoms.

What Tests Do Healthcare Professionals Use to Diagnose a Bladder Infection?

Healthcare professionals typically test a urine sample, which is called "urinalysis," to help to diagnose a bladder infection. A urine culture, which takes longer to come back from the lab, is needed for an accurate diagnosis. In some cases, a healthcare professional may order more tests to look at your child's urinary-tract.

How Do Healthcare Professionals Treat Bladder Infections in Children?

Bladder infections in children are treated with antibiotics, a type of medicine that fights bacteria.

Medicines

Which antibiotic your child takes is based on age, any allergies to antibiotics, and the type of bacteria causing the UTI. Children older than two months usually take an antibiotic by mouth—as a liquid or as a chewable tablet.

Your child may go to a hospital for intravenous (IV) antibiotics if the child is younger than two months old or vomiting. IV medicines are given through a vein.

Your child should start to feel better within a day or two, but it is important to take every dose of the antibiotic on time and to finish all the medicine. The infection could come back if your child stops taking the antibiotic too soon.

The length of treatment depends on:

- How severe the infection is

- Whether a child's symptoms and infection go away

- Whether a child has repeated bladder infections

- Whether the child has vesicoureteral reflux or another problem in the urinary-tract

At-Home Treatments

Children should drink plenty of liquids and urinate often to speed healing. Drinking water is the best. Ask your healthcare professional how much liquid your child should drink.

A heating pad on a child's back or abdomen may help ease pain from a kidney or bladder infection.

How Can You Help Your Child Prevent a Bladder Infection?

Drinking enough liquids, following good bathroom and diapering habits, wearing loose-fitting clothes, and getting treated for related health problems may help prevent a UTI in a child or teen.

Be Sure Your Child Drinks Enough Liquids

Drinking more liquids may help flush bacteria from the urinary-tract. Talk with a healthcare professional about how much liquid your child should drink, and which beverages are best to help prevent a repeat UTI.

Follow Good Bathroom and Diapering Habits

Some children simply do not urinate often enough. Children should urinate often and when they first feel the need to go. Bacteria can grow and cause an infection when urine stays in the bladder too long. Caregivers should change diapers often for infants and toddlers and should clean the genital area well. Gentle cleansers that do not irritate the skin are best.

Your child should always wipe from front to back after urinating or having a bowel movement. This step is most important after a bowel movement to keep bacteria from getting into the urethra and bladder.

Avoid Constipation

Hard stools can press against the urinary-tract and block the flow of urine, allowing bacteria to grow. Helping your child have regular bowel movements can prevent constipation.

Wear Loose-Fitting Clothing

Consider having children wear cotton underwear and loose-fitting clothes so air can keep the area around the urethra dry.

Treat Related Health Problems

When a child's bladder does not work exactly as it should—called "dysfunctional voiding"—treatments may help the bladder work better and prevent repeated infections. The muscles that control urination may be out of sync. Or, your child's bladder may be overactive or underactive.

Healthcare professionals can treat these types of bladder problems with medicines, behavior changes, or both. Children often grow out of these bladder problems naturally over time.

If your child has vesicoureteral reflux, urinary-tract blockage, or an anatomical problem, see a pediatric urologist or other specialists. Treating these conditions may help prevent repeated bladder infections.

Diabetes and other health conditions can increase the risk of bladder infection. Ask your child's healthcare professional on how to reduce the risk of developing a bladder infection.

Can Drinking Liquids Help Prevent or Relieve a Bladder Infection?

Yes. Check with a healthcare professional about how much liquid your child should drink to prevent or relieve a bladder infection. The amount will depend on your child's size, age, and activity level, as well as the weather. If your child lives in a hot climate and is active, she or he may need more liquid to replace fluid lost through sweat.

Can Your Child's Eating, Diet, or Nutrition Help Prevent a Bladder Infection?

Food does not play a role in preventing or treating bladder infections in children. Some research suggests that cranberry products such as juice, extracts, or pills may help prevent these infections in children, but there is not enough evidence to be certain. Cranberry products are not an effective treatment once your child already has a bladder infection.

Children who may have a bladder infection should see a healthcare professional right away for diagnosis and treatment. Cranberry products should not replace medical treatment.

Chapter 24

Liver Disorders in Children

Chapter Contents

Section 24.1

Alpha-1 Antitrypsin Deficiency

This section includes text excerpted from "Alpha-1 Antitrypsin
Deficiency," National Heart, Lung, and Blood Institute (NHLBI),
November 15, 2013. Reviewed September 2019.

What Is Alpha-1 Antitrypsin Deficiency?

Alpha-1 antitrypsin deficiency (AATD), is a condition that raises the
risk for lung disease and other diseases. Those who have severe AATD,
may develop emphysema, cirrhosis and other serious liver diseases,
and a rare skin disease called "necrotizing panniculitis."

Causes of Alpha-1 Antitrypsin Deficiency

Alpha-1 antitrypsin deficiency is an inherited disease. "Inherited"
means it is passed from parents to children through genes.

Children who have AATD inherit two faulty *AAT* genes, one from
each parent. These genes tell cells in the body how to make AAT
proteins.

In AATD, the AAT proteins made in the liver are not the right
shape. Thus, they get stuck in the liver cells. The proteins cannot get to the organs in the body that they protect, such as the
lungs. Without the AAT proteins protecting the organs, diseases
can develop.

The most common faulty gene that can cause AATD is called "PiZ."
If you inherit two *PiZ* genes (one from each parent), you will have
AATD.

If you inherit a *PiZ* gene from one parent and a normal *AAT* gene
from the other parent, you will not have AATD. However, you might
pass the *PiZ* gene to your children.

Even if you inherit two faulty *AAT* genes, you may not have any
related complications. You may never even realize that you have
AATD.

Risk Factors of Alpha-1 Antitrypsin Deficiency

Alpha-1 antitrypsin deficiency occurs in all ethnic groups. However,
the condition occurs most often in Whites of European descent. It is
an inherited condition. "Inherited" means the condition is passed from
parents to children through genes. If you have bloodline relatives with

known AATD, you are at increased risk for the condition. Even so, it does not mean that you will develop one of the diseases related to the condition.

Screening and Prevention of Alpha-1 Antitrypsin Deficiency

You cannot prevent AATD because the condition is inherited. If you inherit two faulty *AAT* genes, you will have AATD. Even so, you may never develop one of the diseases related to the condition.

Check your living and working spaces for things that may irritate your lungs. Examples include flower and tree pollen, ash, allergens, air pollution, wood-burning stoves, paint fumes, and fumes from cleaning products and other household items.

If you have a lung disease related to AATD, ask your doctor whether you might benefit from augmentation therapy. This is a treatment in which you receive infusions of AAT protein. Augmentation therapy raises the level of AAT protein in your blood and lungs.

Signs, Symptoms, and Complications of Alpha-1 Antitrypsin Deficiency

The first lung-related symptoms of AATD may include shortness of breath, less ability to be physically active, and wheezing. These signs and symptoms most often begin between the ages of 20 and 40.

Other signs and symptoms may include repeated lung infections, tiredness, a rapid heartbeat upon standing, vision problems, and weight loss.

Some people who have severe AATD develop emphysema—often when they are only in their forties or fifties. Signs and symptoms of emphysema include problems breathing, wheezing, and a chronic (ongoing) cough.

At first, many people who have AATD are diagnosed with asthma. This is because wheezing also is a symptom of asthma. Also, people who have AATD respond well to asthma medicines.

Diagnosis of Alpha-1 Antitrypsin Deficiency

Alpha-1 antitrypsin deficiency usually is diagnosed after you develop a lung or liver disease that is related to the condition.

Your doctor may suspect AATD if you have signs or symptoms of a serious lung condition, especially emphysema, without any obvious cause. She or he also may suspect AATD if you develop emphysema when you are 45 years old or younger.

Specialists Involved

Many doctors may be involved in the diagnosis of AATD. These include primary care doctors, pulmonologists (lung specialists), and hepatologists (liver specialists).

To diagnose AATD, your doctor will:

- Ask about possible risk factors. Risk factors include smoking and exposure to dust, fumes, and other toxic substances

- Ask about your medical history. A common sign of AATD is if you have a lung or liver disease without any obvious causes or risk factors. Another sign is if you have emphysema at an unusually early age (45 years or younger)

- Ask about your family's medical history. If you have bloodline relatives who have AATD, you are more likely to have the condition

Diagnostic Tests

Your doctor may recommend tests to confirm a diagnosis of AATD. She or he also may recommend tests to check for lung- or liver-related conditions.

- A genetic test is the most certain way to check for AATD. This test will show whether you have faulty *AAT* genes.

- A blood test also may be used. This test checks the level of AAT protein in your blood. If the level is a lot lower than normal, it is likely that you have AATD.

Lung-Related Tests

If you have a lung disease related to AATD, your doctor may recommend lung function tests and high-resolution computed tomography scanning, also called "CT scanning."

Lung function tests measure how much air you can breathe in and out, how fast you can breathe air out, and how well your lungs deliver oxygen to your blood. These tests may show how severe your lung disease is and how well treatment is working.

High-resolution CT scanning uses x-rays to create detailed pictures of parts of the body. A CT scan can show whether you have emphysema or another lung disease and how severe it is.

Treatment of Alpha-1 Antitrypsin Deficiency

Alpha-1 antitrypsin deficiency has no cure, but its related lung diseases have many treatments. Most of these treatments are the same as the ones used for a lung disease called "chronic obstructive pulmonary disease" (COPD).

If you have symptoms related to AATD, your doctor may recommend:

- **Inhaled bronchodilators and inhaled steroids.** These medicines help open your airways and make breathing easier. They also are used to treat asthma and COPD.

- **Flu and pneumococcal vaccines** to protect you from illnesses that could make your condition worse. Prompt treatment of lung infections also can help protect your lungs.

- **Pulmonary rehabilitation (rehab).** Rehab involves treatment by a team of experts at a special clinic. In rehab, you will learn how to manage your condition and function at your best.

- **Extra oxygen**, if needed.

- **A lung transplant.** A lung transplant may be an option if you have severe breathing problems. If you have a good chance of surviving the transplant surgery, you may be a candidate for it.

Augmentation therapy is a treatment used only for people who have AAT-related lung diseases. This therapy involves getting infusions of the AAT protein. The infusions raise the level of the protein in your blood and lungs.

Not enough research has been done to show how well this therapy works. However, some research suggests that this therapy may slow the development of AATD in people who do not have severe disease.

People who have AATD and develop related liver or skin diseases will be referred to doctors who treat those diseases.

Section 24.2

Jaundice and Kernicterus

This section includes text excerpted from "Jaundice and Kernicterus,"
Centers for Disease Control and Prevention (CDC), April 9, 2018.

Jaundice is the yellow color seen in the skin of many newborns. Jaundice happens when a chemical called "bilirubin" builds up in the baby's blood. During pregnancy, the mother's liver removes bilirubin for the baby, but after birth, the baby's liver must remove the bilirubin. In some babies, the liver might not be developed enough to efficiently get rid of bilirubin. When too much bilirubin builds up in a new baby's body, the skin and whites of the eyes might look yellow. This yellow coloring is called "jaundice."

When severe jaundice goes untreated for too long, it can cause a condition called "kernicterus." Kernicterus is a type of brain damage that can result from high levels of bilirubin in a baby's blood. It can cause athetoid cerebral palsy and hearing loss. Kernicterus also causes problems with vision and teeth and sometimes can cause intellectual disabilities. Early detection and management of jaundice can prevent kernicterus.

Signs and Symptoms of Jaundice

Jaundice usually appears first on the face and then moves to the chest, belly, arms, and legs as bilirubin levels get higher. The whites of the eyes can also look yellow. Jaundice can be harder to see in babies with darker skin color. The baby's doctor or nurse can test how much bilirubin is in the baby's blood.

See your baby's doctor the same day if your baby:

- Is very yellow or orange (skin color changes start from the head and spread to the toes)

- Is hard to wake up or will not sleep at all

- Is not breastfeeding or sucking from a bottle well

- Is very fussy

- Does not have enough wet or dirty diapers

Get emergency medical help if your baby:

- Is crying inconsolably or with a high pitch

- Is arched like a bow (the head or neck and heels are bent backward and the body forward)

- Has a stiff, limp, or floppy body

- Has strange eye movements

Diagnosis of Jaundice

Before leaving the hospital with your newborn, you can ask the doctor or nurse about a jaundice bilirubin test.

A doctor or nurse may check the baby's bilirubin using a light meter that is placed on the baby's head. This results in a transcutaneous bilirubin (TcB) level. If it is high, a blood test will likely be ordered.

The best way to accurately measure bilirubin is with a small blood sample from the baby's heel. This results in a total serum bilirubin (TSB) level. If the level is high, based upon the baby's age in hours and other risk factors, treatment will likely follow. Repeat blood samples will also likely be taken to ensure that the TSB decreases with the prescribed treatment.

Bilirubin levels are usually the highest when the baby is 3 to 5 days old. At a minimum, babies should be checked for jaundice every 8 to 12 hours in the first 48 hours of life and again before 5 days of age.

Treatment of Jaundice

No baby should develop brain damage from untreated jaundice.

When being treated for high bilirubin levels, the baby will be undressed and put under special lights. The lights will not hurt the baby. This can be done in the hospital or even at home. The baby's milk intake may also need to be increased. In some cases, if the baby has very high bilirubin levels, the doctor will do a blood exchange transfusion. Jaundice is generally treated before brain damage is a concern.

Putting the baby in sunlight is not recommended as a safe way of treating jaundice.

Risk Factors of Jaundice

About 60 percent of all babies have jaundice. Some babies are more likely to have severe jaundice and higher bilirubin levels than others. Babies with any of the following risk factors need close monitoring and early jaundice management:

Preterm Babies

Babies born before 37 weeks, or 8.5 months, of pregnancy, might have jaundice because their liver is not fully developed. The young liver might not be able to get rid of so much bilirubin.

Babies with Darker Skin Color

Jaundice may be missed or not recognized in a baby with a darker skin color. Checking the gums and inner lips may detect jaundice. If there is any doubt, a bilirubin test should be done.

East Asian or Mediterranean Descent

A baby born to an East Asian or Mediterranean family is at a higher risk of becoming jaundiced. Also, some families inherit conditions, and their babies are more likely to get jaundice.

Feeding Difficulties

A baby who is not eating, wetting, or stooling well in the first few days of life is more likely to get jaundice.

Sibling with Jaundice

A baby with a sister or brother that had jaundice is more likely to develop jaundice.

Bruising

A baby with bruises at birth is more likely to get jaundice. A bruise forms when blood leaks out of a blood vessel and causes the skin to look black and blue. The healing of large bruises can cause high levels of bilirubin and your baby might get jaundice.

Blood Type

Women with an O blood type or Rh-negative blood factor might have babies with higher bilirubin levels. A mother with Rh-incompatibility should be given Rhogam.

If You Are Concerned

If you think your baby has jaundice you should call and visit your baby's doctor right away. Ask your baby's doctor or nurse about a jaundice bilirubin test.

If your baby does have jaundice, it is important to take jaundice seriously and stick to the follow-up plan for appointments and recommended care.

Make sure your baby is getting enough to eat. The process of removing waste also removes bilirubin in your baby's blood. If you are breast-feeding, you should nurse the baby at least 8 to 12 times a day for the first few days. This will help you make enough milk for the baby and will help keep the baby's bilirubin level down. If you are having trouble breastfeeding, ask your doctor, nurse, or a lactation coach for help.

Section 24.3

Viral Hepatitis

This section includes text excerpted from "What Is Viral Hepatitis?" Centers for Disease Control and Prevention (CDC), July 3, 2019.

Hepatitis means inflammation of the liver. The liver is a vital organ that processes nutrients, filters the blood, and fights infections. When the liver is inflamed or damaged, its function can be affected. Heavy alcohol use, toxins, some medications, and certain medical conditions can cause hepatitis. However, hepatitis is often caused by a virus. In the United States, the most common types of viral hepatitis are hepatitis A, hepatitis B, and hepatitis C.

What Causes Viral Hepatitis

The viruses that cause viral hepatitis are:

- **Hepatitis A.** Hepatitis A virus

- **Hepatitis B.** Hepatitis B virus

- **Hepatitis C.** Hepatitis C virus

Statistics on Viral Hepatitis

- **Hepatitis A.** About 4,000 new infections each year

- **Hepatitis B.** About 21,000 new infections each year
- **Hepatitis C.** About 41,000 new infections each year

Key Facts of Viral Hepatitis
Hepatitis A

- Effective vaccine available
- Recent foodborne outbreaks in the United States traced to imported food
- Common in many countries, especially those without modern sanitation

Hepatitis B

- Effective vaccine available
- Hepatitis B is a leading cause of liver cancer

Hepatitis C

- Hepatitis C is a leading cause of liver transplants and liver cancer

How Long Does Viral Hepatitis Last?

Hepatitis A. Hepatitis A can last from a few weeks to several months.

Hepatitis B. Hepatitis B can range from a mild illness lasting a few weeks to a serious, life-long (chronic) condition. More than 90 percent of unimmunized infants who get infected develop a chronic infection, but 6 to 10 percent of older children who get infected develop chronic hepatitis B.

Hepatitis C. Hepatitis C can range from a mild illness lasting a few weeks to a serious, life-long (chronic) infection. Those who get infected with the hepatitis C virus develop chronic hepatitis C.

How Does Viral Hepatitis Spread?

Hepatitis A. Hepatitis A is spread when a person ingests fecal matter—even in microscopic amounts—from contact with objects, food, or drinks contaminated by feces or stool from an infected person.

Hepatitis B. Hepatitis B is primarily spread when blood, semen, or certain other bodily fluids—even in microscopic amounts—from a person infected with the hepatitis B virus enters the body of someone who is not infected. The hepatitis B virus can also be transmitted from:

- Birth to an infected mother

- Sharing equipment that has been contaminated with blood from an infected person, such as needles, syringes, and even medical equipment, such as glucose monitors

- Sharing personal items such as toothbrushes

- Poor-infection control has resulted in outbreaks in healthcare facilities

Hepatitis C. Hepatitis C is spread when blood from a person infected with the Hepatitis C virus—even in microscopic amounts—enters the body of someone who is not infected. The hepatitis C virus can also be transmitted from:

- Sharing equipment that has been contaminated with blood from an infected person, such as needles and syringes

- Poor infection control has resulted in outbreaks in healthcare facilities

- Birth to an infected mother

Who Should Be Vaccinated for Viral Hepatitis?
Hepatitis A

- All children at age one year

- Travelers to countries where hepatitis A is common

- Family and caregivers of adoptees from countries where hepatitis A is common

- People who use drugs, whether injected or not

- People with chronic or long-term liver disease, including hepatitis B or hepatitis C

- People with clotting-factor disorders

- People with direct contact with others who have hepatitis A

- Any person wishing to obtain immunity

- People who are experiencing homelessness

Hepatitis B

- All infants

- All children and adolescents younger than 19 years of age who have not been vaccinated

- People at risk for infection by sexual exposure including those, whose sex partners have hepatitis B, sexually active people who are not in a long-term, mutually monogamous relationship, people seeking evaluation or treatment for an STD, and men who have sex with men

- People at risk for infection by exposure to blood including; people who inject drugs, people who live with a person who has hepatitis B, residents and staff of facilities for people with developmental disablties people, healthcare and public-safety workers at risk for exposure to blood or blood-contaminated body fluids on the job

- International travelers to countries where hepatitis B is common

- People with hepatitis C

- People with chronic liver disease

- People with human immunodeficiency virus (HIV)

- All other people seeking protection from hepatitis B virus infection

Hepatitis C

- There is no vaccine available for hepatitis C.

How Serious Viral Hepatitis Is?
Hepatitis A

- People can be sick for a few weeks to a few months.

- Most recover with no lasting liver damage.

- Although very rare, death can occur.

Hepatitis B

- 15 to 25 percent of chronically infected people develop chronic liver disease, including cirrhosis, liver failure, or liver cancer.

Hepatitis C

- 75 to 85 percent of people who get infected with the hepatitis C virus develop a chronic infection.

- 5 to 20 percent of people with chronic hepatitis C develop cirrhosis.

- 1 to 5 percent will die from cirrhosis or liver cancer.

Treatment of Viral Hepatitis
Hepatitis A

- Supportive treatment for symptoms

Hepatitis B

- **Acute:** No medication available; best addressed through supportive care

- **Chronic:** Regular monitoring for signs of liver disease progression; some patients are treated with antiviral drugs

Hepatitis C

- **Acute:** There is not a recommended treatment for acute hepatitis C. People should be considered for treatment if their infection becomes chronic.

- **Chronic:** There are several medications available to treat chronic hepatitis C. Treatments usually involve 8 to 12 weeks of oral therapy (pills) and cure over 90 percent of people with few side effects

Who Should Be Tested for Viral Hepatitis?
Hepatitis A

- Testing for hepatitis A is not routinely recommended.

Hepatitis B

The Centers for Disease Control and Prevention (CDC) recommends hepatitis B testing for:

- People born in countries with 2 percent or higher HBV prevalence

- Men who have sex with men
- People who inject drugs
- People with human immunodeficiency virus (HIV)
- Household and sexual contacts of people with hepatitis B
- People requiring immunosuppressive therapy
- People with end-stage renal disease (including hemodialysis patients)
- People with hepatitis C
- People with elevated alanine aminotransferase (ALT) levels
- Pregnant women
- Infants born to hepatitis B virus (HBV)-infected mothers

Hepatitis C

The CDC recommends hepatitis C testing for:

- Current or former injection drug users, including those who injected only once many years ago
- Everyone born from 1945 to 1965
- Anyone who received clotting factor concentrates made before 1987
- Recipients of blood transfusions or solid organ transplants before July 1992
- Long-term hemodialysis patients
- People with known exposures to hepatitis C virus, such as healthcare workers or public-safety workers after needle sticks involving blood from someone infected with hepatitis C virus and recipients of blood or organs from a donor who tested positive for the hepatitis C virus
- People with HIV
- Children born to mothers with hepatitis C

The U.S. Preventive Services Task Force (USPSTF) recommends hepatitis C testing for additional groups including:

- People in jails or prisons

- People who use drugs snorted through the nose (in addition to people who inject drugs)

- People who get an unregulated tattoo

Symptoms of Viral Hepatitis

Many people with hepatitis do not have symptoms and do not know they are infected. If symptoms occur with an acute infection, they can appear anytime from two weeks to six months after exposure. Symptoms of chronic viral hepatitis can take decades to develop. Symptoms of hepatitis can include: fever, fatigue, loss of appetite, nausea, vomiting, abdominal pain, dark urine, light-colored stools, joint pain, and jaundice.

Chapter 25

Musculoskeletal Disorders in Children

Chapter Contents

Section 25.1

Knock Knees

"Knock Knees," © 2017 Omnigraphics. Reviewed September 2019.

Knock knees, also known as "genu valgum," is a condition in which an inward-turning alignment of the leg bones creates a large gap between a person's feet when they stand with their knees together. In young children, knock knees is generally considered to be a normal stage in the development of the lower extremities. Children are typically born with an outward-turning alignment of the leg bones due to their position in the womb, and they remain bow-legged until the age of about 18 months. Leg alignment gradually straightens by the age of 2, as children learn to walk. Knock knees usually appear between the ages of 2 and 4, as the alignment of the leg bones continues bending inward. As a result, about 20 percent of 3-year-olds have at least a 2-inch (5 cm) gap between their ankles while standing with their knees together. In about 99 percent of cases, however, the condition corrects itself by the time a child reaches the age of 7 or 8.

Although knock knees affect both genders, the condition is more common among girls. The inward bend is usually symmetrical in both legs, but it is not uncommon for one leg to remain straight. Knock knees are not usually associated with other health problems, although severe cases can cause pain in the knee or hip joints or an altered gait. If the condition persists into adulthood, it may increase the risk of arthritis in the knee joints. In very rare cases—especially when knock knees develop after the age of 6—the condition can be symptomatic of a health condition that requires medical attention.

Causes and Symptoms of Knock Knees

Most cases of knock knees occur as part of the normal development of the leg bones. Cases that appear outside of the usual window of growth may have other causes, including bone diseases related to vitamin deficiencies, such as osteomalacia or rickets. Other possible contributing factors include obesity, injury to the growth plate of the tibia (shin bone), infection in the leg bones (osteomyelitis), and genetic conditions affecting the development of the leg bones or joints.

The main symptom of knock knees is a gap between the ankles when the child is standing with the feet pointed straight ahead and the knees together. Since most children outgrow the condition, it is not necessary to seek medical attention except if the following symptoms appear:

- Knock knees develop before two years of age or after six years of age
- The child has knee pain or difficulty walking
- The gap between the ankles is greater than three inches (eight centimeters)
- The gap seems to be increasing
- Only one leg seems to be affected

Diagnosis of Knock Knees

Observation and measurement of the inward-turning alignment of the child's knees and ankles is the first step in diagnosing knock knees. The doctor is likely to conduct a physical examination that includes measurements of the child's height, weight, body mass index (BMI), leg length, leg symmetry, knee extension, and knee rotation. The doctor will also assess the child's gait and inquire about any knee pain or difficulty walking.

When knock knees appear in a child older than six, or when the condition affects only one leg, the child may be referred to an orthopedic surgeon for further testing. Blood tests may be conducted to check for vitamin deficiencies or other underlying problems. In some cases, standing x-rays may be performed.

Treatment of Knock Knees

Knock knees that occur as part of the normal development of the lower extremities do not require medical treatment. Instead, doctors will usually observe the child's growth to ensure that the condition corrects itself over time. For cases of knock knees that are related to an underlying health condition, such as a vitamin deficiency, the treatment would focus on addressing that condition.

For severe cases of knock knees, or those that do not improve as the child grows, the treatment options include leg braces and surgery. Children whose condition does not resolve itself by the age of eight may need to wear a leg brace at night while they sleep. The brace gradually pulls the knee into a straighter position. Another nonsurgical option is an orthopedic shoe that helps adjust the alignment of the leg.

Surgery is only required in very rare cases where natural growth and leg braces fail to correct severe knock knees. The most common surgical procedure for children is called guided growth. It involves attaching metal plates to the growth centers on the inside of the knee. These plates usually remain in place for about one year. During this time, they prevent the inner part of the knee from growing, which gives the outer part of the knee a chance to catch up. Guided growth surgery is usually performed when a child is approaching puberty, or around age 11 for girls and 13 for boys. Although it requires general anesthesia, it is a minimally invasive procedure that allows children to get back on their feet within a few days.

Osteotomy, on the other hand, is major surgery that entails several months of recovery time. It involves cutting through the bone of the shin or thigh, removing a thin wedge of bone, realigning the legs in a straight position, and inserting metal screws or plates to hold the bones together. Osteotomies are usually performed only to correct severe deformities in adults and children who have stopped growing.

Prognosis of Knock Knees

Most children with knock knees outgrow the condition and have a positive prognosis. Even those who require leg braces or surgery usually heal quickly with good results. When severe knock knees are left untreated, some children may experience difficulty walking or running that interferes with their enjoyment of sports and activities. If the condition continues into adolescence, some teens may experience embarrassment or low self-esteem related to their appearance or gait. Finally, knock knees that persist into adulthood can contribute to knee problems, such as pain, ligament tears, dislocation, or early arthritis.

References

1. Kaneshiro, Neil K. "Knock Knees," MedlinePlus, National Institutes of Health (NIH), 2016.

2. "Knock Knees," NHS Choices, 2016.

3. "Knock Knees: Symptoms and Causes," Boston Children's Hospital, 2016.

Section 25.2

Pediatric Flatfoot

"Flat Feet," © 2017 Omnigraphics. Reviewed September 2019.

What Is Pediatric Flatfoot?

Pediatric flatfoot is a medical condition in which the arch of the child's foot partially or totally collapses when the child is standing. Pediatric flatfoot can be present in one or both of the child's feet. The condition is most often an inherited disorder, although certain injuries and diseases may also cause pediatric flatfoot. There are two main types of pediatric flatfoot: flexible and rigid.

In cases of flexible pediatric flatfoot, the foot arch collapses when the child stands but reappears when the child is standing on tiptoe or sitting. Flexible pediatric flatfoot occurs most often in very young children and generally resolves without treatment by the time the child reaches age five.

Rigid pediatric flatfoot occurs when the foot arch does not appear when the child sits or stands on tiptoe. Rigid flatfoot can occur in children as young as newborn, or the condition may not develop until preadolescence. Tarsal coalition is a type of rigid pediatric flatfoot that is present from birth. In these cases, two or more bones in the child's foot are fused together abnormally. Children with tarsal coalition may not experience any pain or other symptoms, or symptoms may emerge during preadolescence years. Another type of rigid pediatric flatfoot is known as congenital vertical talus. This type of flatfoot is present at birth and is identified by the rigid "rocker bottom" appearance of the child's feet. Most children with this type of flatfoot will begin to experience symptoms at walking age, because the condition makes it painful for the child to walk or wear shoes.

Symptoms of Pediatric Flatfoot

The majority of children with pediatric flatfoot never experience symptoms. Pediatric flatfoot is generally identified by parents or other caregivers through visual observation of the appearance of the child's feet. Among children who do have symptoms of pediatric flatfoot, the most common indications include:

- Discomfort in the legs or bottom of the feet

- Discomfort while walking or a change in the way the child walks

- Discomfort during other physical activities such as sports or games, or voluntary withdrawal from physical activities

- Outward-tilting heels

- Discomfort while wearing shoes

Assessment and Testing of Pediatric Flatfoot

Pediatricians generally diagnose flatfoot in children through visual examination of the child's legs, knees, feet, and the wear patterns on the soles of the child's shoes, along with observation of the child sitting, standing, and walking. x-rays can help the pediatrician classify the type of pediatric flatfoot disorder as well as the severity of the condition. Magnetic resonance imaging (MRI) or other medical imaging tests may also be used in diagnosis of pediatric flatfoot.

Treatment of Pediatric Flatfoot

The majority of cases of pediatric flatfoot resolve untreated. In cases where the affected child complains of pain in their feet, recommendations often include the use of special shoe inserts to provide arch support, stretching exercises, and physical therapy. In severe cases of rigid pediatric flatfoot, surgery may be required. A pediatrician may refer the child to a foot and ankle surgeon for evaluation. Various surgical techniques can be used to correct pediatric flatfoot depending upon a range of factors including the child's age, the severity of the child's condition, the extent of the child's symptoms, and the type of flatfoot disorder.

References

1. "Flatfoot," St. Louis Children's Hospital, 2016.

2. "Flatfoot in Children," Cleveland Clinic, November 27, 2013.

3. "Pediatric Flatfoot," American College of Foot and Ankle Surgeons (ACFAS), 2005.

Section 25.3

Growing Pains

"Growing Pains," © 2018 Omnigraphics. Reviewed September 2019.

What Are Growing Pains?

"Growing pains" is the term used to describe a benign ache or throbbing in the legs commonly experienced by preschool- and school-age children. The condition generally affects kids between the ages of 3 and 4 and those from 8 to 12, and statistics show that at least 10 to 35 percent of children go through this pain at least once during childhood. Both boys and girls can suffer from growing pains, but the condition is seen slightly more often in girls.

Symptoms of Growing Pains

The symptoms of growing pains differ for each child and can range from mild to severe, from infrequent to everyday, and can last from months to years. Some common symptoms of growing pains include:

- Pain in both legs.
- Pain in the muscles rather than the joints, usually in the calves, behind the thighs or knees, and in the shins.
- Pain that often occurs late in the afternoon or at night and fades away in the morning.
- The intensity of pain may sometimes wake a child from her or his sleep.
- Stiffness can accompany pain.
- Some children may also be susceptible to headaches or abdominal pains.

The following symptoms require the attention of a healthcare provider, since they can indicate a more serious problem:

- The pain persists for a long period.
- It does not diminish in the morning.
- The pain affects the joint and not the muscle.
- Symptoms interfere with the child's normal activities.

- Unusual rashes develop.

- The pain only affects one limb.

The symptoms are accompanied by swelling in the legs, loss of appetite, fever, and fatigue.

Causes and Risk Factors of Growing Pains

It was once believed that these pains were linked to the faster growth of bones in comparison with the growth of tendons. However, we now know that growing pains are not related to the process of growing at all. However, despite the new understanding, the name "growing pains" remains the common term for the condition. To date, no single specific cause for growing pains has been identified. One study suggests that children with less bone strength may experience growing pains. In some cases, it is possible that increased physical activity, such as running, jumping, and climbing, may cause the pain. In addition, some studies have linked growing pains to restless leg syndrome (RLS).

Diagnosis of Growing Pains

To diagnose growing pains, a healthcare provider will generally ask a number of questions regarding the symptoms and medical history of the child and will conduct a physical examination. The healthcare provider will rule out other possible reasons for the symptoms before diagnosing the condition as growing pains. For example, since growing pains usually affect both legs, the problem might not be the same if the pain is only in one leg, and it does not fade by morning, and an alternative diagnosis may be necessary.

One method growing pains can be differentiated from other types of pain is by the way a child reacts to touch during the examination. Generally, a child experiencing growing pains will feel better when the area is massaged, whereas many other kinds of pain will increase when touched. In a few cases, blood tests or x-rays may help doctors with a diagnosis.

Treatment of Growing Pains

There is no specific treatment for growing pains, and it generally subsides on its own, usually within one or two years. The healthcare provider will likely help the parents of the child understand that growing pain is not a serious condition, and ask the parents to follow certain steps to ease the child's discomfort. These steps may include:

- **Massage.** Massaging the affected area may help reduce the pain.

- **Heat treatment.** A heating pad can provide relief for aching muscles.

- **Stretching.** Stretching the legs may help ease some of the pain.

- **Medication.** The healthcare provider might prescribe ibuprofen, naproxen, or acetaminophen for pain. Aspirin should be avoided for young children, since it may increase the risk of a condition called Reye syndrome, which could be life-threatening.

Growing pains are generally not serious, and most children outgrow the condition over time. However, proper management of the pain can help relieve the trauma of recurring pain, which can be upsetting to children.

References

1. "Growing Pains," Cleveland Clinic, n.d.

2. "Growing Pains," The Nemours Foundation/KidsHealth®, June 2015.

3. "Growing Pains," WebMD, July 28, 2016.

4. "Patient Care and Health Information: Growing Pains," Mayo Clinic, August 19, 2016.

Section 25.4

Juvenile Idiopathic Arthritis

This section includes text excerpted from "Juvenile Arthritis,"
National Institute of Arthritis and Musculoskeletal and Skin
Diseases (NIAMS), June 30, 2015. Reviewed September 2019.

What Is Juvenile Arthritis?

"Juvenile arthritis" (JA) is the term used to describe arthritis in
children. Children can get arthritis just like adults. Arthritis is caused
by inflammation of the joints. A joint is where two or more bones are
joined together. Arthritis causes:

- Pain

- Swelling

- Stiffness

- Loss of motion

The most common type of arthritis in children is called "juvenile
idiopathic arthritis" (JIA) (idiopathic means "from unknown causes").
There are several other forms of arthritis affecting children.

Juvenile arthritis is a rheumatic disease or one that causes loss
of function due to an inflamed supporting structure or structures
of the body. Some rheumatic diseases also can involve internal
organs.

Who Gets Juvenile Arthritis

Juvenile arthritis affects children of all ages and ethnic backgrounds. About 294,000 American children under age 18 have arthritis
or other rheumatic conditions.

What Are the Symptoms of Juvenile Arthritis?

The most common symptoms of JA are joint swelling, pain, and stiffness that do not go away. Usually, it affects the knees, hands, and feet,
and it is worse in the morning or after a nap. Other signs can include:

- Limping in the morning because of a stiff knee

- Excessive clumsiness

- High fever and skin rash

- Swelling in lymph nodes in the neck and other parts of the body

Most children with arthritis have times when the symptoms get better or go away (remission) and other times when they get worse (flare).

What Causes Juvenile Arthritis

Scientists are looking for possible causes of JA. They are studying both genetic and environmental factors that they think are involved.

Juvenile arthritis is usually an autoimmune disorder. A healthy immune system helps a person fight off harmful bacteria and viruses. But in an autoimmune disorder, the immune system attacks some of the body's own healthy cells and tissues.

Scientists do not know why this happens or what causes the disorder in children. Some think that something in a child's genes (passed from parents to children) makes the child more likely to get arthritis, and then something else, such as a virus, sets off arthritis.

Is There a Test for Juvenile Arthritis?

There is no easy way a doctor can tell if a child has juvenile arthritis. Doctors usually suspect arthritis when a child has symptoms of:

- Constant joint pain or swelling

- Skin rashes that cannot be explained

- Fever along with swelling of lymph nodes or inflammation in the body's organs

To be sure that it is juvenile arthritis, doctors may:

- Perform a physical exam

- Ask about family health history

- Order lab or blood tests

- Order x-rays

How Is Juvenile Arthritis Treated?

Doctors who treat arthritis in children will try to make sure your child can remain physically active. They also try to make sure your child can stay involved in social activities and have an overall good quality of life (QOL).

Doctors can prescribe treatments to reduce swelling, maintain joint movement, and relieve pain. They also try to prevent, identify, and treat problems that result from arthritis. Most children with arthritis need a blend of treatments—some treatments include medicines.

Who Treats Juvenile Arthritis

A team approach is the best way to treat JA. It is best if a doctor trained to treat these types of diseases in children called a "pediatric rheumatologist," manages your child's care. However, many children's doctors and "adult" rheumatologists also treat children with arthritis.

Other members of your child's healthcare team may include:

- Physical therapist

- Occupational therapist

- Counselor or psychologist

- Eye doctor

- Dentist and orthodontist

- Bone surgeon

- Dietitian

- Pharmacist

- Social worker

- Rheumatology nurse

- School nurse

Helping Your Child

Juvenile arthritis can strain your child's ability to take part in social and after-school activities, and it can make schoolwork more difficult. But, all family members can help the child both physically and emotionally by:

- Getting the best care possible

- Learning as much as you can about your child's disease and its treatment

- Joining a support group

- Treating your child as normally as possible
- Encouraging exercise and physical therapy for your child
- Working closely with your child's school
- Talking with your child about her or his condition and feelings
- Working with therapists or social workers

Exercise Is Key to Reducing Symptoms of Juvenile Arthritis

Pain sometimes limits what children with JA can do. However, exercise is key to reducing the symptoms of arthritis and maintaining function and range of motion of the joints. Ask your child's healthcare team for exercise guidelines.

Most children with arthritis can take part in physical activities and certain sports when their symptoms are under control. Swimming is a good activity because it uses many joints and muscles without putting weight on the joints.

During a disease flare, your child's doctor may advise your child to limit certain activities. It will depend on the joints involved. Once the flare is over, your child can return to her or his normal activities.

Section 25.5

Myositis and Dermatomyositis

This section contains text excerpted from the following sources: Text
under the heading "What Is Myositis?" is excerpted from "Myositis,"
MedlinePlus, National Institutes of Health (NIH), April 17, 2016.
Reviewed September 2019; Text beginning with the heading "What Is
Dermatomyositis?" is excerpted from "Dermatomyositis Information
Page," National Institute of Neurological Disorders
and Stroke (NINDS), March 27, 2019.

What Is Myositis?

"Myositis" means inflammation of the muscles that you use to move
your body. An injury, infection, or autoimmune disease can cause it.
Two specific kinds are polymyositis and dermatomyositis. Polymyositis
causes muscle weakness, usually in the muscles closest to the trunk of
your body. Dermatomyositis causes muscle weakness, plus a skin rash.

Other symptoms of myositis may include:

- Fatigue after walking or standing

- Tripping or falling

- Trouble swallowing or breathing

Doctors may use a physical exam, lab tests, imaging tests, and a
muscle biopsy to diagnose myositis. There is no cure for these diseases,
but you can treat the symptoms. Polymyositis and dermatomyositis
are first treated with high doses of a corticosteroid. Other options
include medications, physical therapy, exercise, heat therapy, assistive
devices, and rest.

What Is Dermatomyositis?

Dermatomyositis is one of a group of muscle diseases known as the
"inflammatory myopathies," which are characterized by chronic muscle
inflammation accompanied by muscle weakness.

Dermatomyositis' cardinal symptom is a skin rash that precedes,
accompanies, or follows progressive muscle weakness. The rash looks
patchy, with purple or red discolorations, and characteristically develops on the eyelids and on muscles used to extend or straighten joints,
including knuckles, elbows, knees, and toes. Red rashes may also occur
on the face, neck, shoulders, upper chest, back, and other locations, and

there may be swelling in the affected areas. The rash sometimes occurs without obvious muscle involvement. Children with dermatomyositis may develop calcium deposits, which appear as hard bumps under the skin or in the muscle (called "calcinosis"). Calcinosis most often occurs one to three years after the disease begins. These deposits are seen more often in children with dermatomyositis than in adults. In some cases of dermatomyositis, distal muscles (muscles located away from the trunk of the body, such as those in the forearms and around the ankles and wrists) may be affected as the disease progresses.

Dermatomyositis may be associated with collagen-vascular or autoimmune diseases, such as lupus.

Treatment of Dermatomyositis

There is no cure for dermatomyositis, but the symptoms can be treated. Options include medication, physical therapy, exercise, heat therapy (including microwave and ultrasound), orthotics and assistive devices, and rest. The standard treatment for dermatomyositis is a corticosteroid drug, given either in pill form or intravenously.

Immunosuppressant drugs, such as azathioprine and methotrexate, may reduce inflammation in people who do not respond well to prednisone. Periodic treatment using intravenous immunoglobulin (IVIG) can also improve recovery. Other immunosuppressive agents used to treat the inflammation associated with dermatomyositis include cyclosporine A, cyclophosphamide, and tacrolimus.

Physical therapy is usually recommended to prevent muscle atrophy and to regain muscle strength and range of motion.

Many individuals with dermatomyositis may need a topical ointment, such as topical corticosteroids, for their skin disorder. They should wear a high-protection sunscreen and protective clothing.

Surgery may be required to remove calcium deposits that cause nerve pain and recurrent infections.

Prognosis of Dermatomyositis

Most cases of dermatomyositis respond to therapy. The disease is usually more severe and resistant to therapy in individuals with cardiac or pulmonary problems.

Section 25.6

Marfan Syndrome

This section includes text excerpted from "Marfan Syndrome,"
National Institute of Arthritis and Musculoskeletal and Skin
Diseases (NIAMS), October 30, 2019. Reviewed September 2019.

What Is Marfan Syndrome?

Marfan syndrome (MFS) is a disorder that affects connective tissue.
Connective tissue supports many parts of your body. You can think of
it as a type of "glue" between cells.

Marfan syndrome can affect many parts of the body, such as:

- Skeleton
- Heart and blood vessels
- Eyes
- Skin
- Nervous system
- Lungs

  It is usually passed from parent to child through the genes.

Who Gets Marfan Syndrome

Marfan syndrome is passed down from parents. Children have 50
percent chance of getting the disease if one of their parents has it.
Men, women, and children can have MFS. It is found in people of all
races and ethnic backgrounds.

What Are the Symptoms of Marfan Syndrome?

Marfan syndrome affects people in different ways. Some people
have only mild symptoms, and others have severe problems. Most of
the time, the symptoms get worse as the person gets older. It affects
many parts of the body, including the:

- **Skeleton.** People with MFS are often very tall, thin, and loose-
  jointed. They may have:

  - Bones in the arms, legs, fingers, and toes that are longer than
    normal

- A long, narrow face
- Crowded teeth because the roof of the mouth is arched
- A breastbone that sticks out or caves in
- A curved backbone
- Flat feet

- **Heart and blood vessels.** Most people with MFS have problems with the heart and blood vessels, such as:

  - A weak part of the vessel that carries blood from the heart. This can make the blood vessel tear or break.

  - Heart valves that leak, causing a "heart murmur." Large leaks may cause:

    - Shortness of breath

    - Tiredness

    - Very fast or uneven heart rate

- **Eyes.** Some people with MFS have problems with the eyes, such as:

  - Nearsightedness

  - Glaucoma (high pressure within the eye) at a young age

  - Cataracts (the eye's lens becomes cloudy)

  - A shift in one or both lenses of the eye

  - A detached retina

- **Skin.** Many people with MFS have:

  - Stretch marks on the skin. These are not a health problem.

  - A hernia (part of an organ that pushes out of its space)

- **Nervous system.** When people with Marfan get older, the tissue surrounding the brain and spinal cord may weaken and stretch. This affects the bones in the lower spine. Symptoms of this problem include:

  - Pain in the stomach area

  - Painful, numb, or weak legs

- **Lungs.** People with MFS do not usually have problems with their lungs. If there are symptoms, they include:
  - Stiff air sacs in the lungs
  - A collapsed lung if the air sacs become stretched or swollen
  - Snoring or not breathing for short periods while sleeping

What Causes Marfan Syndrome

Connective tissue is made of many kinds of protein. MFS is caused by a problem with a gene that makes one of these proteins.

Is There a Test for Marfan Syndrome?

There is no single test for MFS. Your doctor may use many tools to see if you have the disease:

- Medical history (whether you have had any symptoms)
- Family history (any family members who have MFS or who died at a young age from heart problems)
- A physical exam, including the length of the bones in the arms and legs
- An eye exam
- Heart tests

How Is Marfan Syndrome Treated?

There is no cure for MFS, but treatment can help. You should see your doctor on a regular basis to treat or even prevent some problems.

- **Skeleton:**
  - Get a yearly exam of the spine and breastbone
  - Use a back brace
  - Have surgery for serious back problems
- **Heart and blood vessels:**
  - Get regular checkups and heart tests
  - See a doctor or go to an emergency room for pain in the chest, back, or stomach area

- Wear a medical alert bracelet
- Take medicine for heart valve problems
- Have surgery to replace a valve or repair the blood vessel from the heart if the problem is severe

- **Eyes:**
  - Get yearly eye exams
  - Wear eyeglasses or contact lenses
  - Have surgery if needed

- **Lungs:**
  - Do not smoke (because it can hurt your lungs)
  - See a doctor if you have any problems breathing during sleep

- **Nervous system:** Take medicine for back pain.

Who Treats Marfan Syndrome

You may need special kinds of doctors to treat MFS. Your health-care team may include:

- Family doctor or pediatrician
- Cardiologist
- Orthopaedist
- Ophthalmologist
- Geneticist

Living with Marfan Syndrome

Advances in medicine now make it possible for people with MFS to live about as long as the average person. However, the disease can cause strong emotions, such as anger and fear. You may also be worried that your children will have the disease. Children with MFS might find it hard that they cannot play some sports.

Women with MFS can have healthy babies. But pregnancy is a high risk since it stresses the heart. If you are planning to become pregnant, talk to your doctor about whether you should have surgery to reduce this risk. If you are already pregnant, see your doctor right away to prevent problems with your heart.

Ways to help live with the disease include:

- Get proper medical care and correct information.

- Find strong social support.

- Eat a balanced diet and maintain a healthy lifestyle.

- Get medium levels of exercise to keep the skeleton and heart-healthy. You should not play contact or competitive sports. You should also not do exercises where you tighten the muscles without moving them ("planks" are an example).

- Get genetic counseling, which may help you learn about the disease and the risk of passing it on to your children.

Section 25.7

Muscular Dystrophy

This section includes text excerpted from "Muscular Dystrophy: Condition Information," *Eunice Kennedy Shriver* National Institute of Child Health and Human Development (NICHD), December 1, 2016. Reviewed September 2019.

What Is Muscular Dystrophy?

"Muscular dystrophy" (MD) refers to a group of more than 30 inherited diseases that cause muscle weakness and muscle loss. Some forms of MD appear in infancy or childhood, while others may not appear until middle age or even later. In addition, the types of MD differ in the areas of the body they affect and in the severity of the symptoms. All forms of MD grow worse as the person's muscles get weaker. Most people with MD eventually lose their ability to walk.

What Causes Muscular Dystrophy

Muscular dystrophy is generally an inherited disease caused by gene mutations (changes in the deoxyribonucleic acid (DNA) sequence) that affect proteins in muscles. In some cases, the mutation was not inherited from a person's parents but instead happened spontaneously. Such a mutation can then be inherited by the affected person's offspring.

Hundreds of genes are involved in making the proteins that affect muscles. Each type of MD is caused by a genetic mutation that is specific to that type. Some of the forms, such as lamb-girdle and distal, are caused by defects in the same gene.

Muscular dystrophy is not contagious and cannot be caused by injury or activity.

What Are the Types of Muscular Dystrophy That Are Prevalent in Children?

There are more than 30 forms of MD, with information on the primary types. Those that are prevalent among them are discussed below.

Duchenne Muscular Dystrophy

The most common and severe form of MD among children, Duchenne Muscular Dystrophy (DMD) accounts for more than 50 percentage of all cases. DMD is caused by a deficiency of dystrophin, a protein that helps strengthen muscle fibers and protect them from injury.

Symptoms of Duchenne Muscular Dystrophy

Weakness begins in the upper legs and pelvis. People with DMD may also:

- Fall down a lot
- Have trouble rising from a lying or sitting position
- Waddle when walking
- Have difficulty running and jumping
- Have calf muscles that appear large because of fat accumulation

Becker

Also caused by a deficiency of dystrophin, and with symptoms similar to those of DMD, Becker can progress slowly or quickly.

Symptoms of Becker

Patients with Becker MD may:

• Walk on their tiptoes

• Fall down a lot

• Have difficulty rising from the floor

• Have cramping in their muscles

Congenital Muscular Dystrophy

About half of all U.S. cases with congenital MD are caused by a defect in the protein merosin, which surrounds muscle fibers. When caused by defects in other proteins, this type of MD may also affect the central nervous system (CNS).

Symptoms of Congenital Muscular Dystrophy

People with congenital MD may:

• Have problems with motor function and muscle control that appear at birth or during infancy

• Develop chronic shortening of muscles or tendons around joints, which prevents joints from moving freely

• Develop scoliosis (curvature of the spine)

• Have trouble breathing and swallowing

• Have foot deformities

• Have intellectual disabilities

Emery-Dreifuss Muscular Dystrophy

Affecting boys primarily, the two forms of Emery-Dreifuss MD are caused by defects in the proteins that surround the nucleus in cells.

Symptoms of Emery-Dreifuss Muscular Dystrophy

Weakness begins in the upper arm and lower leg muscles. Those with this form may also:

• Develop chronic shortening of muscles around joints (preventing them from moving freely), in the spine, ankles, knees, elbows, and back of the neck

- Have elbows locked in a flexed position
- Develop shoulder deterioration
- Have a rigid spine
- Walk on their toes
- Experience mild weakness in their facial muscles

Facioscapulohumeral Muscular Dystrophy

"Facioscapulohumeral" (FSHD) muscular dystrophy refers to the areas affected: the face (facio), the shoulders (scapulo), and the upper arms (humeral). Researchers do not know what gene causes FSHD. They do know where the defect occurs and that it affects specific muscle groups.

Symptoms of Facioscapulohumeral Muscular Dystrophy

Facioscapulohumeral muscular dystrophy often appears first in the eyes (difficulty in opening and shutting) and mouth (inability to smile or pucker). Other symptoms may include:

- Muscle wasting that causes shoulders to appear slanted and shoulder blades to appear "winged"
- Impaired reflexes only at the biceps and triceps
- Trouble swallowing, chewing, or speaking
- Hearing problems
- Swayback curve in the spine, called "lordosis"

Limb-Girdle Muscular Dystrophy

This form of MD can appear in childhood but most often appears in adolescence or young adulthood. Limb-girdle can progress quickly or slowly, but most patients become severely disabled (with muscle damage and inability to walk) within 20 years of developing the disease.

Symptoms of Limb-Girdle Muscular Dystrophy

Patients with limb-girdle MD may:

- First develop weakness around the hips, which then spreads to the shoulders, legs, and neck

- Fall down a lot

- Have trouble rising from chairs, climbing stairs, or carrying things

- Waddle when they walk

- Have a rigid spine

How Many People Are Affected by Muscular Dystrophy?

The incidence of MD in the United States varies, because different kinds of MD are rarer than others. The most common forms in children, Duchenne and Becker, affect approximately 1 in every 5,600 to 7,700 males ages 5 to 24.

What Are Common Symptoms of Muscular Dystrophy?

Muscle weakness that worsens over time is a common symptom of all forms of MD. Each form of MD varies in the order in which symptoms occur and in the parts of the body that are affected.

How Is Muscular Dystrophy Diagnosed?

The first step in diagnosing MD is a visit with a healthcare provider for a physical exam. The healthcare provider will ask a series of questions about the patient's family history and medical history, including any problems affecting the muscles that the patient may be experiencing.

The healthcare provider may order tests to determine whether the problems are a result of MD and, if so, what form of this disorder. The tests may also rule out other problems that could cause muscle weakness, such as surgery, toxic exposure, medications, or other muscle diseases. These tests may include:

- Blood tests

- Muscle biopsies

- Genetic testing

- Neurological tests

- Heart testing

- Exercise assessments

- Imaging tests

What Are the Treatments for Muscular Dystrophy?

No treatment is currently available to stop or reverse any form of MD. Instead, certain therapies and medications aim to treat the various problems that result from MD and improve the quality of life (QOL) for patients.

Section 25.8

Legg-Calvé-Perthes Disease

This section contains text excerpted from the following sources: Text beginning with the heading "What Is Legg-Calvé-Perthes Disease?" is excerpted from Genetics Home Reference (GHR), National Institutes of Health (NIH), September 2014. Reviewed September 2019; Text beginning with the heading "Inheritance of Legg-Calvé-Perthes Disease" is excerpted from "Legg-Calve-Perthes Disease," Genetic and Rare Diseases Information Center (GARD), National Center for Advancing Translational Sciences (NCATS), July 28, 2016. Reviewed September 2019.

What Is Legg-Calvé-Perthes Disease?

Legg-Calvé-Perthes disease (LCPD) is a bone disorder that affects the hips. Usually, only one hip is involved, but in about 10 percent of cases, both hips are affected. LCPD begins in childhood, typically between ages 4 and 8, and affects boys more frequently than girls.

In this condition, the upper end of the thigh bone, known as the "femoral head," breaks down. As a result, the femoral head is no longer round and does not move easily in the hip socket, which leads to hip pain, limping, and restricted leg movement. The bone eventually begins to heal itself through a normal process called "bone remodeling," by which old bone is removed and new bone is created to replace it. This cycle of breakdown and healing can recur multiple times. Affected individuals are often shorter than their peers due to bone abnormalities. Many people with LCPD go on to develop a painful joint disorder called "osteoarthritis" in the hips at an early age.

Frequency of Legg-Calvé-Perthes Disease

The incidence of LCPD varies by population. The condition is most common in White populations, in which it affects an estimated 1 to 3 in 20,000 children under age 15.

Causes of Legg-Calvé-Perthes Disease

Legg-Calvé-Perthes disease is usually not caused by genetic factors. The cause in these cases is unknown. In a small percentage of cases, mutations in *collagen, type II, alpha 1 (COL2A1)* gene cause the bone abnormalities characteristic of LCPD. The *COL2A1* gene provides instructions for making a protein that forms type II collagen. This type of collagen is found mostly in cartilage, a tough but flexible tissue that makes up much of the skeleton during early development. Most cartilage is later converted to bone, except for the cartilage that continues to cover and protect the ends of bones and is present in the nose and external ears. Type II collagen is essential for the normal development of bones and other connective tissues that form the body's supportive framework.

COL2A1 gene mutations involved in LCPD lead to the production of an altered protein; collagen that contains this protein may be less stable than normal. Researchers speculate that the breakdown of bone characteristic of LCPD is caused by impaired blood flow to the femoral head, which leads to death of the bone tissue (osteonecrosis); however, it is unclear how abnormal type II collagen is involved in this process or why the hips are specifically affected.

Inheritance of Legg-Calvé-Perthes Disease

Legg-Calve-Perthes disease is usually not caused by genetic factors (thus is usually not inherited), but there are some cases where LCPD affects more than one family member. In a small percentage of these familial cases, changes or mutations in the *COL2A1* gene have been found to cause LCPD. When mutations in the *COL2A1* gene are the cause of LCPD, the disease is inherited in an autosomal dominant manner. In some cases, it appears that genetic and environmental factors interact to increase a person's chance to develop LCPD.

Diagnosis of Legg-Calvé-Perthes Disease

Making a diagnosis for a genetic or rare disease can often be challenging. Healthcare professionals typically look at a person's medical history, symptoms, physical exam, and laboratory test results in order to make a diagnosis.

Prognosis of Legg-Calvé-Perthes Disease

The prognosis for people with LCPD depends on the extent and severity of bone involvement and residual deformity. Overall, the prognosis for recovery and sports participation after treatment is very good for most people. Generally, younger age at diagnosis is associated with a better outcome.

For people who are younger than age 5 when LCPD develops, the incidence of degenerative arthritis later in life is reportedly very low. The more deformed the femoral head is during healing, the greater the risk of osteoarthritis of the hip later in life. The risk is also higher for those with metaphyseal defects (where the shaft of the bone flares out), and for those who develop LCPD late in childhood (at age 10 or older). Nearly 100 percent of people with complex involvement of the femoral head and residual deformity will develop degenerative arthritis. Total hip replacement in early adulthood may be needed in some cases.

Section 25.9

Scoliosis

This section includes text excerpted from "Scoliosis in Children and Adolescents," National Institute of Arthritis and Musculoskeletal and Skin Diseases (NIAMS), December 30, 2015. Reviewed September 2019.

What Is Scoliosis?

Scoliosis is a disorder in which there is a sideways curve of the spine. Curves are often S-shaped or C-shaped. In most people, there is no known cause for this curve. Curves frequently follow patterns that have been studied in previous patients.

People with milder curves may only need to visit their doctor for regular check-ups. Some people who have scoliosis require treatment.

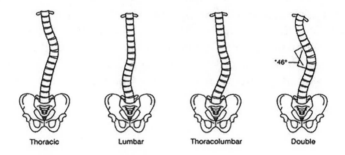

Figure 25.1. *Curved Patterns of the Spine*

Who Gets Scoliosis

People of all ages can have scoliosis. The most common type has no known cause and occurs in children age 10 to 12 and in their early teens. Girls are more likely than boys to have this type of scoliosis. You are more likely to have scoliosis if your parent, brother or sister have it.

What Are the Symptoms of Scoliosis?

Scoliosis is a disorder in which there is a sideways curve of the spine. Signs of scoliosis can include:

- Uneven shoulders

- Head that is not centered
- Sides of the body are not level with each other
- One side of the rib cage is higher than the other when bending forward

What Causes Scoliosis

In most people with scoliosis, the cause is not known. In some cases, there is a known cause.

Doctors classify curves as:

- **Nonstructural,** which is when the spine is structurally normal and the curve is temporary. In these cases, the doctor will try to find and correct the cause.

- **Structural,** which is when the spine has a fixed curve. The cause could be a disease, injury, infection, birth defect, or unknown.

Is There a Test for Scoliosis?

Your doctor may do the following to diagnosis you with scoliosis:

- **Medical history** to look for medical problems that might be causing your spine to curve

- **Physical examination** to look at your back, chest, pelvis, legs, feet, and skin

- **X-rays** to measure the curve of the spine and to determine how to treat scoliosis

How Is Scoliosis Treated?

Your doctor may recommend the following treatments:

- **Observation.** If the curve is mild and you are still growing, your doctor will re-examine you every few months.

- **Bracing.** If the curve is moderate and you are still growing, your doctor may recommend a brace to keep the curve from getting worse. Braces are selected for the specific curve problem and fitted to each patient. Braces must be worn every day for the full number of hours prescribed by the doctor.

- **Surgery.** If you are still growing and have a severe curve that is getting worse, your doctor may suggest surgery. This often involves fusing together two or more bones in the spine. The doctor may also put in a metal rod or other device to help keep the spine straight after surgery. You should seek the advice of at least two experts, and ask about the benefits and risks of the surgery.

The following treatments have not been shown to keep curves from getting worse in scoliosis:

- Chiropractic treatment

- Electrical stimulation

- Nutritional supplements

Living with Scoliosis

Exercise programs have not been shown to keep scoliosis from getting worse. But it is important for all people, including those with scoliosis, to exercise and remain physically fit. Weight-bearing exercise, such as walking, running, soccer, and gymnastics, helps keep bones strong. For both girls and boys, exercising and playing sports can improve their sense of well-being.

Chapter 26

Neurological Disorders in Children

Chapter Contents

Section 26.1

Childhood Brain and Spinal-Cord Tumors

This section includes text excerpted from "Childhood Brain and Spinal Cord Tumors Treatment Overview (PDQ®)—Patient Version," National Cancer Institute (NCI), January 15, 2019.

What Are Childhood Brain and Spinal-Cord Tumors?

A childhood brain or spinal-cord tumor is a disease in which abnormal cells form in the tissues of the brain or spinal cord.

There are many types of childhood brain and spinal-cord tumors. The tumors are formed by the abnormal growth of cells and may begin in different areas of the brain or spinal cord.

The tumors may be benign (not cancer) or malignant (cancer). Benign brain tumors grow and press on nearby areas of the brain. They rarely spread into other tissues. Malignant brain tumors are likely to grow quickly and spread into other brain tissue. When a tumor grows into or presses on an area of the brain, it may stop that part of the brain from working the way it should. Both benign and malignant brain tumors can cause signs or symptoms and need treatment.

Together, the brain and spinal cord make up the central nervous system (CNS).

Part of the Brain

The brain has three major parts:

- The cerebrum is the largest part of the brain. It is at the top of the head. The cerebrum controls thinking, learning, problem-solving, emotions, speech, reading, writing, and voluntary movement.

- The cerebellum is in the lower back of the brain (near the middle of the back of the head). It controls movement, balance, and posture.

- The brainstem connects the brain to the spinal cord. It is in the lowest part of the brain (just above the back of the neck). The brainstem controls breathing, heart rate, and the nerves and muscles used in seeing, hearing, walking, talking, and eating.

Spinal Cord and Its Role

The spinal cord is a column of nerve tissue that runs from the brain stem down the center of the back. It is covered by three thin layers of tissue called "membranes." These membranes are surrounded by the vertebrae (backbones). Spinal-cord nerves carry messages between the brain and the rest of the body, such as a message from the brain to cause muscles to move or a message from the skin to the brain to feel touch.

Spinal-Cord Tumors: A Common Type of Childhood Cancer

Although cancer is rare in children, brain and spinal-cord tumors are the second most common type of childhood cancer, after leukemia. Brain tumors can occur in both children and adults. Treatment for children is usually different than treatment for adults.

This summary describes the treatment of primary brain and spinal cord-tumors (tumors that begin in the brain and spinal cord). Treatment of metastatic brain and spinal-cord tumors is not covered in this summary. Metastatic tumors are formed by cancer cells that begin in other parts of the body and spread to the brain or spinal cord.

The cause of most childhood brain and spinal-cord tumors is unknown.

Signs and Symptoms of Childhood Brain and Spinal-Cord Tumors

Signs and symptoms depend on the following:

- Where the tumor forms in the brain or spinal cord
- The size of the tumor
- How fast the tumor grows
- The child's age and development

Signs and symptoms may be caused by childhood brain and spinal-cord tumors or by other conditions, including cancer that has spread to the brain. Check with your child's doctor if your child has any of the following:

Brain Tumor Signs and Symptoms

- Morning headache or headache that goes away after vomiting

- Frequent nausea and vomiting

- Vision, hearing, and speech problems

- Loss of balance and trouble walking

- Unusual sleepiness or change in activity level

- Unusual changes in personality or behavior

- Seizures

- Increase in the head size (in infants)

Spinal-Cord Tumor Signs and Symptoms

- Back pain or pain that spreads from the back towards the arms or legs

- A change in bowel habits or trouble urinating

- Weakness in the legs

- Trouble walking

In addition to these signs and symptoms of brain and spinal-cord tumors, some children are unable to reach certain growth and development milestones, such as sitting up, walking, and talking in sentences.

Tests to Examine Childhood Brain and Spinal-Cord Tumors

The following tests and procedures may be used:

- **Physical exam and history:** An exam of the body to check general signs of health, including checking for signs of disease, such as lumps or anything else that seems unusual. A history of the patient's health habits and past illnesses and treatments will also be taken.

- **Neurological exam:** A series of questions and tests to check the brain, spinal cord, and nerve function. The exam checks a person's mental status, coordination, and ability to walk normally, and how well the muscles, senses, and reflexes work. This may also be called a "neuro exam" or a "neurologic exam."

- **Magnetic resonance imaging (MRI) with gadolinium:** A procedure that uses a magnet, radio waves, and a computer to make a series of detailed pictures of the brain and spinal cord. A substance called "gadolinium" is injected into a vein. The gadolinium collects around the cancer cells so they show up brighter in the picture. This procedure is also called "nuclear magnetic resonance imaging" (NMRI).

- **Serum tumor marker test:** A procedure in which a sample of blood is examined to measure the amounts of certain substances released into the blood by organs, tissues, or tumor cells in the body. Certain substances are linked to specific types of cancer when found in increased levels in the blood. These are called "tumor markers."

Most Childhood Brain Tumors Are Diagnosed and Removed in Surgery

If doctors think there might be a brain tumor, a biopsy may be done to remove a sample of tissue. For tumors in the brain, the biopsy is done by removing part of the skull and using a needle to remove a sample of tissue. A pathologist views the tissue under a microscope to look for cancer cells. If cancer cells are found, the doctor may remove as much tumor as safely possible during the same surgery. The pathologist checks the cancer cells to find out the type and grade of brain tumor. The grade of the tumor is based on how abnormal the cancer cells look under a microscope and how quickly the tumor is likely to grow and spread.

The following test may be done on the sample of tissue that is removed:

- **Immunohistochemistry:** A test that uses antibodies to check for certain antigens in a sample of tissue. The antibody is usually linked to a radioactive substance or a dye that causes the tissue to light up under a microscope. This type of test may be used to tell the difference between different types of cancer.

Some Childhood Brain and Spinal-Cord Tumors Are Diagnosed by Imaging Tests

Sometimes a biopsy or surgery cannot be done safely because of where the tumor formed in the brain or spinal cord. These tumors are diagnosed based on the results of imaging tests and other procedures.

Prognosis of Childhood Brain and Spinal-Cord Tumors

The prognosis (chance of recovery) depends on the following:

- Whether there are any cancer cells left after surgery

- The type of tumor

- Where the tumor is in the body

- The child's age

- Whether the tumor has just been diagnosed or has recurred (come back)

Staging Childhood Brain and Spinal-Cord Tumors
In Childhood Brain and Spinal-Cord Tumors, Treatment Options Are Based on Several Factors

Staging is the process used to find how much cancer there is and if cancer has spread within the brain, spinal cord, or to other parts of the body. It is important to know the stage in order to plan cancer treatment.

In childhood brain and spinal cord tumors, there is no standard staging system. Instead, the plan for cancer treatment depends on several factors:

- **The type of tumor** and where the tumor formed in the brain

- **Whether the tumor is newly diagnosed or recurrent.**
  A newly diagnosed brain or spinal cord tumor is one that has never been treated. A recurrent childhood brain or spinal cord tumor is one that has recurred (come back) after it has been treated. Childhood brain and spinal-cord tumors may come back in the same place or in another part of the brain, or spinal cord. Sometimes they come back in another part of the body. The tumor may come back many years after first being treated. Tests and procedures, including biopsy, that was done to diagnose and stage the tumor may be done to find out if the tumor has recurred.

- **The grade of the tumor.** The grade of the tumor is based on how abnormal the cancer cells look under a microscope and how quickly the tumor is likely to grow and spread. It is important to know the grade of the tumor and if there were any cancer cells remaining after surgery in order to plan treatment. The grade of the tumor is not used to plan treatment for all types of brain and spinal-cord tumors.

- **The tumor risk group.** Risk groups are either average risk and poor risk or low, intermediate, and high risk. The risk groups are based on the amount of tumor remaining after surgery, the spread of cancer cells within the brain and spinal cord or to other parts of the body, where the tumor has formed, and the age of the child. The risk group is not used to plan treatment for all types of brain and spinal-cord tumors.

Tests and Procedures Done to Detect Childhood Brain and Spinal-Cord Tumors Risk Group

After the tumor is removed in surgery, some of the tests used to detect childhood brain and spinal-cord tumors are repeated to help determine the tumor risk group. This is to find out how much tumor remains after surgery.

Childhood Brain and Spinal-Cord Tumors May Recur after Treatment

A recurrent childhood brain or spinal-cord tumor is one that has recurred (come back) after it has been treated. Childhood brain and spinal-cord tumors may come back in the same place or in another part of the brain. Sometimes they come back in another part of the body. The tumor may come back many years after first being treated. Diagnostic and staging tests and procedures, including biopsy, may be done to make sure that the tumor has recurred.

Treatment of Childhood Brain and Spinal-Cord Tumor

Different types of treatment are available for children with brain and spinal-cord tumors. Some treatments are standard (the currently used treatment), and some are being tested in clinical trials. A treatment clinical trial is a research study meant to help improve current treatments or obtain information on new treatments for patients with cancer. When clinical trials show that a new treatment is better than the standard treatment, the new treatment may become the standard treatment.

Because cancer in children is rare, taking part in a clinical trial should be considered. Clinical trials are taking place in many parts of the country. Some clinical trials are open only to patients who have not started treatment.

Healthcare Providers Who Are Experts in Treating Childhood Brain and Spinal-Cord Tumors

Treatment will be overseen by a pediatric oncologist, a doctor who specializes in treating children with cancer. The pediatric oncologist works with other healthcare providers who are experts in treating children with brain tumors and who specialize in certain areas of medicine. These may include the following specialists:

- Pediatrician
- Neurosurgeon
- Neurologist
- Neuro-oncologist
- Neuropathologist
- Neuroradiologist
- Radiation oncologist
- Endocrinologist
- Psychologist
- Ophthalmologist
- Rehabilitation specialist
- Social worker
- Nurse specialist

Childhood Brain and Spinal-Cord Tumors May Cause Signs or Symptoms That Begin before the Cancer Is Diagnosed and Continue for Months or Years

Childhood brain and spinal-cord tumors may cause signs or symptoms that continue for months or years. Signs or symptoms caused by the tumor may begin before diagnosis. Signs or symptoms caused by treatment may begin during or right after treatment.

Treatment for Childhood Brain and Spinal-Cord Tumors May Cause Side Effects

Side effects from cancer treatment that begin after treatment and continue for months or years are called "late effects."

Late effects of cancer treatment may include the following:

- Physical problems

- Changes in mood, feelings, thinking, learning, or memory

- Second cancers (new types of cancer)

Some late effects may be treated or controlled. It is important to talk with your child's doctors about the effects cancer treatment can have on your child.

Patients May Want to Think about Taking Part in a Clinical Trial

For some patients, taking part in a clinical trial may be the best treatment choice. Clinical trials are part of the cancer research process. Clinical trials are done to find out if new cancer treatments are safe and effective or better than the standard treatment.

Many standard treatments for cancer are based on earlier clinical trials. Patients who take part in a clinical trial may receive the standard treatment or be among the first to receive a new treatment.

Patients who take part in clinical trials also help improve the way cancer will be treated in the future. Even when clinical trials do not lead to effective new treatments, they often answer important questions and help move research forward.

Patients Can Enter Clinical Trials before, during, or after Starting Their Cancer Treatment

Some clinical trials only include patients who have not yet received treatment. Other trials test treatments for patients whose cancer has not gotten better. There are also clinical trials that test new ways to stop cancer from recurring (coming back) or reduce the side effects of cancer treatment.

Follow-Up Tests May Be Needed

Some of the tests that were done to diagnose the cancer or to find out the stage of the cancer may be repeated. Some tests will be repeated in order to see how well the treatment is working. Decisions about whether to continue, change or stop treatment may be based on the results of these tests.

Some of the tests will continue to be done from time to time after treatment has ended. The results of these tests can show if your child's condition has changed or if the cancer has recurred (come back). These tests are sometimes called "follow-up tests" or "check-ups."

Section 26.2

Cerebral Palsy

This section includes text excerpted from "Cerebral Palsy (CP)," Centers for Disease Control and Prevention (CDC), April 18, 2018.

What Is Cerebral Palsy?

Cerebral palsy (CP) is a group of disorders that affect a person's ability to move and maintain balance and posture. CP is the most common motor disability in childhood. Cerebral means having to do with the brain. Palsy means weakness or difficulties with using the muscles. CP is caused by abnormal brain development or damage to the developing brain that affects a person's ability to control her or his muscles.

The symptoms of CP vary from person to person. A person with severe CP might need to use special equipment to be able to walk, or might not be able to walk at all and might need lifelong care. A person with mild CP, on the other hand, might walk a little awkwardly, but might not need any special help. CP does not get worse over time, though the exact symptoms can change over a person's lifetime.

All people with CP have difficulties with movement and posture. Many also have related conditions, such as intellectual disability; seizures; problems with vision, hearing, or speech; changes in the spine (such as scoliosis); or joint problems (such as contractures).

Types of Cerebral Palsy

Doctors classify CP according to the main type of movement disorder involved. Depending on which areas of the brain are affected, one or more of the following movement disorders can occur:

- Stiff muscles (spasticity)

- Uncontrollable movements (dyskinesia)

- Poor balance and coordination (ataxia)

There are four main types of CP.

Spastic Cerebral Palsy

The most common type of CP is spastic CP. Spastic CP affects about 80 percent of people with CP. People with spastic CP have increased muscle tone. This means their muscles are stiff and, as a result, their movements can be awkward.

Dyskinetic Cerebral Palsy (Also Includes Athetoid, Choreoathetoid, and Dystonic Cerebral Palsies)

People with dyskinetic CP have problems controlling the movement of their hands, arms, feet, and legs, making it difficult to sit and walk. The movements are uncontrollable and can be slow and writhing or rapid and jerky. Sometimes the face and tongue are affected and the person has a hard time sucking, swallowing, and talking. A person with dyskinetic CP has muscle tone that can change (varying from too tight to too loose) not only from day to day but even during a single day.

Ataxic Cerebral Palsy

People with ataxic CP have problems with balance and coordination. They might be unsteady when they walk. They might have a hard time with quick movements or movements that need a lot of control, like writing. They might have a hard time controlling their hands or arms when they reach for something.

Mixed Cerebral Palsy

Some people have symptoms of more than one type of CP. The most common type of mixed CP is spastic-dyskinetic CP.

Early Signs of Cerebral Palsy

The signs of CP vary greatly because there are many different types and levels of disability. The main sign that a child might have CP is a delay reaching motor or movement milestones (such as rolling over, sitting, standing, or walking). Following are some other signs of possible CP. It is important to note that some children without CP also might have some of these signs.

In a Baby Younger than Six Months of Age

- The head lags when you pick her or him up from lying on her or his back

- She or he feels stiff

- She or he feels floppy

- When held cradled in your arms, she or he seems to overextend the back and neck, constantly acting as if she or he is pushing away from you

- When you pick your baby up, her or his legs get stiff and cross or scissor

In a Baby Older than Six Months of Age

- Does not roll over in either direction

- Cannot bring her or his hands together

- She or he has difficulty bringing hands up to the mouth

- She or he reaches out with only one hand while keeping the other fisted

In a Baby Older than Ten Months of Age

- She or he crawls in a lopsided manner, pushing off with one hand and leg while dragging the opposite hand and leg

- She or he scoots around on the buttocks or hops on the knees but does not crawl on all fours

Tell your child's doctor or nurse if you notice any of these signs.

Screening and Diagnosis of Cerebral Palsy

Diagnosing CP at an early age is important to the well-being of children and their families. Diagnosing CP can take several steps:

Developmental Monitoring

Developmental monitoring (also called "surveillance") means tracking a child's growth and development over time. If any concerns about the child's development are raised during monitoring, then a developmental screening test should be given as soon as possible.

Developmental Screening

During the developmental screening, a short test is given to see if the child has specific developmental delays, such as motor or movement delays. If the results of the screening test are cause for concern, then the doctor will make referrals for developmental and medical evaluations.

Developmental and Medical Evaluations

The goal of the developmental evaluation is to diagnose the specific type of disorder that affects a child.

Treatments of Cerebral Palsy

There is no cure for CP, but treatment can improve the lives of those who have the condition. It is important to begin a treatment program as early as possible.

After a CP diagnosis is made, a team of health professionals works with the child and family to develop a plan to help the child reach her or his full potential. Common treatments include medicines; surgery; braces; and physical, occupational, and speech therapy. No single treatment is the best one for all children with CP. Before deciding on a treatment plan, it is important to talk with the child's doctor to understand all the risks and benefits.

Causes and Risk Factors of Cerebral Palsy

Cerebral palsy is caused by abnormal development of the brain or damage to the developing brain that affects a child's ability to control her or his muscles. There are several possible causes of abnormal development or damage. People used to think that CP was mainly caused by a lack of oxygen during the birth process. Now, scientists think that this causes only a small number of CP cases.

The brain damage that leads to CP can happen before birth, during birth, within a month after birth, or during the first years of a child's life, while the brain is still developing. CP related to brain damage that occurred before or during birth is called "congenital CP." The majority of CP (85–90%) is congenital. In many cases, the specific cause is not known. A small percentage of CP is caused by brain damage that occurs more than 28 days after birth. This is called "acquired CP," and usually is associated with an infection (such as meningitis) or head injury.

If You Are Concerned

If you think your child is not meeting movement milestones or might have CP, contact your doctor or nurse and share your concerns.

If you or your doctor is still concerned, ask for a referral to a specialist who can do a more in-depth evaluation of your child and assist in making a diagnosis.

At the same time, call your state's public early childhood system to request a free evaluation to find out if your child qualifies for intervention services. This is sometimes called a "Child Find evaluation." You do not need to wait for a doctor's referral or a medical diagnosis to make this call.

Where to call for a free evaluation from the state depends on your child's age:

- If your child is not yet three years old, contact your local early intervention system. You can find the right contact information for your state by calling the Early Childhood Technical Assistance Center (ECTA) at 919-962-2001.

- If your child is three years of age or older, contact your local public school system. Even if your child is not yet old enough for kindergarten or enrolled in a public school, call your local elementary school or board of education and ask to speak with someone who can help you have your child evaluated.

Section 26.3

Epilepsy

This section contains text excerpted from the following sources: Text
beginning with the heading "What Is Epilepsy?" is excerpted from
"Epilepsy Information Page," National Institute of Neurological
Disorders and Stroke (NINDS), May 22, 2019; Text under the
heading "Sudden Unexpected Death in Epilepsy Information for
Parents of Children with Epilepsy" is excerpted from "Epilepsy,"
Centers for Disease Control and Prevention (CDC), May 8, 2018.

What Is Epilepsy?

The epilepsies are a spectrum of brain disorders ranging from
severe, life-threatening and disabling, to ones that are much more
benign. In epilepsy, the pattern of neuronal activity common in people
who are not disabled becomes disturbed, causing strange sensations,
emotions, and behavior or sometimes convulsions, muscle spasms, and
loss of consciousness.

The epilepsies have many possible causes and there are several
types of seizures. Anything that disturbs the predominant pattern
of neuron activity—from illness to brain damage to abnormal brain
development—can lead to seizures. Epilepsy may develop because of an
abnormality in brain wiring, an imbalance of nerve signaling chemicals
called "neurotransmitters," changes in important features of brain
cells called "channels," or some combination of these and other factors.
Having a single seizure as the result of a high fever (called "febrile
seizure") or head injury does not necessarily mean that a person has
epilepsy. Only when a person has had two or more seizures is she or he
considered to have epilepsy. A measurement of electrical activity in the
brain and brain scans, such as magnetic resonance imaging (MRI) or
computed tomography (CT) are common diagnostic tests for epilepsy.

Treatment of Epilepsy

Once epilepsy is diagnosed, it is important to begin treatment
as soon as possible. For about 70 percent of those diagnosed with
epilepsy, seizures can be controlled with modern medicines and surgical techniques. Some drugs are more effective for specific types of
seizures. An individual with seizures, particularly those that are not
easily controlled, may want to see a neurologist specifically trained
to treat epilepsy. In some children, special diets may help to control

seizures when medications are either not effective or cause serious side effects.

Prognosis of Epilepsy

While epilepsy cannot be cured, for some people the seizures can be controlled with medication, diet, assistive devices, and/or surgery. Most seizures do not cause brain damage, but ongoing uncontrolled seizures may cause brain damage. It is not uncommon for people with epilepsy, especially children, to develop behavioral and emotional problems in conjunction with seizures. Issues may also arise as a result of the stigma attached to having epilepsy, which can lead to embarrassment and frustration or bullying, teasing, or avoidance in school and other social settings. For many people with epilepsy, the risk of seizures restricts their independence (some states refuse drivers licenses to people with epilepsy) and recreational activities.

Epilepsy can be a life-threatening condition. Some people with epilepsy are at special risk for abnormally prolonged seizures or sudden unexplained death caused by epilepsy.

Sudden Unexpected Death in Epilepsy
Sudden Unexpected Death in Epilepsy in Children

Watching a child deal with the day-to-day challenge of epilepsy can be hard for any parent. Researchers have found that sudden unexpected death in epilepsy (SUDEP) is uncommon among younger-aged children, but it is still an important concern for some children. "SUDEP" refers to deaths in people with epilepsy that are not caused by injury, drowning, or other known causes. Most, but not all, cases of SUDEP occur during or immediately after a seizure. The exact cause is not known, but these are possible factors:

- **Breathing.** A seizure may cause a person to have pauses in breathing (apnea). If these pauses last too long, they can reduce the oxygen in the blood to a life-threatening level. In addition, during a convulsive seizure, a person's airway sometimes may get covered or obstructed, leading to suffocation.

- **Heart rhythm.** Rarely, a seizure may cause a dangerous heart rhythm or even heart failure.

- **Other causes and mixed causes.** SUDEP may result from more than one cause or a combination involving both breathing difficulty and abnormal heart rhythm.

Risk Factors for Sudden Unexpected Death in Epilepsy in Children

Children with uncontrolled epilepsy or frequent seizures are at the highest risk for SUDEP.

In addition, other risk factors may include the following:

- Early-onset of epilepsy

- Developmental disabilities

Steps You Can Take to Reduce the Risk of Sudden Unexpected Death in Epilepsy for Your Child

If your child has epilepsy, ask her or his doctor to discuss the risk of SUDEP with you. The first and most important step to reduce your child's risk of SUDEP is to make sure she or he takes seizure medicine as prescribed.

If your child is taking seizure medicine and still having seizures, discuss options for adjusting the medicine with the doctor. If seizures continue, consider consulting an epilepsy specialist, if you are not already seeing one.

Other possible steps you can take to reduce your child's risk of SUDEP may include:

- Avoid seizure triggers, if these are known.

- Get enough sleep.

- Train adults in the house in seizure first aid.

How Do I Talk to My Child's Healthcare Provider about Sudden Unexpected Death in Epilepsy?

When you decide to talk to your child's healthcare provider about SUDEP, you may want to ask:

- What risk does my child have for SUDEP?

- If my child's risk for SUDEP is increased, what can I do to reduce this risk?

- What should I do if my child forgets to take her or his antiepileptic drug (AED)?

- What steps should I take if it is decided to change my child's seizure medicine?

- What medicines provide the best seizure control for my child?

- Are there any specific activities my child should avoid?

- What instructions should I give family and friends if my child has a seizure?

Section 26.4

Headache

This section includes text excerpted from "Headache: Hope through Research," National Institute of Neurological Disorders and Stroke (NINDS), August 13, 2019.

Why Headaches Hurt

Information about touch, pain, temperature, and vibration in the head and neck is sent to the brain by the trigeminal nerve, one of 12 pairs of cranial nerves that start at the base of the brain.

The nerve has three branches that conduct sensations from the scalp, the blood vessels inside and outside of the skull, the lining around the brain (the meninges), and the face, mouth, neck, ears, eyes, and throat.

The brain tissue itself lacks pain-sensitive nerves and does not feel pain. Headaches occur when pain-sensitive nerve endings called "nociceptors" react to headache triggers (such as stress, certain foods or odors, or use of medicines) and send messages through the trigeminal nerve to the thalamus, the brain's "relay station" for pain sensation from all over the body. The thalamus controls the body's sensitivity to light and noise and sends messages to parts of the brain that manage awareness of pain and emotional response to it. Other parts of the brain may also be part of the process, causing nausea, vomiting, diarrhea, trouble concentrating, and other neurological symptoms.

When to See a Doctor

Not all headaches require a physician's attention. But headaches can signal a more serious disorder that requires prompt medical care.

Immediately call or see a physician if you or someone you are with experience any of these symptoms:

- Sudden, severe headache that may be accompanied by a stiff neck

- Severe headache accompanied by fever, nausea, or vomiting that is not related to another illness

- "First" or "worst" headache, often accompanied by confusion, weakness, double vision, or loss of consciousness

- Headache that worsens over days or weeks or has changed in pattern or behavior

- Recurring headache in children

- Headache following a head injury

- Headache and a loss of sensation or weakness in any part of the body, which could be a sign of a stroke

- Headache associated with convulsions

- Headache associated with shortness of breath

- Two or more headaches a week

- Persistent headache in someone who has been previously headache-free, particularly in someone over age 50

- New headaches in someone with a history of cancer or human immunodeficiency virus (HIV)/acquired immune deficiency syndrome (AIDS)

Diagnosing Your Headache

How and under what circumstances a person experiences a headache can be key to diagnosing its cause. Keeping a headache journal can help a physician better diagnose your type of headache and determine the best treatment. After each headache, note the time of day when it occurred; its intensity and duration; any sensitivity to light, odors, or sound; activity immediately prior to the headache; use of prescription and nonprescription medicines; amount of sleep the previous night; any stressful or emotional conditions; any influence from weather or daily activity; foods and fluids consumed in the past 24 hours; and any known health conditions at that time. Women should record the days of their menstrual cycles. Include notes about other family members who have a history of headache or other disorders. A pattern may emerge that can be helpful in reducing or preventing headaches.

Once your doctor has reviewed your medical and headache history and conducted a physical and neurological exam, lab screening and diagnostic tests may be ordered to either rule out or identify conditions that might be the cause of your headaches. Blood tests and urinalysis can help diagnose brain or spinal-cord infections, blood-vessel damage, and toxins that affect the nervous system. Testing a sample of the fluid that surrounds the brain and spinal cord can detect infections, bleeding in the brain (called a "brain hemorrhage"), and measure any buildup of pressure within the skull. Diagnostic imaging, such as with computed tomography (CT) and magnetic resonance imaging (MRI), can detect irregularities in blood vessels and bones, certain brain tumors and cysts, brain damage from a head injury, brain hemorrhage, inflammation, infection, and other disorders. Neuroimaging also gives doctors a way to see what is happening in the brain during headache attacks. An electroencephalogram (EEG) measures brain wave activity and can help diagnose brain tumors, seizures, head injury, and inflammation that may lead to headaches.

Children and Headache

Headaches are common in children. Headaches that begin early in life can develop into migraines as the child grows older. Migraines in children or adolescents can develop into tension-type headaches at any time. In contrast to adults with migraine, young children often feel migraine pain on both sides of the head and have headaches that usually last less than two hours. Children may look pale and appear restless or irritable before and during an attack. Other children may become nauseous, lose their appetite, or feel pain elsewhere in the body during the headache.

Headaches in children can be caused by a number of triggers, including emotional problems, such as the tension between family members, stress from school activities, weather changes, irregular eating and sleep, dehydration, and certain foods and drinks. Of special concern among children are headaches that occur after a head injury or those accompanied by rash, fever, or sleepiness.

It may be difficult to identify the type of headache because children often have problems describing where it hurts, how often the headaches occur, and how long they last. Asking a child with a headache to draw a picture of where the pain is and how it feels can make it easier for the doctor to determine the proper treatment.

Migraine, in particular, is often misdiagnosed in children. Parents and caretakers sometimes have to be detectives to help determine that a child has a migraine. Clues to watch for include sensitivity to light and noise, which may be suspected when a child refuses to watch television or use the computer, or when the child stops playing to lie down in a dark room. Observe whether or not a child is able to eat during a headache. Very young children may seem cranky or irritable and complain of abdominal pain (abdominal migraine).

Headache treatment in children and teens usually includes rest, fluids, and over-the-counter (OTC) pain relief medicines. Always consult with a physician before giving headache medicines to a child. Most tension-type headaches in children can be treated with OTC medicines that are marked for children with usage guidelines based on the child's age and weight. Headaches in some children may also be treated effectively using relaxation/behavioral therapy. Children with cluster headache may be treated with oxygen therapy early in the initial phase of the attacks.

Coping with Headache

Headache treatment is a partnership between you and your doctor, and honest communication is essential. Finding a quick fix to your headache may not be possible. It may take some time for your doctor or specialist to determine the best course of treatment. Avoid using OTC medicines more than twice a week, as they may actually worsen headache pain and the frequency of attacks. Visit a local headache support group meeting (if available) to learn how others with headache cope with their pain and discomfort. Relax whenever possible to ease stress and related symptoms, get enough sleep, regularly perform aerobic exercises, and eat a regularly scheduled and healthy diet that avoids food triggers. Gaining more control over your headache, stress, and emotions will make you feel better and let you embrace daily activities as much as possible.

Section 26.5

Neurofibromatosis

This section includes text excerpted from "Neurofibromatosis
Fact Sheet," National Institute of Neurological Disorders
and Stroke (NINDS), August 13, 2019.

What Are Neurofibromatoses?

The neurofibromatoses are a group of three genetically distinct
disorders that cause tumors to grow in the nervous system. Tumors
begin in the supporting cells that make up the nerve and the myelin
sheath (the thin membrane that envelops and protects the nerves),
rather than the cells that actually transmit information. The type of
tumor that develops depends on the type of supporting cells involved.

Scientists have classified the disorders as neurofibromatosis type
1 (NF1, also called "von Recklinghausen disease"), neurofibromatosis
type 2 (NF2), and a type that was once considered to be a variation
of NF2 but is now called "schwannomatosis." An estimated 100,000
Americans have a neurofibromatosis disorder, which occurs in both
sexes and in all races and ethnic groups.

The most common nerve-associated tumors in NF1 are neurofibromas (tumors of the peripheral nerves), whereas schwannomas (tumors
that begin in Schwann cells that help form the myelin sheath) are
most common in NF2 and schwannomatosis. Most tumors are benign,
although occasionally they may become cancerous.

Why these tumors occur still is not completely known, but it
appears to be related mainly to mutations in genes that play key roles
in suppressing cell growth in the nervous system. These mutations
keep the genes—identified as *NF1, NF2,* and *SMARCB1 / INI1*—from
making normal proteins that control cell production. Without the
normal function of these proteins, cells multiply out of control and
form tumors.

What Is Neurofibromatosis Type 1?

Neurofibromatosis type 1 is the most common neurofibromatosis, occurring in 1 in 3,000 to 4,000 individuals in the United States.
Although many affected people inherit the disorder, between 30 and
50 percent of new cases result from a spontaneous genetic mutation
of unknown cause. Once this mutation has taken place, the mutant
gene can be passed to succeeding generations.

What Are the Signs and Symptoms of Neurofibromatosis Type 1?

To diagnose NF1, a doctor looks for two or more of the following:

- 6 or more light brown spots on the skin, measuring more than 5 millimeters in diameter in children or more than 15 millimeters across in adolescents
- 2 or more neurofibromas, or one plexiform neurofibroma (a neurofibroma that involves many nerves)
- Freckling in the area of the armpit or the groin
- 2 or more growths on the iris of the eye (known as "Lisch nodules" or "iris hamartomas")
- A tumor on the optic nerve (called an "optic nerve glioma")
- Abnormal development of the spine (scoliosis), the temple (sphenoid) bone of the skull, or the tibia (one of the long bones of the shin)
- A parent, sibling, or child with NF1

What Other Symptoms or Conditions Are Associated with Neurofibromatosis Type 1?

Many children with NF1 have larger than normal head circumference and are shorter than average. Hydrocephalus, an abnormal buildup of fluid in the brain, is a possible complication of the disorder. Headache and epilepsy are also more likely in individuals with NF1 than in the healthy population. Cardiovascular complications associated with NF1 include congenital heart defects, high blood pressure (hypertension), and constricted, blocked, or damaged blood vessels (vasculopathy). Children with NF1 may have poor language and visual-spatial skills, and perform less well on academic achievement tests, including those that measure reading, spelling, and math skills. Learning disabilities, such as attention deficit hyperactivity disorder (ADHD), are common in children with NF1. An estimated three to five percent of tumors may become cancerous, requiring aggressive treatment. These tumors are called "malignant peripheral nerve sheath tumors."

When Do Symptoms Appear?

Symptoms, particularly the most common skin abnormalities-café-au-lait spots, neurofibromas, Lisch nodules, and freckling in the armpit and groin are often evident at birth or shortly afterward, and almost always by the time a child is 10 years old. Because many features of these disorders are age-dependent, a definitive diagnosis may take several years.

What Is the Prognosis for Someone with Neurofibromatosis Type 1?

Neurofibromatosis type 1 is a progressive disorder, which means most symptoms will worsen over time, although a small number of people may have symptoms that remain constant. It is not possible to predict the course of an individual's disorder. In general, most people with NF1 will develop mild to moderate symptoms. Most people with NF1 have a normal life expectancy. Neurofibromas on or under the skin can increase with age and cause cosmetic and psychological issues.

How Is Neurofibromatosis Type 1 Treated?

Scientists do not know how to prevent neurofibromas from growing. Surgery is often recommended to remove tumors that become symptomatic and may become cancerous, as well as for tumors that cause significant cosmetic disfigurement. Several surgical options exist, but there is no general agreement among doctors about when surgery should be performed or which surgical option is best. Individuals considering surgery should carefully weigh the risks and benefits of all their options to determine which treatment is right for them. Treatment for neurofibromas that become malignant may include surgery, radiation, or chemotherapy. Surgery, radiation and/or chemotherapy may also be used to control or reduce the size of optic nerve gliomas when vision is threatened. Some bone malformations, such as scoliosis, can be corrected surgically.

Treatments for other conditions associated with NF1 are aimed at controlling or relieving symptoms. Headache and seizures are treated with medications. Since children with NF1 have a higher than average risk for learning disabilities, they should undergo a detailed neurological exam before they enter school. Once these children are in school, teachers or parents who suspect there is evidence of one or more learning disabilities should request an evaluation that includes an IQ test and the standard range of tests to evaluate verbal and spatial skills.

What Is Neurofibromatosis Type 2?

This rare disorder affects about one in 25,000 people. Approximately 50 percent of affected people inherit the disorder; in others, the disorder is caused by a spontaneous genetic mutation of unknown cause. The hallmark finding in NF2 is the presence of slow-growing tumors on the eighth cranial nerves. These nerves have two branches: the acoustic branch helps people hear by transmitting sound sensations to the brain, and the vestibular branch helps people maintain their balance. The characteristic tumors of NF2 are called "vestibular schwannomas" because of their location and the types of cells involved. As these tumors grow, they may press against and damage nearby structures, such as other cranial nerves and the brain stem, the latter which can cause serious disability. Schwannomas in NF2 may occur along any nerve in the body, including the spinal nerves, other cranial nerves, and peripheral nerves in the body. These tumors may be seen as bumps under the skin (when the nerves involved are just under the skin surface) or can also be seen on the skin surface as small (less than 1 inch), dark, rough areas of hairy skin. In children, tumors may be smoother, less pigmented, and less hairy.

Although individuals with NF2 may have schwannomas that resemble small, flesh-colored skin flaps, they rarely have the café-au-lait spots that are seen in NF1.

Individuals with NF2 are at risk for developing other types of nervous system tumors, such as ependymomas and gliomas (two tumor types that grow in the spinal cord) and meningiomas (tumors that grow along the protective layers surrounding the brain and spinal cord). Affected individuals may develop cataracts at an earlier age or changes in the retina that may affect vision. Individuals with NF2 may also develop problems with nerve function independent of tumors, usually symmetric numbness and weakness in the extremities, due to the development of peripheral neuropathy.

What Are the Signs and Symptoms of Neurofibromatosis Type 2?

To diagnose NF2, a doctor looks for the following:

- Bilateral vestibular schwannomas; or
- A family history of NF2 (parent, sibling, or child) plus a unilateral vestibular schwannoma before age 30; or
- Any two of the following:
  - Glioma
  - Meningioma

631

- Schwannoma, or

- Juvenile posterior subcapsular/lenticular opacity (cataract) or juvenile cortical cataract

When Do Symptoms Appear?

Signs of NF2 may be present in childhood but are so subtle that they can be overlooked, especially in children who do not have a family history of the disorder. Typically, symptoms of NF2 are noticed between 18 and 22 years of age. The most frequent first symptom is hearing loss or ringing in the ears (tinnitus). Less often, the first visit to a doctor will be because of disturbances in balance, visual impairment (such as vision loss from cataracts), weakness in an arm or leg, seizures, or skin tumors.

What Is the Prognosis for Someone with Neurofibromatosis Type 2?

Because NF2 is so rare, few studies have been done to look at the natural progression of the disorder. The course of NF2 varies greatly among individuals, although inherited NF2 appears to run a similar course among affected family members. Generally, vestibular schwannomas grow slowly, and balance and hearing deteriorate over a period of years. A study suggests that an earlier age of onset and the presence of meningiomas are associated with greater mortality risk.

How Is Neurofibromatosis Type 2 Treated?

Neurofibromatosis type 2 is best managed at a specialty clinic with an initial screening and annual follow-up evaluations (more frequent if the disease is severe).

Surgical options depend on tumor size and the extent of hearing loss. There is no general agreement among doctors about when surgery should be performed or which surgical option is best. Individuals considering surgery should carefully weigh the risks and benefits of all options to determine which treatment is right for them. Surgery to remove the entire tumor while it is still small might help preserve hearing. If the hearing is lost during this surgery, but the auditory nerve is maintained, the surgical placement of a cochlear implant (a device placed in the inner ear, or cochlea, that processes electronic signals from sound waves to the auditory nerve) may be an option to improve hearing.

What Is Schwannomatosis?

Schwannomatosis is a rare form of neurofibromatosis that is genetically and clinically distinct from NF1 and NF2. Inherited forms of the disorder account for only 15 percent of all cases. Researchers have identified a mutation of the *SMARCB1/INI1* gene that is associated with the familial form of the disease but does not fully understand what causes the intense pain that characterizes this disorder.

What Are the Signs and Symptoms of Schwannomatosis?

The distinguishing feature of schwannomatosis is the development of multiple schwannomas everywhere in the body except on the vestibular nerve. The dominant symptom is a pain, which develops as a schwannoma enlarges, compressed nerves, or presses on adjacent tissue. Some people experience additional neurological symptoms, such as numbness, tingling, or weakness in the fingers and toes. Individuals with schwannomatosis do not have neurofibromas.

About one-third of individuals with schwannomatosis have tumors limited to a single part of the body, such as an arm, leg, or a segment of the spine. Some people develop many schwannomas, while others develop only a few.

What Is the Prognosis for Someone with Schwannomatosis?

Anyone with schwannomatosis experiences some degree of pain, but the intensity varies. A small number of people have such mild pain that they are never diagnosed with the disorder. Most people have significant pain, which can be managed with medications or surgery. In some extreme cases, the pain will be so severe and disabling it will keep people from working or leaving the house.

How Is Schwannomatosis Treated?

There is no currently accepted medical treatment or drug for schwannomatosis, but surgical management is often effective. The pain usually subsides when tumors are removed completely, although it may recur should new tumors form. When surgery is not possible, ongoing monitoring and management of pain in a multidisciplinary pain clinic is advisable.

Are There Prenatal Tests for the Neurofibromatoses?

Clinical genetic testing can confirm the presence of a mutation in the *NF1* gene. Prenatal testing for the NF1 mutation is also possible using amniocentesis or chorionic villus sampling procedures. Genetic testing for the NF2 mutation is sometimes available but is accurate only in about 65 percent of those individuals tested. Prenatal or genetic testing for schwannomatosis currently does not exist.

Section 26.6

Tourette Syndrome

This section includes text excerpted from "Tourette Syndrome (TS),"
Centers for Disease Control and Prevention (CDC), July 18, 2019.

What Is Tourette Syndrome?

Tourette syndrome (TS) is a condition of the nervous system. TS causes people to have "tics."

Tics are sudden twitches, movements, or sounds that people do repeatedly. People who have tics cannot stop their bodies from doing these things. For example, a person might keep blinking over and over again. Or, a person might make a grunting sound unwillingly.

Having tics is a little bit like having hiccups. Even though you might not want to hiccup, your body does it anyway. Sometimes people can stop themselves from doing a certain tic for a while, but it is hard. Eventually, the person has to do the tic.

Types of Tics
Motor Tics

Motor tics are movements of the body. Examples of motor tics include blinking, shrugging the shoulders, or jerking an arm.

Vocal Tics

Vocal tics are sounds that a person makes with her or his voice. Examples of vocal tics include humming, clearing the throat, or yelling out a word or phrase.

Tics can be either simple or complex:

Simple Tics

Simple tics involve just a few parts of the body. Examples of simple tics include squinting the eyes or sniffing.

Complex Tics

Complex tics usually involve several different parts of the body and can have a pattern. An example of a complex tic is bobbing the head while jerking an arm and then jumping up.

Symptoms of Tourette Syndrome

The main symptoms of TS are tics. Symptoms usually begin when a child is 5 to 10 years of age. The first symptoms often are motor tics that occur in the head and neck area. Tics usually are worse during times that are stressful or exciting. They tend to improve when a person is calm or focused on an activity.

The types of tics and how often a person has tics changes a lot over time. Even though the symptoms might appear, disappear, and reappear, these conditions are considered chronic.

In most cases, tics decrease during adolescence and early adulthood, and sometimes disappear entirely. However, many people with TS experience tics into adulthood and, in some cases, tics can become worse during adulthood.

Although the media often portray people with TS as involuntarily shouting out swear words (called "coprolalia") or constantly repeating the words of other people (called "echolalia"), these symptoms are rare and are not required for a diagnosis of TS.

Diagnosis of Tourette Syndrome

There is no single test, such as a blood test, to diagnose TS. Health professionals look at the person's symptoms to diagnose TS and other tic disorders. The tic disorders differ from each other in terms of the type of tic present (motor or vocal, or combination of the both), and how long the symptoms have lasted. TS can be diagnosed if a person has both motor and vocal tics, and has had tic symptoms for at least a year.

Treatments of Tourette Syndrome

Although there is no cure for TS, there are treatments available to help manage the tics. Many people with TS have tics that do not get in the way of their daily lives and, therefore, do not need any treatment. However, medication and behavioral treatments are available if tics cause pain or injury; interfere with school, work, or social life; or cause stress.

Other Concerns and Conditions

Tourette syndrome often occurs with other conditions (called "co-occurring conditions"). Almost 9 out of 10 children diagnosed with TS 86 percent also have been diagnosed with at least one additional mental, behavioral, or developmental condition. The two most common conditions are attention deficit hyperactivity disorder (ADHD) and obsessive-compulsive disorder (OCD). It is important to find out if a person with TS has any other conditions, and treat those conditions properly.

Risk Factors and Causes of Tourette Syndrome

Doctors and scientists do not know the exact cause of TS. Research suggests that it is an inherited genetic condition. That means it is passed on from parent to child through genes.

Who Is Affected by Tourette Syndrome?

Studies that included children with diagnosed and undiagnosed TS have estimated that 1 of every 162 children have TS. In the United States, 1 of every 360 children 6 through 17 years of age has been diagnosed with TS, based on parent reports. This suggests that about half of children with TS are not diagnosed.

Chapter 27

Respiratory and Lung Conditions in Children

Chapter Contents

Section 27.1

Asthma

This section contains text excerpted from the following
sources: Text in this section begins with excerpts from "Asthma in
Children," MedlinePlus, National Institutes of Health (NIH),
May 18, 2018; Text beginning with the heading "Asthma in Children"
is excerpted from "Vital Signs," Centers for Disease
Control and Prevention (CDC), May 10, 2018.

Asthma is a chronic disease that affects your airways. Your airways
are tubes that carry air in and out of your lungs. If you have asthma,
the inside walls of your airways become sore and swollen.

In the United States, about 20 million people have asthma. Nearly
nine million of them are children. Children have smaller airways than
adults, which makes asthma especially serious for them. Children
with asthma may experience wheezing, coughing, chest tightness, and
trouble breathing, especially early in the morning or at night.

Many things can cause asthma, including:

• Allergens-mold, pollen, animals

• Irritants-cigarette smoke, air pollution

• Weather-cold air, changes in weather

• Exercise

• Infections-flu, the common cold

When asthma symptoms become worse than usual, it is called
an "asthma attack." Asthma is treated with two kinds of medicines:
quick-relief medicines to stop asthma symptoms and long-term control
medicines to prevent symptoms.

Asthma in Children

Asthma is a serious disease causing wheezing, difficulty breathing,
and coughing. Over a lifetime, it can cause permanent lung damage.
About 16 percent of Black children and 7 percent of White children
have asthma. While we do not know what causes asthma, we do know
how to prevent asthma attacks or at least make them less severe.
Today, children with asthma and their caregivers report fewer attacks,
missed school days, and hospital visits. More children with asthma are
learning to control their asthma using an asthma action plan. Still,

more than half of children with asthma had one or more attacks in 2016. Every year, 1 in 6 children with asthma visits the Emergency Department with about 1 in 20 children with asthma hospitalized for asthma.

Prevalence of Asthma in Children

- Attacks have gone down in children of all races and ethnicities from 2001 through 2016.

- About 50 percent of children with asthma had an attack in 2016.

- Asthma attacks occurred most frequently among children younger than age 5 in 2016.

- Emergency department and urgent care center visits related to asthma attacks were highest among children ages 0 to 4 years and nonHispanic Black children.

Your asthma is well controlled if:

- You have symptoms no more than two days a week, and these symptoms do not wake you from sleep more than 1 or 2 nights a month.

- You can do all of your normal activities.

- You have no more than one asthma attack a year that requires you to take a pill or liquid for several days to treat the attack.

- Your peak flow, a measurement of how well air moves in and out of your lungs, does not drop below 80 percent of your personal best number.

- You need to take quick-relief medicines no more than two days a week.

Asthma Medication

- Inhaled corticosteroids and other control medicines can prevent asthma attacks.

- Rescue inhalers or nebulizers can give quick relief of symptoms

- But about half of children who are prescribed asthma control medicines do not use them regularly.

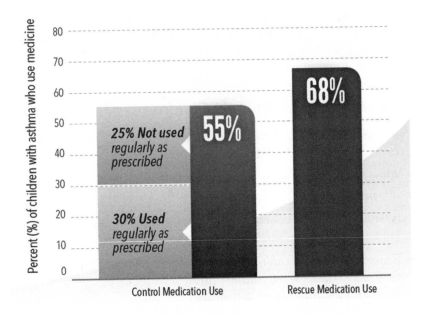

Figure 27.1. *Medication Use among Children with Asthma in 2013* (Source: National Health Interview Survey (NHIS), 2013.)

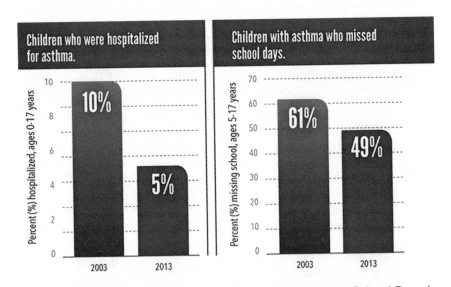

Figure 27.2. *Asthma-Related Hospitalizations and Missed School Days in 2013* (Source: National Health Interview Survey (NHIS), 2003 and 2013.)

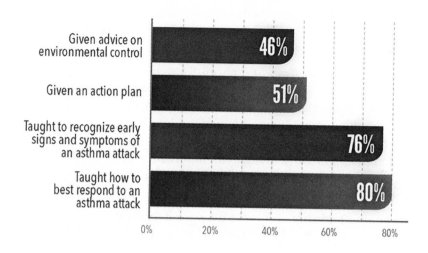

Figure 27.3. *Asthma Education of Children in 2013* (Source: National Health Interview Survey (NHIS), 2013.)

What Can Be Done

The federal government is:

- Working with state, territorial, private and nongovernment partners to support medical management, asthma-self management education, and, for people at high risk, home visits to reduce triggers and help with asthma management

- Providing guidelines, tools such as asthma action plans, and educational messages to help children, their caregivers, and healthcare professionals better manage asthma

- Promoting policies and best practices to reduce exposure to indoor and outdoor asthma triggers such as tobacco smoke and air pollution

- Tracking asthma rates and assuring efficient and effective use of resources invested in asthma services

Doctors, nurses, and other healthcare providers are:

- Teaching children and parents to manage asthma by using a personalized action plan shared with school staff and other caregivers. Such a plan helps children use medicine properly and avoid asthma triggers like tobacco smoke, pet dander, and air pollution.

- Working with community-health workers, pharmacists, and others to ensure that children with asthma receive needed services

- Working with children and parents to assess each child's asthma, prescribe appropriate medicines, and determine whether home health visits would help prevent attacks

Some payers/health-insurance plans are:

- Reimbursing healthcare providers for the education of children with asthma, including the development of their personalized asthma action plans

- Providing training and incentives for healthcare providers to practice guidelines-based medical management

- Taking actions to improve access to and proper use of asthma medications and devices

- Providing each child with asthma with the medical and community-based services needed to control her or his asthma

Parents and children are:

- Learning about asthma, how to manage it, and how to recognize the warning signs of an asthma attack

- Taking steps to reduce asthma triggers such as tobacco smoke, mold, and pet dander in the home. If caregivers smoke, they should try to quit or at least never smoke around children.

- Making sure children use their asthma-controller medicine as prescribed

- Communicating with schools, other family members, caregivers, and healthcare providers about the child's asthma action plan and about asthma symptoms

Schools are:

- Educating school nurses and other school staff about asthma and how to help children control it

- Carrying out asthma-friendly policies to help children follow their action plans, including stocking quick-relief medications, letting older children carry controller and rescue medicines, and helping children take part in school activities, such as exercising indoors when air quality is poor

Section 27.2

Bronchitis

This section includes text excerpted from "Bronchitis," Centers for Disease Control and Prevention (CDC), April 7, 2017.

What Is Acute Bronchitis?

Bronchitis occurs when the airways of the lungs swell and produce mucus. That is what makes you cough. Acute bronchitis often called a "chest cold," is the most common type of bronchitis. The symptoms last less than three weeks. Antibiotics are not indicated to treat acute bronchitis. Using antibiotics, when not needed, could do more harm than good.

If you are a healthy person without underlying heart or lung problems or a weakened immune system, this information is for you.

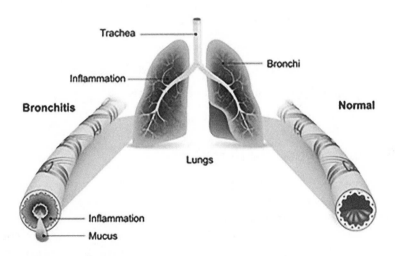

Figure 27.4. *Lungs with Bronchitis*

Symptoms of Acute Bronchitis

- Coughing with or without mucus production

You may also experience:

- Soreness in the chest
- Fatigue (feeling tired)

- Mild headache

- Mild body aches

- Watery eyes

- Sore throat

Causes of Acute Bronchitis

Acute bronchitis is usually caused by a virus and often occurs after an upper respiratory infection.

Bacteria can sometimes cause acute bronchitis, but even in these cases, antibiotics are not recommended and will not help you get better.

When to Seek Medical Care

See a healthcare professional if you or your child have any of the following:

- Temperature higher than 100.4°F

- Cough with bloody mucus

- Shortness of breath or trouble breathing

- Symptoms that last more than three weeks

- Repeated episodes of bronchitis

Recommended Treatment

Acute bronchitis almost always gets better on its own—without antibiotics. Using antibiotics when they are not needed can do more harm than good. Unintended consequences of antibiotics include side effects, such as rash and diarrhea, as well as more serious consequences, such as an increased risk for an antibiotic-resistant infection or *Clostridium difficile* (*C. difficile*) infection, sometimes deadly diarrhea.

To feel better:

- Get plenty of rest

- Drink plenty of fluids

- Use a clean humidifier or cool mist vaporizer

- Breathe in steam from a bowl of hot water or shower

- Use lozenges (do not give lozenges to children younger than four years of age)

- Ask your healthcare professional or pharmacist about over-the-counter (OTC) medicines that can help you feel better

Prevention of Acute Bronchitis

- Practice good hand hygiene.

- Keep you and your child up to date with recommended vaccines.

- Do not smoke and avoid secondhand smoke, chemicals, dust, or air pollution.

- Always cover your mouth and nose when coughing or sneezing.

- Make sure you and your child are to up-to-date with all recommended vaccines.

And remember, antibiotics will not treat acute bronchitis. Using antibiotics when not needed could do more harm than good.

Section 27.3

Cystic Fibrosis

This section includes text excerpted from "Cystic Fibrosis," National Heart, Lung, and Blood Institute (NHLBI), August 1, 2019.

Cystic fibrosis (CF) is a genetic condition that affects a protein in the body. People who have CF have a faulty protein that affects the body's cells, tissues, and glands that make mucus and sweat.

Mucus is normally slippery and protects the linings of the airways, digestive tract, and other organs and tissues. People who have CF make thick, sticky mucus that can build up and lead to blockages, damage, or infections in the affected organs. Inflammation also causes damage to organs such as the lungs and the pancreas.

Some people who have CF have few or no signs or symptoms, while others experience severe symptoms or life-threatening complications. Symptoms of CF depend on which organs are affected and the severity of the condition. The most serious and common complications of CF are problems with the lungs, also known as "pulmonary" or "respiratory problems," which may include serious lung infections. People who have CF often also have problems maintaining good nutrition, because they have a hard time absorbing the nutrients from food. This is a problem that can delay growth.

Your doctor may recommend treatments to improve lung function and manage other complications. Early treatment can improve your quality of life and help you live longer.

Causes of Cystic Fibrosis

Cystic fibrosis is an inherited disease caused by mutations in a gene called the "cystic fibrosis transmembrane conductance regulator (*CFTR*) gene." The *CFTR* gene provides instructions for the CFTR protein. The CFTR protein is located in every organ of the body that makes mucus, including the lungs, liver, pancreas, and intestines, as well as sweat glands. The CFTR protein has also been found in other cells in the body, such as cells of the heart and the immune system. The mutations in the *CFTR* gene cause the CFTR protein to not work properly. This causes thick, sticky mucus and blockages in the lungs and digestive system.

Normally, mucus coats tiny hair-like structures called "cilia" in the airways of your lungs, which sweep the mucus particles up to the nose and mouth where your body can get rid of them. In people who have CF, this process does not work properly.

Risk Factors of Cystic Fibrosis

A person may have an increased risk for CF because of her or his family history and genetics, and race or ethnicity.

Family History and Genetics

A person is at higher risk for having CF if one or both parents is a carrier of a mutated *CFTR* gene or has CF. A person is also at higher risk if a sibling, half-sibling, or first cousin has CF. More than 10 million Americans are carriers of a *CFTR* gene mutation, yet many of them do not know it.

Race or Ethnicity

Cystic fibrosis is most common in people of northern European ancestry and less common in Hispanics and African Americans. It is relatively uncommon in Asian Americans.

646

Screening and Prevention for Cystic Fibrosis
Screening

Genetic testing may be performed to look for carriers, as well as to screen relatives of people who have CF. Genetic testing may also be used as a prenatal screening tool to look for a mutated *CFTR* gene. All newborns in the United States are now screened for CF. Since universal screening for CF began relatively recently, there are still young people and adults who have not been screened.

Prevention Strategies

There is no way to prevent whether or not you have CF. Couples who are planning to have children and know that they are at risk of having a child with CF may want to meet with a genetic counselor. A genetic counselor can answer questions about the risk and explain the choices that are available.

Signs and Symptoms of Cystic Fibrosis

Cystic fibrosis most commonly affects the lungs. Some people who have CF may have wheezing and a cough that may produce mucus or blood.

Other signs and symptoms depend on the organs affected and may include:

- **Blockage of the intestine** in a baby soon after birth
- **Clubbing of fingers and toes** due to less oxygen getting to the hands and feet
- **Fever,** which may include night sweats
- **Gastrointestinal symptoms,** such as severe abdominal pain, chronic diarrhea, or constipation
- **Jaundice,** or yellow skin, for an abnormally long time after birth
- **Low body mass index (BMI)** or being underweight
- **Muscle and joint pain**
- **Delayed growth or puberty**
- **Salty skin** and saltier than normal sweat
- **Sinus** infections

Diagnosis of Cystic Fibrosis

To diagnose CF, your doctor may recommend some of the following tests and procedures:

- **Genetic testing to detect mutated *CFTR* genes.** This test can confirm a positive CF screening test and a sweat test. If genetic testing is done as part of newborn or other screening, it may not be repeated during the newborn stage.

- **Prenatal diagnostic tests** to diagnose CF in an unborn baby, using mutated *CFTR* genes. This is done with procedures that take either a sample of amniotic fluid, the liquid in the sac surrounding your unborn baby, or tissue from the placenta. Cells from these samples are checked for gene mutations. Infants with positive prenatal testing for CF will be further tested after birth to confirm the diagnosis of CF.

- **Sweat test for high sweat chloride** to see if you have high levels of chloride in your sweat. The sweat test is the standard test for diagnosing CF. It may be used if you have symptoms that may indicate CF, or to confirm a positive diagnosis from a screening of your newborn baby. A normal sweat chloride test alone does not mean you do not have CF. Lower levels of chloride may indicate the need for further testing to diagnose or rule out CF.

Treatment of Cystic Fibrosis

While there is not yet a cure for CF, advances in treatment are helping people live longer, healthier lives. After early diagnosis, the goal is a proactive treatment to slow down lung disease as much as possible. You or your child will work with CF specialists. In newborns with a positive screening result, treatment may begin while the diagnosis is being confirmed. Treatment for CF is focused on airway clearance, medicines to prevent and fight infections, and surgery if needed.

Your Healthcare Team

Your healthcare team will likely include a CF specialist. This is a doctor who is familiar with the complex nature of CF. Your doctor may work with a medical team that specializes in CF, often at major medical centers. The United States has more than 100 CF Care Centers, with medical teams that include:

- Doctors specializing in the lungs, diabetes, and the digestive system

- Genetic counselors

- Nurses

- Nutritionists and dietitians

- Pharmacists

- Physical therapists

- Psychologists

- Respiratory therapists

- Social workers

Airway Clearance Techniques

Airway clearance techniques help loosen lung mucus so it can be cleared, reducing infections and improving breathing. The techniques include special ways of breathing and coughing, devices used by mouth and therapy vests that use vibrations to loosen mucus, and chest physical therapy. These techniques are often used along with medicines such as bronchodilators and mucus thinners.

Medicines

Medicines to treat CF include those used to maintain and improve lung function, fight infections, clear mucus and help breathing, and work on the faulty CFTR protein. Your doctor may prescribe some of the following medicines to treat CF:

- **Antibiotics** to prevent or treat lung infections and improve lung function. Your doctor may prescribe oral, inhaled, or intravenous (IV) antibiotics.

- **Anti-inflammatory medicines,** such as ibuprofen or corticosteroids, to reduce inflammation. Inflammation causes many of the changes in CF, such as lung disease. Ibuprofen is especially beneficial for children, but the side effects can include kidney and stomach problems. Corticosteroids can cause bone thinning and increased blood sugar and blood pressure.

- **Bronchodilators** to relax and open airways. These treatments are taken by inhaling them.

- **Mucus thinners** to make it easier to clear the mucus from your airways. These treatments are taken by inhaling them.

- **CFTR modulators** that help improve the function of the faulty CFTR protein. They improve lung function and help with weight gain. Examples include ivacaftor and lumacaftor.

Surgery

Surgery may be an option for people with advanced conditions.

Chapter 28

Skin Conditions in Children

Chapter Contents

Section 28.1

Eczema

This section contains text excerpted from the following sources:
Text in this section begins with excerpts from "Eczema,"
MedlinePlus, National Institutes of Health (NIH), August 15, 2016.
Reviewed September 2019; Text beginning with the heading "Eczema
Causes and Strategies for Prevention" is excerpted from "Eczema
(Atopic Dermatitis) Causes and Strategies for Prevention," National
Institute of Allergy and Infectious Diseases (NIAID),
June 30, 2016. Reviewed September 2019.

"Eczema" is a term for several different types of skin swelling.
Eczema is also called "dermatitis." Most types cause dry, itchy skin
and rashes on the face, inside the elbows and behind the knees, and
on the hands and feet. Scratching the skin can cause it to turn red,
and to swell and itch even more.

Eczema is not contagious. The cause is not known. It is likely caused
by both genetic and environmental factors. Eczema may get better or
worse over time, but it is often a long-lasting disease. People who have
it may also develop hay fever and asthma.

The most common type of eczema is atopic dermatitis. It is most
common in babies and children but adults can have it too. As children
who have atopic dermatitis grow older, this problem may get better
or go away. But sometimes the skin may stay dry and get irritated
easily.

Eczema Causes and Strategies for Prevention

A combination of genetic and environmental factors appears to be
involved in the development of eczema. The condition often is associated with other allergic diseases, such as asthma, hay fever, and food
allergies. Children whose parents have asthma and allergies are more
likely to develop atopic dermatitis than children of parents without
allergic diseases. Approximately 30 percent of children with atopic
dermatitis have food allergies, and many develop asthma or respiratory allergies. People who live in cities or drier climates also appear
more likely to develop the disease.

The condition tends to worsen when a person is exposed to certain
triggers, such as:

- Pollen, mold, dust mites, animals, and certain foods (for allergic
  individuals)

- Cold and dry air
- Colds or the flu
- Skin contact with irritating chemicals
- Skin contact with rough materials, such as wool
- Emotional factors, such as stress
- Fragrances or dyes added to skin lotions or soaps

Taking too many baths or showers and not moisturizing the skin properly afterward may also make eczema worse.

Eczema Treatment
Skin Care at Home

You and your doctor should discuss the best treatment plan and medications for your atopic dermatitis. But taking care of your skin at home may reduce the need for prescription medications. Some recommendations include:

- Avoid scratching the rash or skin.

- Relieve the itch by using a moisturizer or topical steroids. Take antihistamines to reduce severe itching.

- Keep your fingernails cut short. Consider light gloves if nighttime scratching is a problem.

- Lubricate or moisturize the skin two to three times a day using ointments, such as petroleum jelly. Moisturizers should be free of alcohol, scents, dyes, fragrances, and other skin-irritating chemicals. A humidifier in the home also can help.

- Avoid anything that worsens symptoms, including:
  - Irritants, such as wool and lanolin (an oily substance derived from sheep wool used in some moisturizers and cosmetics)
  - Strong soaps or detergents
  - Sudden changes in body temperature and stress, which may cause sweating

- When washing or bathing:
  - Keep water contact as brief as possible and use gentle body washes and cleansers instead of regular soaps. Lukewarm baths are better than long, hot baths.

- Do not scrub or dry the skin too hard or for too long.

- After bathing, apply lubricating ointments to damp skin. This will help trap moisture in the skin.

Wet Wrap Therapy

Researchers at the National Institute of Allergy and Infectious Diseases (NIAID) and other institutions are studying an innovative treatment for severe eczema called "wet wrap therapy." It includes three lukewarm baths a day, each followed by an application of topical medicines and moisturizer that is sealed in by a wrap of wet gauze.

Treatment may include wet wrap therapy to bring the condition under control. Patients and their caregivers also receive training on home-based skincare to properly manage flare-ups once they leave the hospital.

Eczema Complications

The skin of people with atopic dermatitis lacks infection-fighting proteins, making them susceptible to skin infections caused by bacteria and viruses. Fungal infections also are common in people with atopic dermatitis.

Bacterial Infections

A major health risk associated with atopic dermatitis is skin colonization or infection by bacteria, such as *Staphylococcus aureus*. Sixty to ninety percent of people with atopic dermatitis are likely to have staph bacteria on their skin. Many eventually develop an infection, which worsens atopic dermatitis.

Viral Infections

People with atopic dermatitis are highly vulnerable to certain viral infections of the skin. For example, if infected with herpes simplex virus (HSV), they can develop a severe skin condition called "atopic dermatitis with eczema herpeticum."

Those with atopic dermatitis should not receive the licensed smallpox vaccine, even if their disease is in remission because they are at risk of developing a severe infection called "eczema vaccinatum." This infection is caused when the live vaccinia virus in the smallpox vaccine reproduces and spreads throughout the body. Furthermore, those in close contact with people who have atopic dermatitis or a history of the disease should not receive the smallpox vaccine because of the risk of transmitting the live vaccine virus to the person with atopic dermatitis.

Section 28.2

Psoriasis

This section includes text excerpted from "Psoriasis," National Institute of Arthritis and Musculoskeletal and Skin Diseases (NIAMS), March 30, 2019.

What Is Psoriasis?

Psoriasis is a skin disease that causes red, scaly skin that may feel painful, swollen or hot.

If your child have psoriasis, they are more likely to get some other conditions, including:

- Psoriatic arthritis, a condition that causes joint pain and swelling

- Cardiovascular problems, which affect the heart and blood circulation system

- Obesity

- High blood pressure

- Diabetes

Some treatments for psoriasis can have serious side effects, so be sure to talk about them with your child's doctor.

Who Gets Psoriasis

Anyone can get psoriasis, but it is more common in adults. Certain genes have been linked to psoriasis, so you are more likely to get it if someone else in your family has it.

What Are the Types of Psoriasis?

There are several different types of psoriasis. Here are a few examples:

- **Plaque psoriasis,** which causes patches of skin that are red at the base and covered by silvery scales.

- **Guttate psoriasis,** which causes small, drop-shaped lesions on your trunk, limbs, and scalp. This type of psoriasis is most often triggered by upper respiratory infections, such as strep throat.

- **Pustular psoriasis,** which causes pus-filled blisters. Attacks or flares can be caused by medications, infections, stress, or certain chemicals.

- **Inverse psoriasis,** which causes smooth, red patches in folds of skin near the genitals, under the breasts or in the armpits. Rubbing and sweating can make this type of psoriasis worse.

- **Erythrodermic psoriasis,** which causes red and scaly skin over much of your body. This can be a reaction to a bad sunburn or taking certain medications, such as corticosteroids. It can also happen if you have a different type of psoriasis that is not well controlled. This type of psoriasis can be very serious, so if you have it, you should see a doctor immediately.

What Are the Symptoms of Psoriasis?

Psoriasis usually causes patches of thick, red skin with silvery scales that itch or feel sore. These patches can show up anywhere on your body, but they usually occur on the elbows, knees, legs, scalp, lower back, face, palms, and soles of feet. They can also show up on your fingernails and toenails, genitals, and inside your mouth. You may find that your skin gets worse for a while, which is called a "flare," and then improves.

What Causes Psoriasis

Psoriasis is an autoimmune disease, which means that your body's immune system—which protects you from diseases—starts overacting and causing problems. If you have psoriasis, a type of white blood cells (WBCs) called the "T cells" become so active that they trigger other immune system responses, including swelling and fast turnover of skin cells.

Your skin cells grow deep in the skin and rise slowly to the surface. This is called "cell turnover," and it usually takes about a month. If you have psoriasis, though, cell turnover can take only a few days. Your skin cells rise too fast and pile up on the surface, causing your skin to look red and scaly.

Some things may cause a flare, meaning your psoriasis becomes worse for a while, including:

- Infections

- Stress

- Changes in the weather that dry out your skin

- Certain medicines

- Cuts, scratches, or sunburns

Certain genes have been linked to psoriasis, meaning it runs in families.

Is There a Test for Psoriasis?

Psoriasis can be hard to diagnose because it can look like other skin diseases. Your doctor may look at a small sample of your skin under a microscope to help them figure out if psoriasis is causing your skin condition.

How Is Psoriasis Treated?

There are several different types of treatment for psoriasis. Your doctor may recommend that you try one of these or a combination of them:

- **Topical treatment,** which means putting creams on your skin.

- **Light therapy,** which involves a doctor shining an ultraviolet light on your skin or getting more sunlight. It is important that a doctor controls the amount of light you are getting from this therapy, because too much ultraviolet light may make your psoriasis worse.

- **Systemic treatment,** which can include taking prescription medicines or getting shots of medicine.

Who Treats Psoriasis

Several types of healthcare professionals may treat you, including:

- Dermatologists, who treat skin problems.
- Internists, who diagnose and treat adults.

Chapter 29

Vision and Eye Problems in Children

Chapter Contents

Amblyopia

This section includes text excerpted from "Facts about Amblyopia," National Eye Institute (NEI), September 2013. Reviewed September 2019.

Amblyopia Defined
What Is Amblyopia?

The brain and the eyes work together to produce vision. The eye focuses light on the back part of the eye known as the "retina." Cells of the retina then trigger nerve signals that travel along the optic nerves to the brain. "Amblyopia" is the medical term used when the vision of one eye is reduced because it fails to work properly with the brain. The eye itself looks normal, but for various reasons, the brain favors the other eye. This condition is also sometimes called "lazy eye."

How Common Is Amblyopia?

Amblyopia is the most common cause of visual impairment among children, affecting approximately 2 to 3 out of every 100 children. Unless it is successfully treated in early childhood, amblyopia usually persists into adulthood. It is also the most common cause of monocular (one eye) visual impairment among young and middle-aged adults.

Cause of Amblyopia

Amblyopia can result from any condition that prevents the eye from focusing clearly. Amblyopia can be caused by the misalignment of the two eyes—a condition called "strabismus." With strabismus, the eyes can cross in (esotropia) or turn out (exotropia). Occasionally, amblyopia is caused by a clouding of the front part of the eye, a condition called "cataract."

A common cause of amblyopia is the inability of one eye to focus as well as the other one. Amblyopia can occur when one eye is more "nearsighted," "more farsighted," or has more "astigmatism." These terms refer to the ability of the eye to focus light on the retina. Farsightedness, or hyperopia, occurs when the distance from the front to the back of the eye is too short. Eyes that are farsighted tend to focus better at a distance but have more difficulty focusing on near objects.

Nearsightedness, or myopia, occurs when the eye is too long from front to back. Eyes with nearsightedness tend to focus better on near objects. Eyes with astigmatism have difficulty focusing on far and near objects because of their irregular shape.

Treatment of Amblyopia
How Is Amblyopia Treated in Children?

Treating amblyopia involves forcing the child to use the eye with weaker vision. There are two common ways to treat amblyopia:

Patching

An adhesive patch is worn over the stronger eye for weeks to months. This therapy forces the child to use the eye with amblyopia. Patching stimulates vision in the weaker eye and helps parts of the brain involved in vision develop more completely.

A National Eye Institute (NEI)-funded study showed that patching the unaffected eye of children with moderate amblyopia for two hours daily work as well as patching for six hours daily. Shorter patching time can lead to better compliance with treatment and improved quality of life for children with amblyopia. However, a study showed that children whose amblyopia persists despite two hours of daily patching may improve if daily patching is extended to 6 hours.

Previously, eye care professionals thought that treating amblyopia would be of little benefit to older children. However, results from a nationwide clinical trial showed that many children from ages seven to 17 years old benefited from treatment for amblyopia. This study shows that age alone should not be used as a factor to decide whether or not to treat a child for amblyopia.

Atropine

A drop of a drug called "atropine" is placed in the stronger eye to temporarily blur vision so that the child will use the eye with amblyopia, especially when focusing on near objects. The NEI-supported research has shown that atropine eye drops when placed in the unaffected eye once a day, work as well as eye patching. Atropine eye drops are sometimes easier for parents and children to use.

661

Section 29.2

Pink Eye

This section includes text excerpted from "Facts about
Pink Eye," National Eye Institute (NEI), November 2015.
Reviewed September 2019.

What Is Pink Eye?

Pink eye, also known as "conjunctivitis," involves inflammation of
the conjunctiva, the thin, clear tissue that lines the inside of the eyelid
and covers the white part of the eye, or sclera. The inflammation makes
blood vessels more visible, giving the eye a pink or reddish appearance.
The affected eye(s) may be painful, itchy or have a burning sensation.
The eyes can also tear or have a discharge that forms a crust during
sleep causing the eyes to be "stuck shut" in the morning. Other signs
or symptoms that may accompany pink eye include:

- Swelling of the conjunctiva

- Feeling like a foreign body is in the eye(s)

- Sensitivity to bright light

- Enlargement and/or tenderness of the lymph node in front of the
  ear. This enlargement may feel like a small lump when touched.
  (Lymph nodes act as filters in the body, collecting and destroying
  viruses and bacteria.)

- Contact lenses that do not stay in place on the eye and/or feel
  uncomfortable due to bumps that may form under the eyelid

What Causes Pink Eye

Pink eye is most often caused by bacterial or viral infections. Allergic reactions or exposure to irritants can also cause pink eye. Pinpointing the cause may be difficult because the signs and symptoms tend
to be similar regardless of the underlying cause.

Viral conjunctivitis is caused by a wide variety of viruses, but
adenovirus and herpesvirus are the most common viruses that cause
pink eye. Viral conjunctivitis may also occur along with an upper
respiratory tract infection (URTI), cold, or a sore throat.

Bacterial conjunctivitis is caused by infection of the eye with
bacteria, such as *Staphylococcus aureus, Streptococcus pneumonia,*

or Haemophilus. It is a common reason for children to stay homesick from daycare or school.

Allergic conjunctivitis can be caused by allergies to pollen, dust mites, molds, or animal dander.

Irritants, such as contact lenses and lens solutions, chlorine in the swimming pool, smog or cosmetics may also be an underlying cause of conjunctivitis.

How Is Pink Eye Diagnosed?

Conjunctivitis can be diagnosed with an eye examination by a health-care provider. In some cases, the type of conjunctivitis can be determined by assessing the person's signs, symptoms, and recent health history (such as whether the person has recently been exposed to someone with conjunctivitis or has a pattern of seasonal allergy). Most cases resolve with time, and there is usually no need for treatment or laboratory tests unless the person's history suggests bacterial conjunctivitis.

Viral Conjunctivitis

Viral conjunctivitis is often diagnosed based on a person's history and symptoms. It tends to occur in both eyes and often accompanies a common cold or respiratory tract infection. Laboratory tests usually are not needed to diagnose viral conjunctivitis; however, testing may be done if a more severe form of viral conjunctivitis is suspected. More severe causes include herpes simplex virus (HSV) (which usually involves blisters on the skin), varicella-zoster virus (VZV) (chickenpox and shingles), rubella or rubeola (measles). This testing is performed using a sample of the discharge from an infected eye.

Bacterial Conjunctivitis

Bacterial conjunctivitis tends to occur in one eye and may accompany an ear infection. A sample of the discharge from the affected eye may be obtained for laboratory tests to determine which type of bacteria is causing the pink eye and how best to treat it.

Allergic Conjunctivitis

Allergic conjunctivitis tends to occur in both eyes and often accompanies allergy symptoms, such as an itchy nose, sneezing, and scratchy throat. Allergic conjunctivitis may occur seasonally when pollen counts are high, and it can cause the person's eyes to itch intensely. A detailed health history may help determine the source of the allergic reaction.

How Is Pink Eye Treated?

Most cases of pink eye are mild and will resolve on their own without prescription treatment. In many cases, symptom relief can be achieved by using artificial tears for the dryness and cold packs for the inflammation. (Artificial tears can be purchased without a doctor's prescription.)

However, you should seek medical attention if you have any of the following symptoms:

- Moderate to severe pain in the eye(s)

- Vision problems, such as sensitivity to light or blurred vision, that do not improve when any discharge present is wiped from the eye(s)

- Intense redness in the eye(s)

- Symptoms that become worse or persist when severe viral conjunctivitis is suspected

Also seek medical attention if you have signs of conjunctivitis and you have a weakened immune system from HIV infection, cancer treatment, or other medical conditions or treatments.

Viral Conjunctivitis

Most cases of viral conjunctivitis are mild and will clear up in 7 to 14 days without treatment and without any long-term consequences. In some cases, however, viral conjunctivitis can take two or more weeks to resolve, especially if complications arise.

Antiviral medication can be prescribed by a physician to treat more serious forms of conjunctivitis, such as those caused by HSV or VZV. Antibiotics will not improve viral conjunctivitis as these drugs are not effective against viruses.

Bacterial Conjunctivitis

Mild bacterial conjunctivitis may get better without antibiotic treatment and without causing any severe complications.

Antibiotics can help shorten the illness and reduce the spread of infection to others. Your healthcare provider may prescribe antibiotic eye drops or ointment, which should resolve the infection within several days.

Consult your healthcare provider if you have been given antibiotics for bacterial conjunctivitis and symptoms have not improved after 24 hours of treatment.

Allergic Conjunctivitis

Conjunctivitis caused by an allergy usually improves by eliminating or significantly reducing contact with the allergen (such as pollen or animal dander). Allergy medications and certain eye drops can also provide relief.

Conjunctivitis caused by an irritant often clears up by eliminating the irritant. If you develop conjunctivitis and you wear contacts, stop using them temporarily until conjunctivitis resolves. In some cases, your healthcare provider may also prescribe drug treatments to improve symptoms.

What Steps Can You Take to Prevent Pink Eye?

Viral and bacterial conjunctivitis are highly contagious and can be easily spread from person to person. Allergic conjunctivitis is not contagious.

If you or someone around you has infectious (viral or bacterial) conjunctivitis, limit its spread by following these steps:

- Wash your hands often with soap and warm water. And wash up immediately if you have touched an affected person's eyes, linens or clothes (for example, when caring for a child who has pink eye). If soap and water are not available, use an alcohol-based hand sanitizer that contains at least 60 percent alcohol.

- Avoid touching or rubbing your eyes.

- If you have conjunctivitis, wash any discharge from around the eyes several times a day.

- Do not use the same eye drop dispenser/bottle for infected and noninfected eyes—even for the same person.

- Avoid sharing articles like towels, blankets, and pillowcases.

- Clean your eyeglasses.

- Clean, store, and replace your contact lenses as instructed by your eye health professional.

- Do not share eye makeup, face makeup, makeup brushes, contact lenses or containers, or eyeglasses.

There are also steps you can take to avoid reinfection once the infection goes away:

- Throw away any eye or face makeup or applicators you used while infected.

- Throw away contact lens solutions you used while infected.

- Throw away contact lenses and cases you used.

- Clean your eyeglasses and cases.

Can Newborns Get Pink Eye?

Newborns can develop pink eye, which is called "neonatal conjunctivitis," or less commonly, ophthalmia neonatorum. Common symptoms include eye discharge and puffy, red eyelids within one day to two weeks after birth. Newborn conjunctivitis may be caused by infection, irritation, or a blocked tear duct. A mother can pass on infectious conjunctivitis to her newborn during childbirth, even if she has no symptoms herself, because she may carry bacteria or viruses in the birth canal. When caused by an infection, neonatal conjunctivitis can be very serious. The most common types of neonatal conjunctivitis include:

- **Chlamydial (or inclusion) conjunctivitis** is caused by the bacterium *Chlamydia trachomatis* and can cause swelling of the eyelids with purulent (pus) discharge. Symptoms often appear 5 to 12 days after birth but may present at any time during the first month of life.

- **Gonococcal conjunctivitis** is caused by *Neisseria gonorrhoeae*, the bacterium that causes gonorrhea. Gonococcal conjunctivitis causes pus discharge and swelling of eyelids, which may appear 2 to 4 days after birth.

- **Chemical conjunctivitis** can be caused by eye drops or ointment given to newborns to help prevent bacterial eye infections. Symptoms include red eyes and eyelid swelling and usually resolve in 24 to 36 hours. Most hospitals are required by state law to put drops or ointment in a newborn's eyes to prevent disease. The benefits of preventing a more serious type of conjunctivitis are thought to outweigh the risks of chemical conjunctivitis.

- Other bacteria and viruses can also cause conjunctivitis in a newborn. Bacteria that normally live in a woman's vagina and that are not sexually transmitted can cause neonatal conjunctivitis. The viruses that cause genital and oral herpes can also cause neonatal conjunctivitis and severe eye damage. Such viruses may be passed to the baby during childbirth.

How Is Pink Eye Treated in Newborns?

Bacterial conjunctivitis may be treated with topical antibiotic eye drops and ointments, oral antibiotics, or intravenous (given through a vein) antibiotics.

A combination of topical and oral, or topical and intravenous treatments are sometimes used at the same time. A saline solution may be prescribed for rinsing the baby's eye(s) to remove pus, if necessary.

- **Chlamydial conjunctivitis** in newborns is usually treated with oral antibiotics such as erythromycin. Parents are usually treated as well.

- **Gonococcal conjunctivitis** in newborns is usually treated with intravenous antibiotics. If untreated, this condition can lead to corneal ulcers and blindness.

- **Other types of bacterial and viral conjunctivitis** are usually treated with antibiotic eye drops or ointments. A warm compress to the eye may also help relieve swelling and irritation.

- **Blocked tear ducts may cause conjunctivitis.** If a tear duct is blocked, a gentle warm massage between the eye and nasal area may help. If the blocked tear duct is not cleared by one year of age, surgery may be required.

- **Chemical Conjunctivitis** usually resolves in 24 to 36 hours without treatment.

Section 29.3

Refractive Disorders

This section includes text excerpted from "Refractive Errors," National Eye Institute (NEI), June 11, 2015. Reviewed September 2019.

What Are Refractive Errors?

Refractive errors occur when the shape of the eye prevents light from focusing directly on the retina. The length of the eyeball (longer or shorter), changes in the shape of the cornea, or aging of the lens can cause refractive errors.

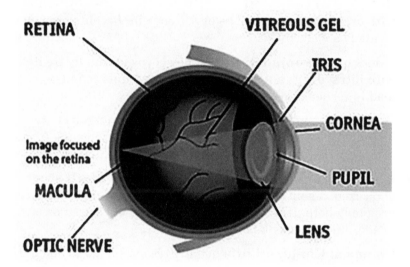

Figure 29.1. *A Normal Eye*

The cornea and lens bend (refract) incoming light rays so they focus precisely on the retina at the back of the eye.

What Is Refraction?

Refraction is the bending of light as it passes through one object to another. Vision occurs when light rays are bent (refracted) as they pass through the cornea and the lens. The light is then focused on the retina. The retina converts the light rays into messages that are sent through the optic nerve to the brain.

What Are the Different Types of Refractive Errors?

The most common types of refractive errors are nearsightedness, farsightedness, astigmatism, and presbyopia.

Nearsightedness (also called "myopia") is a condition where objects up close appear clearly, while objects far away appear blurry. With nearsightedness, the light comes to focus in front of the retina instead of on the retina.

Farsightedness (also called "hyperopia") is a common type of refractive error where distant objects may be seen more clearly than objects that are near. However, people experience farsightedness differently. Some people may not notice any problems with their vision, especially when they are young. For people with significant farsightedness, vision can be blurry for objects at any distance, near or far.

Astigmatism is a condition in which the eye does not focus light evenly onto the retina, the light-sensitive tissue at the back of the eye. This can cause images to appear blurry and stretched out.

Presbyopia is an age-related condition in which the ability to focus up close becomes more difficult. As the eye ages, the lens can no longer change shape enough to allow the eye to focus close objects clearly.

Who Is at Risk for Refractive Errors?

Presbyopia affects most adults over age 35. Other refractive errors can affect both children and adults. Individuals who have parents with certain refractive errors may be more likely to get one or more refractive errors.

What Are the Signs and Symptoms of Refractive Errors?

Blurred vision is the most common symptom of refractive errors. Other symptoms may include the following:

- Double vision
- Haziness
- Glare or halos around bright lights
- Squinting

- Headaches

- Eyestrain

How Are Refractive Errors Diagnosed?

An eye-care professional can diagnose refractive errors during a comprehensive dilated eye examination. People with a refractive error often visit their eye-care professional with complaints of visual discomfort or blurred vision. However, some people do not know they are not seeing as clearly as they could.

How Are Refractive Errors Corrected?

Refractive errors can be corrected with eyeglasses, contact lenses, or refractive surgery.

Eyeglasses are the simplest and safest way to correct refractive errors. Your eye-care professional can prescribe appropriate lenses to correct your refractive error and give you optimal vision.

Contact lenses work by becoming the first refractive surface for light rays entering the eye, causing more precise refraction or focus. In many cases, contact lenses provide clearer vision, a wider field of vision, and greater comfort. They are a safe and effective option if fitted and used properly. It is very important to wash your hands and clean your lenses as instructed in order to reduce the risk of infection.

If you have certain eye conditions, you may not be able to wear contact lenses. Discuss this matter with your eye-care professional.

Refractive surgery aims to change the shape of the cornea permanently. This change in eye shape restores the focusing power of the eye by allowing the light rays to focus precisely on the retina for improved vision. There are many types of refractive surgeries. Your eye-care professional can help you decide if surgery is an option for you.

Section 29.4

Retinitis Pigmentosa

This section includes text excerpted from "Facts about Retinitis Pigmentosa," National Eye Institute (NEI), December 2015. Reviewed September 2019.

What Is Retinitis Pigmentosa?

Retinitis pigmentosa (RP) is a group of rare, genetic disorders that involve a breakdown and loss of cells in the retina—which is the light-sensitive tissue that lines the back of the eye. Common symptoms include difficulty seeing at night and a loss of side (peripheral) vision.

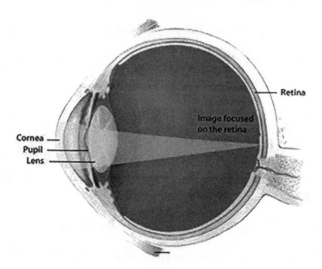

Figure 29.2. *An Eye with Retinitis Pigmentosa*

The retina is the light-sensitive tissue at the back of the eye that contains photoreceptors and other cell types.

What Causes Retinitis Pigmentosa

Retinitis pigmentosa is an inherited disorder that results from harmful changes in any one of more than 50 genes. These genes carry the instructions for making proteins that are needed in cells within the retina, called "photoreceptors." Some of the changes, or mutations, within genes are so severe that the gene cannot make the required protein, limiting the cell's function. Other mutations produce a protein

671

that is toxic to the cell. Still, other mutations lead to an abnormal protein that does not function properly. In all three cases, the result is damage to the photoreceptors.

What Are Photoreceptors?

Photoreceptors are cells in the retina that begin the process of seeing. They absorb and convert light into electrical signals. These signals are sent to other cells in the retina and ultimately through the optic nerve to the brain where they are processed into the images we see. There are two general types of photoreceptors, called "rods" and "cones." Rods are in the outer regions of the retina, and allow us to see in dim and dark light. Cones reside mostly in the central portion of the retina and allow us to perceive fine visual detail and color.

How Does Retinitis Pigmentosa Affect Vision?

In the early stages of RP, rods are more severely affected than cones. As the rods die, people experience night blindness and a progressive loss of the visual field, the area of space that is visible at a given instant without moving the eyes. The loss of rods eventually leads to a breakdown and loss of cones. In the late stages of RP, as cones die, people tend to lose more of the visual field, developing tunnel vision. They may have difficulty performing essential tasks of daily living, such as reading, driving, walking without assistance, or recognizing faces and objects.

How Is Retinitis Pigmentosa Inherited?

To understand how RP is inherited, it is important to know a little more about genes and how they are passed from parent to child. Genes are bundled together on structures called "chromosomes." Each cell in your body contains 23 pairs of chromosomes. One copy of each chromosome is passed by a parent at conception through egg and sperm cells. The X and Y chromosomes, known as "sex chromosomes," determine whether a person is born female (XX) or male (XY). The 22 other paired chromosomes, called "autosomes," contain the vast majority of genes that determine nonsex traits. RP can be inherited in one of three ways:

Autosomal Recessive Inheritance

In autosomal recessive inheritance, it takes two copies of the mutant gene to give rise to the disorder. An individual with a recessive gene mutation is known as a "carrier." When two carriers have a child, there is a:

- One in four chance the child will have the disorder

- One in two chance the child will be a carrier

- One in four chance the child will neither have the disorder nor be a carrier

Autosomal Dominant Inheritance

In this inheritance pattern, it takes just one copy of the gene with a disorder-causing mutation to bring about the disorder. When a parent has a dominant gene mutation, there is a one in two chance that any children will inherit this mutation and the disorder.

X-Linked Inheritance

In this form of inheritance, mothers carry the mutated gene on one of their X chromosomes and pass it to their sons. Because females have two X chromosomes, the effect of a mutation on one X chromosome is offset by the normal gene on the other X chromosome. If a mother is a carrier of an X-linked disorder there is a:

- One in two chance of having a son with the disorder

- One in two chance of having a daughter who is a carrier

How Common Is Retinitis Pigmentosa?

Retinitis pigmentosa is considered a rare disorder. Although current statistics are not available, it is generally estimated that the disorder affects roughly 1 in 4,000 people, both in the United States and worldwide.

How Does Retinitis Pigmentosa Progress?

The symptoms of RP typically appear in childhood. Children often have difficulty getting around in the dark. It can also take abnormally long periods of time to adjust to changes in lighting. As their visual field becomes restricted, patients often trip over things and appear clumsy. People with RP often find bright lights uncomfortable, a condition is known as "photophobia." Because there are many gene mutations that cause the disorder, its progression can differ greatly from person to person. Some people retain central vision and a restricted visual field into their 50s, while others experience significant vision loss in early adulthood. Eventually, most individuals with RP will lose most of their sight.

How Is Retinitis Pigmentosa Diagnosed?

Retinitis pigmentosa is diagnosed in part through an examination of the retina. An eye-care professional will use an ophthalmoscope, a tool that allows for a wider, clear view of the retina. This typically reveals abnormal, dark pigment deposits that streak the retina. These pigment deposits are in part why the disorder was named RP. Other tests for RP include:

- **Electroretinogram (ERG).** An ERG measures the electrical activity of photoreceptor cells. This test uses gold foil or a contact lens with electrodes attached. A flash of light is sent to the retina and the electrodes measure rod and cone cell responses. People with RP have a decreased electrical activity, reflecting the declining function of photoreceptors.

- **Visual field testing.** To determine the extent of vision loss, a clinician will give a visual field test. The person watches as a dot of light moves around the half-circle (180 degrees) of space directly in front of the head and to either side. The patient pushes a button to indicate that she or he can see the light. This process results in a map of their visual field and their central vision.

- **Genetic testing.** In some cases, a clinician takes a DNA sample from the person to give a genetic diagnosis. In this way, a person can learn about the progression of their particular form of the disorder.

Are There Treatments for Retinitis Pigmentosa?
Living with Vision Loss

A number of services and devices are available to help people with vision loss carry out daily activities and maintain their independence. In addition to an eye-care professional, it is important to have help from a team of experts, which may include occupational therapists, orientation and mobility specialists, certified low-vision therapists, and others.

Children with RP may benefit from low vision aids that maximize existing vision. For example, there are special lenses that magnify the central vision to expand the visual field and eliminate glare. Computer programs that read text are readily available. Closed-circuit televisions with a camera can adjust the text to suit one's vision. Portable lighting devices can adjust a dark or dim environment. Mobility training can teach people to use a cane or a guide dog, and eye-scanning techniques can help people to optimize remaining vision. Once a child is diagnosed, she or he will be referred to as a low-vision specialist for a comprehensive evaluation. Parents may also want to meet with the child's school administrators and teachers to make sure that necessary accommodations are put in place.

For parents of children with RP, one challenge is to determine when a child might need to learn to use a cane or a guide dog. Having regular eye examinations to measure the progress of the disorder will help parents make informed decisions regarding low-vision services and rehabilitation.

Targeted Therapies for Retinitis Pigmentosa

A National Eye Institute (NEI)-sponsored clinical trial found that a daily dose of 15,000 international units of vitamin A palmitate modestly slowed the progression of the disorder in adults. Because there are so many forms of RP, it is difficult to predict how any one patient will respond to this treatment. Talk to an eye-care professional to determine if taking vitamin A is right for you or your child.

An artificial vision device called the "Argus II" has also shown promise for restoring some vision to people with late-stage RP. The Argus II, developed by Second Sight with NEI support, is a prosthetic device that functions in place of lost photoreceptor cells. It consists of a light-sensitive electrode that is surgically implanted on the retina. A pair of glasses with a camera wirelessly transmits signals to the electrode that are then relayed to the brain. Although it does not restore 20/20 vision, in clinical studies, the Argus II enabled people with RP to read large letters and navigate environments without the use of a cane or guide dog. In 2012, the U.S. Food and Drug Administration (FDA) granted a humanitarian device exemption for use of the Argus II to treat late-stage RP. This means the device has not proven effective, but the FDA has determined that its probable benefits outweigh its risks to health. The Argus II is eligible for Medicare payment.

Part Four

Developmental and Pediatric Mental-Health Concerns

Chapter 30

Autism Spectrum Disorders

What Is Autism Spectrum Disorder?

Autism spectrum disorder (ASD) is a developmental disability that can cause significant social, communication, and behavioral challenges. There is often nothing about how children with ASD look that sets them apart from other children, but children with ASD may communicate, interact, behave, and learn in ways that are different from most other children. The learning, thinking, and problem-solving abilities of children with ASD can range from gifted to severely challenged. Some children with ASD need a lot of help in their daily lives; others need less.

A diagnosis of ASD now includes several conditions that used to be diagnosed separately: autistic disorder, pervasive developmental disorder-not otherwise specified (PDD-NOS), and Asperger syndrome. These conditions are now called as "autism spectrum disorder."

Signs and Symptoms of Autism Spectrum Disorder

The social, emotional, and communication skills of children with ASD often differ significantly from those of people who do not have this disorder. They might repeat certain behaviors and might not want change in their daily activities. Many children with ASD also have

This chapter includes text excerpted from "Autism Spectrum Disorder (ASD)," Centers for Disease Control and Prevention (CDC), May 3, 2018.

different ways of learning, paying attention, or reacting to things. Signs of ASD begin during early childhood and typically last throughout a child's life.

Children with ASD might:

- Not point at objects to show interest (for example, not point at an airplane flying over)

- Not look at objects when another person points at them

- Have trouble relating to others or have no interest in other people at all

- Avoid eye contact and want to be alone

- Have trouble understanding other people's feelings or talking about their own feelings

- Prefer not to be held or cuddled, or might cuddle only when they want to

- Appear to be unaware when people talk to them, but respond to other sounds

- Be very interested in people, but not know how to talk, play, or relate to them

- Repeat or echo words or phrases said to them, or repeat words or phrases in place of language use common to people who do not have this disorder

- Have trouble expressing their needs using typical words or motions

- Not play "pretend" games (for example, not pretend to "feed" a doll)

- Repeat actions over and over again

- Have trouble adapting when a routine changes

- Have unusual reactions to the way things smell, taste, look, feel, or sound

- Lose skills they once had (for example, stop saying words they were using)

Diagnosis of Autism Spectrum Disorder

Diagnosing ASD can be difficult since there is no medical test, such as a blood test, to diagnose the disorders. Doctors look at the child's behavior and development to make a diagnosis.

Autism spectrum disorders can sometimes be detected at 18 months or younger. By the age of 2, a diagnosis by an experienced professional can be considered very reliable. However, many children do not receive a final diagnosis until they are much older. This delayed diagnosis means that children with ASD might not get the early intervention that can enhance their development.

Treatment of Autism Spectrum Disorder

As of now there is no cure for ASD. However, research shows that early-intervention treatment services can improve a child's development. Early-intervention services help children from birth to 3 years old (36 months) learn important skills. Services can include therapy to help the child talk, walk, and interact with others. Therefore, it is important to talk to your child's doctor as soon as possible if you think your child has ASD or other developmental symptoms.

Even if your child has not been diagnosed with an ASD, she or he may be eligible for early-intervention treatment services. The Individuals with Disabilities Education Act (IDEA) says that children under the age of three years (36 months) who are at risk of having developmental delays may be eligible for services. These services are provided through an early-intervention system in your state. Through this system, you can ask for an evaluation.

In addition, treatment for particular symptoms, such as speech therapy for language delays, often does not need to wait for a formal ASD diagnosis.

Causes and Risk Factors of Autism Spectrum Disorder

All of the causes of ASD are not yet known. However, the Centers for Disease Control and Prevention (CDC) has learned that there are likely many causes for multiple types of ASD. There may be many different factors that make a child more likely to have an ASD, including environmental, biologic, and genetic factors.

- Most scientists agree that genes are one of the risk factors that can make a person more likely to develop ASD.

- Children who have a sibling with ASD are at a higher risk of also having ASD.

- Autism spectrum disorder tends to occur more often in people who have certain genetic or chromosomal conditions, such as fragile X syndrome or tuberous sclerosis.

- When taken during pregnancy, the prescription drugs valproic acid and thalidomide have been linked with a higher risk of ASD.

- There is some evidence that the critical period for developing ASD occurs before, during, and immediately after birth.

- Children born to older parents are at greater risk of having ASD.

Autism spectrum disorders continue to be an important public-health concern. Like the many families living with ASD, the CDC wants to find out what causes the disorder. Understanding the factors that make a person more likely to develop ASD will help the CDC to learn more about the causes. The CDC is working on one of the largest studies to date in the United States, called "Study to Explore Early Development (SEED)." SEED is looking at many possible risk factors for ASD, including genetic, environmental, pregnancy, and behavioral factors.

Who Is Affected with Autism Spectrum Disorder?

Autism spectrum disorders occur in all racial, ethnic, and socio-economic groups, but is about four times more common among boys than among girls.

For over a decade, the CDC's Autism and Developmental Disabilities Monitoring (ADDM) Network has been estimating the number of children with ASD in the United States. The CDC has learned a lot about how many U.S. children have ASD. It will be important to use the same methods to track how the number of children with ASD is changing over time in order to learn more about the disorder.

If You Are Concerned about Autism Spectrum Disorder

If you think your child might have ASD or you think the way your child plays, learns, speaks, or acts may be symptomatic of ASD, contact your child's doctor, and share your concerns.

If you or the doctor is still concerned, ask the doctor for a referral to a specialist who can do a more in-depth evaluation of your child. Specialists who can do a more in-depth evaluation and make a diagnosis include:

- Developmental pediatricians (doctors who have special training in child development and children with special needs)

- Child neurologists (doctors who work on the brain, spine, and nerves)

- Child psychologists or psychiatrists (doctors who specialize in the human mind)

At the same time, call your state's public early-childhood system to request a free evaluation to find out if your child qualifies for intervention services. This is sometimes called a "Child Find" evaluation. You do not need to wait for a doctor's referral or a medical diagnosis to make this call.

Where to call for a free evaluation from the state depends on your child's age:

- If your child is not yet three years old, contact your local early-intervention system.

- You can find the right contact information for your state by calling the Early-Childhood Technical Assistance Center (ECTA) at 919-962-2001.

- If your child is three years old or older, contact your local public-school system.

- Even if your child is not yet old enough for kindergarten or enrolled in a public school, call your local elementary school or board of education and ask to speak with someone who can help you have your child evaluated.

Research shows that early-intervention services can greatly improve a child's development. In order to make sure your child reaches her or his full potential, it is very important to seek specialized services for an ASD as soon as possible.

Chapter 31

Attention Deficit Hyperactivity Disorder

What Is Attention Deficit Hyperactivity Disorder?

Attention deficit hyperactivity disorder (ADHD) is one of the most common neurodevelopmental disorders of childhood. It is usually first diagnosed in childhood and often lasts into adulthood. Children with ADHD may have difficulty paying attention, controlling impulsive behaviors (may act without thinking about what the result will be), or be overly active.

Signs and Symptoms of Attention Deficit Hyperactivity Disorder

It is normal for children to have trouble focusing and behaving at one time or another. However, children with ADHD do not just grow out of these behaviors. The symptoms continue, can be severe, and can cause difficulty at school, at home, or with friends.

A child with ADHD might:

- Daydream a lot

- Forget or lose things a lot

This chapter includes text excerpted from "Attention-Deficit/Hyperactivity Disorder (ADHD)," Centers for Disease Control and Prevention (CDC), December 14, 2018.

- Squirm or fidget

- Talk too much

- Make careless mistakes or take unnecessary risks

- Have a hard time resisting temptation

- Have trouble taking turns

- Have difficulty getting along with others

Types of Attention Deficit Hyperactivity Disorder

There are three different types of ADHD, depending on which types of symptoms are strongest in the individual:

- **Predominantly inattentive presentation:** It is hard for the individual to organize or finish a task, to pay attention to details, or to follow instructions or conversations. The person is easily distracted or forgets details of daily routines.

- **Predominantly hyperactive-impulsive presentation:** The person fidgets and talks a lot. It is hard to sit still for long (e.g., for a meal or while doing homework). Smaller children may run, jump, or climb constantly. The individual feels restless and has trouble with impulsivity. Someone who is impulsive may interrupt others a lot, grab things from people, or speak at inappropriate times. It is hard for the person to wait their turn or listen to directions. A person with impulsiveness may have more accidents and injuries than others.

- **Combined presentation:** Symptoms of the above two types are equally present in the person.

Because symptoms can change over time, the presentation may change over time as well.

Causes of Attention Deficit Hyperactivity Disorder

Scientists are studying causes and risk factors in an effort to find better ways to manage and reduce the chances of a person having ADHD. The causes and risk factors for ADHD are unknown, but current research shows that genetics plays an important role. Recent studies of twins link genes with ADHD.

In addition to genetics, scientists are studying other possible causes and risk factors including:

- Brain injury
- Premature delivery
- Low birth weight

Research does not support the popularly held views that ADHD is caused by eating too much sugar, watching too much television, parenting, or social and environmental factors, such as poverty or family chaos. Of course, many things, including these, might make symptoms worse, especially in certain people. But the evidence is not strong enough to conclude that they are the main causes of ADHD.

Diagnosis of Attention Deficit Hyperactivity Disorder

Deciding if a child has ADHD is a process with several steps. There is no single test to diagnose ADHD, and many other characteristics, such as anxiety, depression, sleep problems, and certain types of learning disabilities, can have similar symptoms. One step of the process involves having a medical exam, including hearing and vision tests, to rule out other diagnoses. Another part of the process may include a checklist for rating ADHD symptoms and taking a history of the child from parents, teachers, and sometimes, the child.

Treatments of Attention Deficit Hyperactivity Disorder

In most cases, ADHD is best treated with a combination of behavior therapy and medication. For preschool-aged children (four to five years of age) with ADHD, behavior therapy, particularly training for parents, is recommended as the first line of treatment. What works best can depend on the child and family. Good treatment plans will include close monitoring, follow-ups, and making changes, if needed, along the way.

Managing Attention Deficit Hyperactivity Disorder Symptoms

Being healthy is important for all children and can be especially important for children with ADHD. In addition to behavioral therapy and medication, maintaining a healthy lifestyle can make it easier for your child to deal with ADHD symptoms. Here are some healthy behaviors that may help:

- Eating a healthful diet centered on fruits, vegetables, whole grains, legumes (for example, beans, peas, and lentils), lean protein sources, and nuts and seeds

- Participating in physical activity for at least 60 minutes each day

- Limiting the amount of daily screen time from TVs, computers, phones, etc.

- Getting the recommended amount of sleep each night based on age

Chapter 32

Behavior or Conduct Issues in Children

Children sometimes argue, are aggressive, or act angry or defiant around adults. A behavior disorder may be diagnosed when these disruptive behaviors are uncommon for the child's age at the time, persist over time, or are severe. Because disruptive behavior disorders involve acting out and showing unwanted behavior towards others, they are often called "externalizing disorders."

Oppositional Defiant Disorder

When children act out persistently to the point that it causes serious problems at home, in school, or with peers, they may be diagnosed with oppositional defiant disorder (ODD). ODD usually starts before 8 years of age, but no later than by about 12 years of age. Children with ODD are more likely to act oppositional or defiant around people they know well, such as family members, a regular care provider, or a teacher. Children with ODD show these behaviors more often than other children their age.

This chapter contains text excerpted from the following sources: Text in this chapter begins with excerpts from "Behavior or Conduct Problems in Children," Centers for Disease Control and Prevention (CDC), March 12, 2019; Text under the heading "Behavior Therapy for Behavior or Conduct Problems" is excerpted from "Behavior Therapy for Behavior or Conduct Problems," Centers for Disease Control and Prevention (CDC), March 12, 2019.

Examples of ODD behaviors include:

- Often being angry or losing one's temper
- Often arguing with adults or refusing to comply with adults' rules or requests
- Often resentful or spiteful
- Deliberately annoying others or becoming annoyed with others
- Often blaming other people for one's own mistakes or misbehavior

Conduct Disorder

Conduct disorder (CD) is diagnosed when children show an ongoing pattern of aggression toward others, and serious violations of rules and social norms at home, in school, and with peers. These rule violations may involve breaking the law and result in arrest. Children with CD are more likely to get injured and may have difficulties getting along with peers.

Examples of CD behaviors include:

- Breaking serious rules, such as running away, staying out at night when told not to, or skipping school
- Being aggressive in a way that causes harm, such as bullying, fighting, or being cruel to animals
- Lying, stealing, or damaging other people's property on purpose

Treatment of Disruptive Behavior Disorders

Starting treatment early is important. Treatment is most effective if it fits the needs of the specific child and family. The first step to treatment is to talk with a healthcare provider. A comprehensive evaluation by a mental-health professional may be needed to get the right diagnosis. Some of the signs of behavior problems, such as not following rules in school, could be related to learning problems that may need additional intervention.

For younger children, the treatment with the strongest evidence is behavior therapy training for parents, where a therapist helps the parent learn effective ways to strengthen the parent–child relationship and respond to the child's behavior. For school-age children and teens, an often-used effective treatment is a combination of training and therapy that includes the child, the family, and the school.

Managing Disruptive Behavior Disorders Symptoms

Being healthy is important for all children and can be especially important for children with behavior or conduct problems. In addition to behavioral therapy and medication, practicing certain healthy lifestyle behaviors may reduce challenging and disruptive behaviors your child might experience. Here are some healthy behaviors that may help:

- Engaging in regular physical activity, including aerobic and vigorous exercise

- Eating a healthful diet centered on fruits, vegetables, whole grains, legumes (for example, beans, peas, and lentils), lean protein sources, and nuts and seeds

- Getting the recommended amount of sleep each night based on age

- Strengthening relationships with family members

Prevention of Disruptive Behavior Disorders

It is not known exactly why some children develop disruptive behavior disorders (DBDs). Many factors may play a role, including biological and social factors. It is known that children are at greater risk when they are exposed to other types of violence and criminal behavior, when they experience maltreatment or harsh or inconsistent parenting, or when their parents have mental-health conditions such as substance-use disorder (SUD), depression, or attention deficit hyperactivity disorder (ADHD). The quality of early-childhood care also can impact whether a child develops behavior problems.

Although these factors appear to increase the risk for DBDs, there are ways to decrease the chance that children experience them.

Behavior Therapy for Behavior or Conduct Problems
What Is Behavior Therapy?

Behavior therapy is an effective treatment for behavior or conduct problems that can improve a child's behavior, self-control, and self-esteem. The goals of behavior therapy are to learn or strengthen positive behaviors and eliminate disruptive behaviors. Behavior therapy can include the parent, the child, or both together. It is most effective in younger children when it is delivered by parents.

When parents become trained in behavior therapy, they learn skills and strategies to help their child succeed at school, at home, and in relationships. Parent behavior therapy means that parents learn how to teach and guide their children and to manage their behavior. Parent training in behavior therapy has been shown to strengthen the relationship between the parent and child and to decrease children's negative or problem behaviors. Parent training programs include practicing new skills with the child, either during the therapy or at home.

Behavior therapy training for parents is effective for managing disruptive behavior in young children through age 12. A review of treatment in children aged 12 years and under found that the best evidence was for parent behavior therapy when delivered either as group therapy or individually with child participation.

Finding a Therapist
How Do Families Find a Therapist Who Trains Parents in Behavior Therapy?

Psychologists, social workers, and licensed counselors can provide this kind of training to parents. Therapists may be found through professional association directories or through health-insurance provider directories. Parents can review the therapist's online profile or call and ask the therapist to describe their approach to behavior treatment.

What Should Parents Look For?

Families should look for a therapist who focuses on training parents. Some therapists will have training or certification in a program that has been proven to work in children with behavior problems. The following list of questions can be used to find a therapist who uses a proven approach:

Does this therapist:

- Teach parents skills and strategies that use positive reinforcement, structure, and consistent discipline to manage their child's behavior?

- Teach parents positive ways to interact and communicate with their child?

- Assign activities for parents to practice with their child?

- Meet regularly with the family to monitor progress and provide coaching and support?

- Re-evaluate and remain flexible enough to adjust strategies as needed?

What Can Parents Expect?

Parents typically attend eight or more sessions with a therapist. Sessions may involve groups or individual families. The therapist meets regularly with the family to review their progress, provide support, and adjust strategies as needed to ensure improvement. Parents practice with their child during or between sessions.

- The therapist meets regularly with the family to monitor progress and provide support.

- Between sessions, parents practice using the skills they have learned from the therapist.

- After therapy ends, families continue to experience improved behavior and reduced stress.

Chapter 33

Developmental Disorders and Disorders That Affect Learning

Chapter Contents

Section 33.1

Developmental Disabilities

This section includes text excerpted from "Facts about
Developmental Disabilities," Centers for Disease
Control and Prevention (CDC), April 17, 2018.

Developmental disabilities are a group of conditions due to an impairment in physical, learning, language, or behavior areas. These conditions begin during the developmental period, may impact day-to-day functioning, and usually last throughout a person's lifetime.

Developmental Milestones

Skills such as taking the first step, smiling for the first time, and waving "bye-bye" are called "developmental milestones." Children reach milestones in how they play, learn, speak, behave, and move (for example, crawling and walking).

Children develop at their own pace, so it is impossible to tell exactly when a child will learn a given skill. However, the developmental milestones give a general idea of the changes to expect as a child gets older.

As a parent, you know your child best. If your child is not meeting the milestones for her or his age, or if you think there could be a problem with your child's development, talk with your child's doctor or healthcare provider and share your concerns. Do not wait.

If You Are Concerned

If your child is not meeting the milestones for her or his age, or you are concerned about your child's development, talk with your child's doctor and share your concerns. Do not wait!

Developmental Monitoring and Screening

A child's growth and development are followed through a partnership between parents and healthcare professionals. At each well-child visit, the doctor looks for developmental delays or problems and talks with the parents about any concerns the parents might have. This is called "developmental monitoring."

Any problems noticed during developmental monitoring should be followed up with developmental screening. Developmental screening is a short test to tell if a child is learning basic skills when she or he should, or if there are delays.

If a child has a developmental delay, it is important to get help as soon as possible. Early identification and intervention can have a significant impact on a child's ability to learn new skills, as well as reduce the need for costly interventions over time.

Causes and Risk Factors of Developmental Disabilities

Developmental disabilities begin anytime during the developmental period and usually last throughout a person's lifetime. Most developmental disabilities begin before a baby is born, but some can happen after birth because of injury, infection, or other factors.

Most developmental disabilities are thought to be caused by a complex mix of factors. These factors include genetics; parental health and behaviors (such as smoking and drinking) during pregnancy; complications during birth; infections the mother might have during pregnancy or the baby might have very early in life; and exposure of the mother or child to high levels of environmental toxins, such as lead. For some developmental disabilities, such as fetal alcohol syndrome, which is caused by drinking alcohol during pregnancy, the cause is known. But for most, not much is known.

Following are some examples of what we know about specific developmental disabilities:

- At least 25 percent of hearing loss among babies is due to maternal infections during pregnancy, such as cytomegalovirus (CMV) infection, complications after birth, and head trauma.

- Some of the most common known causes of intellectual disability include fetal alcohol syndrome; genetic and chromosomal conditions, such as Down syndrome and fragile X syndrome; and certain infections during pregnancy.

- Children who have a sibling with autism are at a higher risk of also having autism spectrum disorder (ASD).

- Low birth weight, premature birth, multiple birth, and infections during pregnancy are associated with an increased risk for many developmental disabilities.

- Untreated newborn jaundice (high levels of bilirubin in the blood during the first few days after birth) can cause a type of brain damage known as "kernicterus." Children with kernicterus are more likely to have cerebral palsy, hearing and vision problems, and problems with their teeth. Early detection and treatment of newborn jaundice can prevent kernicterus.

The Study to Explore Early Development (SEED) is a multiyear study funded by the Centers for Disease Control and Prevention (CDC). As of now, it is the largest study in the United States to help identify factors that may put children at risk for ASD and other developmental disabilities.

Who Is Affected by Developmental Disabilities?

Developmental disabilities occur among all racial, ethnic, and socio-economic groups. Estimates in the United States show that about 1 in 6, or about 15 percent of children aged 3 through 17 years have 1 or more developmental disabilities, such as:

- Attention deficit hyperactivity disorder (ADHD)
- Autism spectrum disorder (ASD)
- Cerebral palsy (CP)
- Hearing loss
- Intellectual disability
- Learning disability
- Vision impairment
- Other developmental delays

For over a decade, the CDC's Autism and Developmental Disabilities Monitoring (ADDM) Network has been tracking the number and characteristics of children with ASD, CP, and intellectual disability in several diverse communities throughout the United States.

Living with a Developmental Disability

Children with disabilities need healthcare and health programs for the same reasons anyone else does—to stay well, active, and be a part of the community.

Having a disability does not mean a child is not healthy or that she or he cannot be healthy. Being healthy means the same thing for all of us—getting and staying well so we can lead full, active lives. That includes having the tools and information to make healthy choices and knowing how to prevent illness. Some health conditions, such as asthma, gastrointestinal symptoms, eczema and skin allergies, and migraine headaches, have been found to be more common among children with developmental disabilities. Thus, it is especially important for children with developmental disabilities to see a healthcare provider regularly.

Section 33.2

Learning Disabilities

This section includes text excerpted from "About Learning Disabilities," *Eunice Kennedy Shriver* National Institute of Child Health and Human Development (NICHD), September 11, 2018.

What Are Learning Disabilities?

Learning disabilities affect how a person learns to read, write, speak, and do math. They are caused by differences in the brain, most often in how it functions but also sometimes in its structure. These differences affect the way the brain processes information.

Learning disabilities are often discovered once a child is in school and has learning difficulties that do not improve over time. A person can have more than one learning disability. Learning disabilities can last a person's entire life, but she or he can still be successful with the right educational supports.

A learning disability is not an indication of a person's intelligence. Learning disabilities are different from learning challenges due to intellectual and developmental disabilities, or emotional, vision, hearing, or motor skills problems.

Different groups may define "learning disability" differently, often depending on the focus of the organization.

Types of Learning Disabilities

Some of the most common learning disabilities are the following:

- **Dyslexia.** Children with dyslexia have problems with reading words accurately and with ease (sometimes called "fluency") and may have a hard time spelling, understanding sentences, and recognizing words they already know.

- **Dysgraphia.** Children with dysgraphia have problems with their handwriting. They may have trouble forming letters, writing within a defined space, and writing down their thoughts.

- **Dyscalculia.** Children with this math learning disability may have difficulty understanding arithmetic concepts and doing addition, multiplication, and measuring.

- **Apraxia of speech.** This disorder involves problems with speaking. Children with this disorder have trouble saying what they want to say. It is sometimes called "verbal apraxia."

- **Central auditory processing disorder (CAPD).** Children with this condition have trouble understanding and remembering language-related tasks. They have difficulty explaining things, understanding jokes, and following directions. They confuse words and are easily distracted.

- **Nonverbal learning disorders.** Children with these conditions have strong verbal skills but difficulty understanding facial expressions and body language. They are clumsy and have trouble generalizing and following multistep directions.

Because there are many different types of learning disabilities, and some children may have more than one, it is hard to estimate how many people might have learning disabilities.

What Are Some Signs of Learning Disabilities?

Many children have trouble reading, writing, or performing other learning-related tasks at some point. This does not mean they have learning disabilities. A child with a learning disability often has several related signs, and they do not go away or get better over time. The signs of learning disabilities vary from person to person.

Please note that the generally common signs included here are for informational purposes only; the information is not intended to screen for learning disabilities in general or for a specific type of learning disability.

Common signs that a person may have learning disabilities include the following:

- Problems reading and/or writing

- Problems with math

- Poor memory

- Problems paying attention

- Trouble following directions

- Clumsiness

- Trouble telling time

- Problems staying organized

A child with a learning disability also may have one or more of the following:

- Acting without really thinking about possible outcomes (impulsiveness)

- "Acting out" in school or social situations

- Difficulty staying focused; being easily distracted

- Difficulty saying a word correctly out loud or expressing thoughts

- Problems with school performance from week to week or day-to-day

- Speaking like a younger child; using short, simple phrases; or leaving out words in sentences

- Having a hard time listening

- Problems dealing with changes in schedule or situations

- Problems understanding words or concepts

These signs alone are not enough to determine that a person has a learning disability. Only a professional can diagnose a learning disability.

Each learning disability has its own signs. A person with a particular disability may not have all of the signs of that disability.

Children being taught in a second language may show signs of learning problems or a learning disability. The learning disability assessment must take into account whether a student is bilingual or facing a second language learner. In addition, for English-speaking children, the assessment should be sensitive to differences that may be due to dialect, a form of a language that is specific to a region or group.

701

Below are some common learning disabilities and the signs associated with them.

Dyslexia

People with dyslexia usually have trouble making the connection between letters and sounds and with spelling and recognizing words.

People with dyslexia often show other signs of the condition. These may include:

- Having a hard time understanding what others are saying
- Difficulty organizing written and spoken language
- Delay in being able to speak
- Difficulty expressing thoughts or feelings
- Difficulty learning new words (vocabulary), either while reading or hearing
- Trouble learning foreign languages
- Difficulty learning songs and rhymes
- Slow rate of reading, both silently and out loud
- Giving up on longer reading tasks
- Difficulty understanding questions and following directions
- Poor spelling
- Problems remembering numbers in the sequence (for example, telephone numbers and addresses)
- Trouble telling left from right

Dysgraphia

A child who has trouble writing or has very poor handwriting and does not outgrow it may have dysgraphia. This disorder may cause a child to be tense and twist awkwardly when holding a pen or pencil.

Other signs of this condition may include:

- A strong dislike of writing and/or drawing
- Problems with grammar
- Trouble writing down ideas
- Losing energy or interest as soon as they start writing

- Trouble writing down thoughts in a logical sequence

- Saying words out loud while writing

- Leaving words unfinished or omitting them when writing sentences

Dyscalculia

Signs of this disability include problems understanding basic arithmetic concepts, such as fractions, number lines, and positive and negative numbers.

Other symptoms may include:

- Difficulty with math-related word problems

- Trouble making change in cash transactions

- Messiness in putting math problems on paper

- Trouble with logical sequences (for example, steps in math problems)

- Trouble understanding the time sequence of events

- Trouble describing math processes

What Causes Learning Disabilities

Researchers do not know all of the possible causes of learning disabilities, but they have found a range of risk factors during their work to find potential causes. Research shows that risk factors may be present from birth and tend to run in families. In fact, children who have a parent with a learning disability are more likely to develop a learning disability themselves. To better understand learning disabilities, researchers are studying how children's brains learn to read, write, and develop math skills. Researchers are working on interventions to help address the needs of those who struggle with reading the most, including those with learning disabilities, to improve learning and overall health.

Factors that affect a fetus developing in the womb, such as alcohol or drug use, can put a child at higher risk for a learning problem or disability. Other factors in an infant's environment may play a role, too. These can include poor nutrition or exposure to lead in water or in paint. Young children who do not receive the support they need for their intellectual development may show signs of learning disabilities once they start school.

Sometimes a person may develop a learning disability later in life due to injury. Possible causes in such a case include dementia or a traumatic brain injury (TBI).

How Are Learning Disabilities Diagnosed?

Learning disabilities are often identified once a child is in school. The school may use a process called "response to intervention" to help identify children with learning disabilities. Special tests are required to make a diagnosis.

Response to Intervention

Response to intervention usually involves the following:

- Monitoring all students' progress closely to identify possible learning problems

- Providing children who are having problems with the help on different levels, or tiers

- Moving children to tiers that provide increasing support if they do not show sufficient progress

Students who are struggling in school can also have individual evaluations. An evaluation can:

- Identify whether a child has a learning disability

- Determine a child's eligibility under federal law for special education services

- Help develop an individualized education plan (IEP) that outlines help for a child who qualifies for special education services

- Establish benchmarks to measure the child's progress

A full evaluation for a learning disability includes the following:

- A medical exam, including a neurological exam, to rule out other possible causes of the child's difficulties. These might include emotional disorders, intellectual and developmental disabilities, and brain diseases.

- Reviewing the child's developmental, social, and school performance

- A discussion of family history
- Academic and psychological testing

Usually, several specialists work as a team to do the evaluation. The team may include a psychologist, a special-education expert, and a speech-language pathologist. Many schools also have reading specialists who can help diagnose a reading disability.

Role of School Psychologists

School psychologists are trained in both education and psychology. They can help diagnose students with learning disabilities and help the student and her or his parents and teachers come up with plans to improve learning.

Role of Speech-Language Pathologists

All speech-language pathologists are trained to diagnose and treat speech and language disorders. A speech-language pathologist can do a language evaluation and assess the child's ability to organize her or his thoughts and possessions. The speech-language pathologist may evaluate the child's learning skills, such as understanding directions, manipulating sounds, and reading and writing.

What Are the Treatments for Learning Disabilities?

Learning disabilities have no cure, but early intervention can lessen their effects. People with learning disabilities can develop ways to cope with their disabilities. Getting help earlier increases the chance of success in school and later in life. If learning disabilities remain untreated, a child may begin to feel frustrated, which can lead to low self-esteem and other problems.

Experts can help a child learn skills by building on the child's strengths and finding ways to compensate for the child's weaknesses. Interventions vary depending on the nature and extent of the disability.

Special Education Services

Children diagnosed with learning disabilities can receive special-education services. The Individuals with Disabilities Education Act (IDEA) requires that public schools provide free special-education supports to children with disabilities.

In most states, each child is entitled to these services beginning at age 3 years and extending through high school or until age 21, whichever comes first. The rules of IDEA for each state are available from the Early Childhood Technical Assistance (ECTA) Center.

IDEA requires that children be taught in the least restrictive environment appropriate for them. This means the teaching environment should meet a child's needs and skills while minimizing restrictions to dominant learning experiences.

Individualized Education Programs

Children who qualify for special-education services will receive an Individualized Education Program, or IEP. This personalized and written education plan:

- Lists goals for the child

- Specifies the services the child will receive

- Lists the specialists who will work with the child

Qualifying for Special Education

To qualify for special-education services, a child must be evaluated by the school system and meet federal and state guidelines. Parents and caregivers can contact their school principal or special-education coordinator to find out how to have their child evaluated.

Interventions for Specific Learning Disabilities

Below are just a few of the ways schools help children with specific learning disabilities.

Dyslexia

- **Intensive teaching techniques.** These can include specific, step-by-step, and very methodical approaches to teaching reading with the goal of improving both spoken language and written-language skills. These techniques are generally more intensive in terms of how often they occur and how long they last and often involve small group or one-on-one instruction.

- **Classroom modifications.** Teachers can give students with dyslexia extra time to finish tasks and provide taped tests that allow the child to hear the questions instead of reading them.

- **Use of technology.** Children with dyslexia may benefit from listening to audiobooks or using word-processing programs.

Dysgraphia

- **Special tools.** Teachers can offer oral exams, provide a note-taker, or allow the child to videotape reports instead of writing them. Computer software can facilitate children being able to produce written text.
- **Use of technology.** A child with dysgraphia can be taught to use word-processing programs, including those incorporating speech-to-text translation, or an audio recorder instead of writing by hand.
- **Reducing the need for writing.** Teachers can provide notes, outlines, and preprinted study sheets.

Dyscalculia

- **Visual techniques.** Teachers can draw pictures of word problems and show the students how to use colored pencils to differentiate parts of problems.
- **Memory aids.** Rhymes and music can help a child remember math concepts.
- **Computers.** A child with dyscalculia can use a computer for drills and practice.

Section 33.3

Dyslexia

This section includes text excerpted from "Dyslexia
Information Page," National Institute of Neurological
Disorders and Stroke (NINDS), March 27, 2019.

What Is Dyslexia?

Dyslexia is a brain-based type of learning disability that specifically impairs a child's ability to read. These individuals typically read at levels significantly lower than expected despite having standard intelligence. Although the disorder varies from child to child, common characteristics among people with dyslexia are difficulty with phonological processing (the manipulation of sounds), spelling, and/or rapid visual–verbal responding. Dyslexia can be inherited in some families, and studies have identified a number of genes that may predispose an individual to developing dyslexia.

Treatment of Dyslexia

The main focus of treatment should be on the specific learning problems of affected individuals. The usual course is to modify teaching methods and the educational environment to meet the specific needs of the individual with dyslexia.

Prognosis of Dyslexia

For those with dyslexia, the prognosis is mixed. The disability affects such a wide range of people and produces such different symptoms and varying degrees of severity that predictions are hard to make. The prognosis is generally good, however, for individuals whose dyslexia is identified early, who have supportive family and friends and a strong self-image, and who are involved in a proper remediation program.

Section 33.4

Language and Speech Disorders

This section includes text excerpted from "Language and
Speech Disorders in Children," Centers for Disease
Control and Prevention (CDC), February 6, 2019.

Children are born ready to learn a language, but they need to learn the language or languages that their family and environment use. Learning a language takes time, and children vary in how quickly they master milestones in language and speech development. Typically developing children may have trouble with some sounds, words, and sentences while they are learning. However, most children can use language easily around five years of age.

Helping Children Learn Language

Parents and caregivers are the most important teachers during a child's early years. Children learn language by listening to others speak and by practicing. Even young babies notice when others repeat and respond to the noises and sounds they make. Children's language and brain skills get stronger if they hear many different words. Parents can help their child learn in many different ways, such as:

- Responding to the first sounds, gurgles, and gestures a baby makes

- Repeating what the child says and adding to it

- Talking about the things that a child sees

- Asking questions and listening to the answers

- Looking at or reading books

- Telling stories

- Singing songs and sharing rhymes

This can happen both during playtime and during daily routines. Parents can also observe the following:

- How their child hears and talks and compare it with typical milestones for communication skills

- How their child reacts to sounds and have their hearing tested if they have concerns

What to Do If There Are Concerns Regarding Language and Speech Disorders in Your Children

Some children struggle with understanding and speaking and they need help. They may not master the language milestones at the same time as other children, and it may be a sign of a language or speech delay or disorder.

Language development has different parts, and children might have problems with one or more of the following:

- Understanding what others say (receptive language). This could be due to:

  - Not hearing the words (hearing loss)

  - Not understanding the meaning of the words

- Communicating thoughts using language (expressive language). This could be due to:

  - Not knowing the words to use

  - Not knowing how to put words together

- Knowing the words to use but not being able to express them

Language and speech disorders can exist together or by themselves. Examples of problems with language and speech development include the following:

- Speech disorders:

  - Difficulty with forming specific words or sounds correctly

  - Difficulty with making words or sentences flow smoothly, such as stuttering or stammering

  - Language delay—the ability to understand and speak develops more slowly than is typical

- Language disorder:

  - Aphasia (difficulty understanding or speaking parts of language due to a brain injury or how the brain works)

  - Auditory processing disorder (APD) (difficulty understanding the meaning of the sounds that the ear sends to the brain)

Language or speech disorders can occur with other learning disorders that affect reading and writing. Children with language disorders may feel frustrated that they cannot understand others or make themselves understood, and they may act out, act helpless, or withdraw. Language or speech disorders can also be present with emotional or behavioral disorders, such as attention deficit hyperactivity disorder (ADHD) or anxiety. Children with developmental disabilities including autism spectrum disorder (ASD) may also have difficulties with speech and language. The combination of challenges can make it particularly hard for a child to succeed in school. Properly diagnosing a child's disorder is crucial so that each child can get the right kind of specialized support.

Detecting Language or Speech Challenges

If a child faces challenges with language or speech development, talk to a healthcare provider about an evaluation. An important first step is to find out if the child may have a hearing loss. Hearing loss may be difficult to notice particularly if a child has a hearing loss only in one ear or has partial hearing loss, which means they can hear some sounds but not others.

A language development specialist such as a speech-language pathologist will conduct a careful assessment to determine what type of problem with language or speech the child may have.

Overall, learning more than one language does not cause language disorders, but children may not follow exactly the same developmental milestones as those who learn only one language. Developing the ability to understand and speak in two languages depends on how much practice the child has using both languages, and the kind of practice. If a child who is learning more than one language has difficulty with language development, careful assessment by a specialist who understands the development of skills in more than one language may be needed.

Treatment for Language or Speech Disorders and Delays

Children with language challenges often need extra help and special instruction. Speech-language pathologists can work directly with children and their parents, caregivers, and teachers.

Having a language or speech delay or disorder can qualify a child for early intervention (for children up to three years of age) and special-education services (for children aged three years and older). Schools can do their own testing for language or speech disorders to see if a child needs intervention. An evaluation by a healthcare professional is needed if there are other concerns about the child's hearing, behavior, or emotions. Parents, healthcare providers, and the school can work together to find the right referrals and treatment.

What Every Parent Should Know

Children with specific learning disabilities, including language or speech disorders, are eligible for special-education services or accommodations at school under the Individuals with Disabilities in Education Act (IDEA) and Section 504, an antidiscrimination law.

The Role of Healthcare Providers

Healthcare providers can play an important part in collaborating with schools to help a child with speech or language disorders and delays or other disabilities get the special services they need. The American Academy of Pediatrics (AAP) has created a report that describes the roles that healthcare providers can have in helping children with disabilities, including language or speech disorders.

Section 33.5

Developmental Apraxia of Speech

This section includes text excerpted from "Apraxia of
Speech," National Institute on Deafness and Other
Communication Disorders (NIDCD), October 31, 2017.

What Is Apraxia of Speech?

Apraxia of speech (AOS)—also known as "acquired apraxia of speech," "verbal apraxia," or "childhood apraxia of speech (CAS)" when diagnosed in children—is a speech–sound disorder. Someone with AOS has trouble saying what she or he wants to say correctly and consistently. AOS is a neurological disorder that affects the brain pathways involved in planning the sequence of movements involved in producing speech. The brain knows what it wants to say, but cannot properly plan and sequence the required speech sound movements.

Apraxia of speech is not caused by weakness or paralysis of the speech muscles (the muscles of the jaw, tongue, or lips). Weakness or paralysis of the speech muscles results in a separate speech disorder, known as "dysarthria." Some people have both dysarthria and AOS, which can make the diagnosis of the two conditions more difficult.

The severity of AOS varies from person to person. It can be so mild that it causes trouble with only a few speech sounds or with the pronunciation of words that have many syllables. In the most severe cases, someone with AOS might not be able to communicate effectively by speaking and may need the help of alternative communication methods.

What Are the Types and Causes of Apraxia of Speech?

There are two main types of AOS: acquired apraxia of speech and childhood apraxia of speech.

- **Acquired AOS** can affect someone at any age, although it most typically occurs in adults. Acquired AOS is caused by damage to the parts of the brain that are involved in speaking and involves the loss or impairment of existing speech abilities. It may result from a stroke, head injury, tumor, or other illness affecting the brain. Acquired AOS may occur together with other conditions that are caused by damage to the nervous system. One of these is dysarthria, as mentioned earlier. Another is aphasia, which is a language disorder.

- **Childhood AOS** is present from birth. This condition is also known as "developmental apraxia of speech," "developmental verbal apraxia," or "articulatory apraxia." Childhood AOS is not the same as developmental delays in speech, in which a child follows the typical path of speech development but does so more slowly than is typical. The causes of childhood AOS are not well understood. Imaging and other studies have not been able to find evidence of brain damage or differences in the brain structure of children with AOS. Children with AOS often have family members who have a history of a communication disorder or a learning disability. This observation and recent research findings suggest that genetic factors may play a role in the disorder. Childhood AOS appears to affect more boys than girls.

713

What Are the Symptoms of Apraxia of Speech?

Children with either form of AOS may have a number of different speech characteristics or symptoms:

- **Distorting sounds.** Children with AOS may have difficulty pronouncing words correctly. Sounds, especially vowels, are often distorted. Because the speaker may not place the speech structures (e.g., tongue, jaw) quite in the right place, the sound comes out wrong. Longer or more complex words are usually harder to say than shorter or simpler words. Sound substitutions might also occur when AOS is accompanied by aphasia.

- **Making inconsistent errors in speech.** For example, someone with AOS may say a difficult word correctly but then have trouble repeating it, or may be able to say a particular sound one day and have trouble with the same sound the next day.

- **Groping for sounds.** Children with AOS often appear to be groping for the right sound or word and may try saying a word several times before they say it correctly.

- **Making errors in tone, stress, or rhythm.** Another common characteristic of AOS is the incorrect use of prosody. Prosody is the rhythm and inflection of speech that we use to help express meaning. Someone who has trouble with prosody might use equal stress, segment syllables in a word, omit syllables in words and phrases, or pause inappropriately while speaking.

Children with AOS generally understand language much better than they are able to use it. Some children with the disorder may also have other speech problems, expressive language problems, or motor-skill problems.

How Is Apraxia of Speech Diagnosed?

Professionals known as "speech-language pathologists" play a key role in diagnosing and treating AOS. Because there is no single symptom or test that can be used to diagnose AOS, the person making the diagnosis generally looks for the presence of several of a group of symptoms, including those described earlier. Ruling out other conditions, such as muscle weakness or language production problems (e.g., aphasia), can help with the diagnostic process.

In formal testing for both acquired and childhood AOS, a speech-language pathologist may ask the patient to perform speech tasks such as repeating a particular word several times or repeating a list of words of increasing length (for example, love, loving, lovingly). For acquired AOS, a speech-language pathologist may also examine the patient's ability to converse, read, write, and perform nonspeech movements. To diagnose childhood AOS, parents and professionals may need to observe a child's speech over a period of time.

How Is Apraxia of Speech Treated?

In some cases, children with acquired AOS recover some or all of their speech abilities on their own. This is called "spontaneous recovery."

Children with AOS will not outgrow the problem on their own. They also do not acquire the basics of speech just by being around other children, such as in a classroom. Therefore, speech-language therapy is necessary for children with AOS as well as for people with acquired AOS who do not spontaneously recover all of their speech abilities.

Speech-language pathologists use different approaches to treat AOS, and no single approach has been proven to be the most effective. Therapy is tailored to the individual and is designed to treat other speech or language problems that may occur together with AOS. Frequent, intensive, one-on-one speech-language therapy sessions are needed for both children and adults with AOS. (The repetitive exercises and personal attention needed to improve AOS are difficult to deliver in group therapy.) Children with severe AOS may need intensive speech-language therapy for years, in parallel with normal schooling, to obtain adequate speech abilities.

In severe cases, children with AOS may need to find other ways to express themselves. These might include formal or informal sign language; a notebook with pictures or written words that can be pointed to and shown to other people; or an electronic communication device— such as a smartphone, tablet, or laptop computer—that can be used to write or produce speech. Such assistive communication methods can also help children with AOS learn to read and better understand spoken language by stimulating areas of the brain involved in language and literacy.

Some children will make more progress during treatment than others. Support and encouragement from family members and friends and extra practice in the home environment are important.

Section 33.6

Stuttering

This section includes text excerpted from "Stuttering,"
National Institute on Deafness and Other Communication
Disorders (NIDCD), March 6, 2017.

What Is Stuttering?

Stuttering is a speech disorder characterized by the repetition of sounds, syllables, or words; prolongation of sounds; and interruptions in speech known as "blocks." An individual who stutters exactly knows what she or he would like to say but has trouble producing a normal flow of speech. These speech disruptions may be accompanied by struggle behaviors, such as rapid eye blinks or tremors of the lips. Stuttering can make it difficult to communicate with other people, which often affects a child's quality of life (QOL) and interpersonal relationships. Stuttering can also negatively influence job performance and opportunities, and treatment can come at a high financial cost.

Symptoms of stuttering can vary significantly throughout a child's day. In general, speaking before a group or talking on the telephone may make a child's stuttering more severe, while singing, reading, or speaking in unison may temporarily reduce stuttering.

Who Stutters

Roughly three million Americans stutter. Stuttering affects people of all ages. It occurs most often in children between the ages of 2 and 6 as they are developing their language skills. Approximately 5 to 10 percent of all children will stutter for some period in their life, lasting from a few weeks to several years. Boys are 2 to 3 times as likely to stutter as girls and as they get older this gender difference increases; the number of boys who continue to stutter is 3 to 4 times larger than the number of girls. Most children outgrow stuttering. Approximately 75 percent of children recover from stuttering. For the remaining 25 percent who continue to stutter, stuttering can persist as a lifelong communication disorder.

How Is Speech Normally Produced?

We make speech sounds through a series of precisely coordinated muscle movements involving breathing, phonation (voice production), and articulation (movement of the throat, palate, tongue, and lips).

Muscle movements are controlled by the brain and monitored through our senses of hearing and touch.

Causes and Types of Stuttering

The precise mechanisms that cause stuttering are not understood. Stuttering is commonly grouped into two types identified as "developmental" and "neurogenic."

Developmental Stuttering

Developmental stuttering occurs in young children while they are still learning speech and language skills. It is the most common form of stuttering. Some scientists and clinicians believe that developmental stuttering occurs when children's speech and language abilities are unable to meet the child's verbal demands. Most scientists and clinicians believe that developmental stuttering stems from complex interactions of multiple factors. Brain imaging studies have shown consistent differences in those who stutter compared to nonstuttering peers. Developmental stuttering may also run in families and research has shown that genetic factors contribute to this type of stuttering. Starting in 2010, researchers at the National Institute on Deafness and Other Communication Disorders (NIDCD) have identified four different genes in which mutations are associated with stuttering.

Neurogenic Stuttering

Neurogenic stuttering may occur after a stroke, head trauma, or other types of brain injury. With neurogenic stuttering, the brain has difficulty coordinating the different brain regions involved in speaking, resulting in problems in the production of clear, fluent speech.

At one time, all stuttering was believed to be psychogenic, caused by emotional trauma, but nowadays we know that psychogenic stuttering is rare.

How Is Stuttering Diagnosed?

Stuttering is usually diagnosed by a speech-language pathologist, a health professional who is trained to test and treat individuals with voice, speech, and language disorders. The speech-language pathologist will consider a variety of factors, including the child's case history (such as when the stuttering was first noticed and under what circumstances), an analysis of the child's stuttering behaviors, and an evaluation of the child's speech and language abilities and the impact of stuttering on her or his life.

When evaluating a young child for stuttering, a speech-language pathologist will try to determine if the child is likely to continue her or his stuttering behavior or outgrow it. To determine this difference, the speech-language pathologist will consider such factors as the family's history of stuttering, whether the child's stuttering has lasted six months or longer, and whether the child exhibits other speech or language problems.

How Is Stuttering Treated?

Although there is no cure for stuttering, there are a variety of treatments available. The nature of the treatment will differ, based upon a person's age, communication goals, and other factors. If you or your child stutters, it is important to work with a speech-language pathologist to determine the best treatment options.

Therapy for Children

For very young children, early treatment may prevent developmental stuttering from becoming a lifelong problem. Certain strategies can help children learn to improve their speech fluency while developing positive attitudes toward communication. Health professionals generally recommend that a child be evaluated if she or he has stuttered for three to six months, exhibits struggle behaviors associated with stuttering, or has a family history of stuttering or related communication disorders. Some researchers recommend that a child be evaluated every three months to determine if the stuttering is increasing or decreasing. Treatment often involves teaching parents about ways to support their child's production of fluent speech. Parents may be encouraged to:

- Provide a relaxed home environment that allows many opportunities for the child to speak. This includes setting aside time to talk to one another, especially when the child is excited and has a lot to say.

- Listen attentively when the child speaks and focuses on the content of the message, rather than responding to how it is said or interrupting the child.

- Speak in a slightly slowed and relaxed manner. This can help reduce the time pressures the child may be experiencing.

- Listen attentively when the child speaks and wait for her or him to say the intended word. Do not try to complete the child's sentences. Also, help the child learn that a person can communicate successfully even when stuttering occurs.

Talk openly and honestly to the child about stuttering if she or he brings up the subject. Let the child know that it is okay for some disruptions to occur.

Stuttering Therapy

Many of the current therapies for teens and adults who stutter focus on helping them learn ways to minimize stuttering when they speak, such as by speaking more slowly, regulating their breathing, or gradually progressing from single-syllable responses to longer words and more complex sentences. Most of these therapies also help address the anxiety a person who stutters may feel in certain speaking situations.

Drug Therapy

The U.S. Food and Drug Administration (FDA) has not approved any drug for the treatment of stuttering. However, some drugs that are approved to treat other health problems—such as epilepsy, anxiety, or depression—have been used to treat stuttering. These drugs often have side effects that make them difficult to use over a long period of time.

Electronic Devices

Some people who stutter use electronic devices to help control fluency. For example, one type of device fits into the ear canal, much like a hearing aid, and digitally replays a slightly altered version of the wearer's voice into the ear so that it sounds as if she or he is speaking in unison with another person. In some people, electronic devices may help improve fluency in a relatively short period of time. Additional research is needed to determine how long such effects may last and whether people are able to easily use and benefit from these devices in real-world situations. For these reasons, researchers are continuing to study the long-term effectiveness of these devices.

Self-Help Groups

Many people find that they achieve their greatest success through a combination of self-study and therapy. Self-help groups provide a way for people who stutter to find resources and support as they face the challenges of stuttering.

Chapter 34

Fragile X Syndrome

What Is Fragile X Syndrome?

Fragile X syndrome (FXS) is a genetic disorder. A genetic disorder means that there are changes to the person's genes. FXS is caused by changes in the *fragile X mental retardation 1* (*FMR1*) gene. The *FMR1* gene usually makes a protein called "fragile X mental retardation protein" (FMRP). FMRP is needed for normal brain development. People who have FXS do not make this protein. People who have other fragile X-associated disorders have changes in their *FMR1* gene but usually, make some of the protein.

Fragile X syndrome affects both males and females. However, females often have milder symptoms than males. The exact number of people who have FXS is unknown, but it has been estimated that about 1.4 per 10,000 males and 0.9 per 10,000 females have FXS.

Signs and Symptoms of Fragile X Syndrome

Signs that a child might have FXS include:

- Developmental delays (not sitting, walking, or talking at the same time as other children the same age)

- Learning disabilities (trouble learning new skills)

This chapter includes text excerpted from "What Is Fragile X Syndrome (FXS)?" Centers for Disease Control and Prevention (CDC), May 30, 2019.

- Social and behavior problems (such as not making eye contact, anxiety, trouble paying attention, hand flapping, acting and speaking without thinking, and being very active)

Males who have FXS usually have some degree of intellectual disability that can range from mild to severe. Females with FXS can have normal intelligence or some degree of intellectual disability. Autism spectrum disorders (ASDs) also occur more frequently in people with FXS.

Testing and Diagnosis of Fragile X Syndrome

Fragile X syndrome can be diagnosed by testing a person's deoxyribonucleic acid (DNA) from a blood test. A doctor or genetic counselor can order the test. Testing also can be done to find changes in the *FMR1* gene that can lead to fragile X-associated disorders.

A diagnosis of FXS can be helpful to the family because it can provide a reason for a child's intellectual disabilities and behavior problems. This allows the family and other caregivers to learn more about the disorder and manage care so that the child can reach her or his full potential. However, the results of DNA tests can affect other family members and raise many issues. So, anyone who is thinking about FXS testing should consider having genetic counseling prior to getting tested.

Treatments of Fragile X Syndrome

There is no cure for FXS. However, treatment services can help people learn important skills. Services can include therapy to learn to talk, walk, and interact with others. In addition, medicine can be used to help control some issues, such as behavior problems. To develop the best treatment plan, people with FXS, parents, and healthcare providers should work closely with one another, and with everyone involved in treatment and support—which may include teachers, childcare providers, coaches, therapists, and other family members.

Early-Intervention Services

Early-intervention services help children from birth to 3 years old (36 months) learn important skills. These services may improve a child's development. Even if the child has not been diagnosed with FXS, she or he may be eligible for services. These services are provided through an early-intervention system in each state. Through this system, you can ask for an evaluation. In addition, treatment for particular symptoms, such as speech therapy for language delays, often does not need to wait for a formal diagnosis. While early intervention is extremely important, treatment services at any age can be helpful.

Finding Support to Address Fragile X Syndrome

Having support and community resources can help increase confidence in managing FXS, enhance the quality of life (QOL), and assist in meeting the needs of all family members. It might be helpful for parents of children with FXS to talk with one another. One parent might have learned how to address some of the same concerns another parent has. Often, parents of children with special needs can give advice about good resources for these children.

Remember that the choices of one family might not be best for another family, so it is important that parents understand all options and discuss them with their child's healthcare providers.

You can contact the National Fragile X Foundation at 800-688-8765 to get information about treatments, educational strategies, therapies, and intervention.

Chapter 35

Mental-Health Disorders in Children

Chapter Contents

Section 35.1

Anxiety and Panic Disorders

This section contains text excerpted from the following
sources: Text in this section begins with excerpts from "Anxiety
and Depression in Children," Centers for Disease Control and
Prevention (CDC), April 15, 2019; Text beginning with the heading
"What Is Panic Disorder?" is excerpted from "Panic Disorder: When
Fear Overwhelms," National Institute of Mental Health (NIMH),
March 15, 2016. Reviewed September 2019; Text under the heading
"Supportive Parenting Can Reduce Child's Anxiety" is excerpted
from "Supportive Parenting Can Reduce Child's Anxiety," National
Institutes of Health (NIH), March 19, 2019.

Many children have fears and worries and may feel sad and hopeless from time to time. Strong fears may appear at different times
during development. For example, toddlers are often very distressed
about being away from their parents, even if they are safe and cared
for. Although fears and worries are typical in children, persistent or
extreme forms of fear and sadness could be due to anxiety or depression. Because the symptoms primarily involve thoughts and feelings,
they are called "internalizing disorders."

What Is Anxiety?

When children do not outgrow the fears and worries that are typical
in young children, or when there are so many fears and worries that
they interfere with school, home, or play activities, the child may be
diagnosed with an anxiety disorder. Examples of different types of
anxiety disorders include

- Being very afraid when away from parents (separation anxiety)

- Having extreme fear about a specific thing or situation, such as
  dogs, insects, or going to the doctor (phobias)

- Being very afraid of school and other places where there are
  people (social anxiety)

- Being very worried about the future and about bad things
  happening (general anxiety)

- Having repeated episodes of sudden, unexpected, intense fear
  that come with symptoms, such as heart pounding, having trouble
  breathing, or feeling dizzy, shaky, or sweaty (panic disorder)

Anxiety may present as fear or worry, but can also make children irritable and angry. Anxiety symptoms can also include trouble sleeping, as well as physical symptoms, such as fatigue, headaches, or stomachaches. Some anxious children keep their worries to themselves and, thus, the symptoms can be missed.

Treatment of Anxiety

The first step to treatment is to talk with a healthcare provider such as your child's primary-care provider, or a mental-health specialist, about getting an evaluation. The American Academy of Child and Adolescent Psychiatry (AACAP) recommends that healthcare providers routinely screen children for behavioral and mental-health concerns. Some of the signs and symptoms of anxiety in children could be caused by other conditions, such as trauma. Specific symptoms such as having a hard time focusing could be a sign of attention deficit hyperactivity disorder (ADHD). It is important to get a careful evaluation to get the best diagnosis and treatment.

Consultation with a health provider can help determine if medication should be part of the treatment. A mental-health professional can develop a therapy plan that works best for the child and family. Behavior therapy includes child therapy, family therapy, or a combination of both. The school can also be included in the treatment plan. For very young children, involving parents in treatment is key. Cognitive-behavioral therapy (CBT) is one form of therapy that is used to treat anxiety, particularly in older children. It helps the child change negative thoughts into more positive, effective ways of thinking, leading to more effective behavior. Behavior therapy for anxiety may involve helping children cope with and manage anxiety symptoms while gradually exposing them to their fears so as to help them learn that bad things do not occur.

Treatments can also include a variety of ways to help the child feel less stressed and be healthier, such as nutritious food, physical activity, sufficient sleep, predictable routines, and social support.

Managing Symptoms: Staying Healthy

Being healthy is important for all children and can be especially important for children with anxiety. In addition to getting the right treatment, leading a healthy lifestyle can play a role in managing symptoms of anxiety.

Here are some healthy behaviors that may help:

- Having a healthy eating plan centered on fruits, vegetables, whole grains, legumes (for example, beans, peas, and lentils), lean protein sources, and nuts and seeds

- Participating in physical activity for at least 60 minutes each day

- Getting the recommended amount of sleep each night based on age

- Practicing mindfulness or relaxation techniques

Prevention of Anxiety

It is not known exactly why some children develop anxiety or depression. Many factors may play a role, including biology and temperament. But it is also known that some children are more likely to develop anxiety or depression when they experience trauma or stress, when they are maltreated, when they are bullied or rejected by other children, or when their own parents have anxiety.

Although these factors appear to increase the risk of anxiety, there are ways to decrease the chance that children experience them.

What Is Panic Disorder?

Children with panic disorder have sudden and repeated attacks of fear that last for several minutes or longer. These are called "panic attacks." Panic attacks are characterized by a fear of disaster or of losing control even when there is no real danger. A child may also have a strong physical reaction during a panic attack. It may feel like having a heart attack. Panic attacks can occur at any time, and many people with panic disorder worry about and dread the possibility of having another attack.

A child with panic disorder may become discouraged and feel ashamed because she or he cannot carry out normal routines, such as going to school or work, going to the grocery store, or driving.

Panic disorder often begins in the late teens or early adulthood. Not everyone who experiences panic attacks will develop panic disorder.

What Causes Panic Disorder

Panic disorder sometimes runs in families, but no one knows for sure why some family members have it while others do not. Researchers have found that several parts of the brain, as well as biological processes, play a key role in fear and anxiety.

Some researchers think that people with panic disorder misinterpret harmless bodily sensations as threats. By learning more about how the brain and body functions in people with panic disorder, scientists may be able to create better treatments. Researchers are also looking for ways in which stress and environmental factors may play a role.

What Are the Signs and Symptoms of Panic Disorder?

Children with panic disorder may have:

- Sudden and repeated panic attacks of overwhelming anxiety and fear

- A feeling of being out of control, or a fear of death or impending doom during a panic attack

- Physical symptoms during a panic attack, such as a pounding or racing heart, sweating, chills, trembling, breathing problems, weakness or dizziness, tingly or numb hands, chest pain, stomach pain, and nausea

- An intense worry about when the next panic attack will happen

- A fear or avoidance of places where panic attacks have occurred in the past

How Is Panic Disorder Treated?

First, talk to your child's doctor about their symptoms. The doctor should do an exam and ask about the child's health history to make sure that an unrelated physical problem is not causing these symptoms. The doctor may refer to your child to a mental-health specialist, such as a psychiatrist or psychologist.

Panic disorder is generally treated with psychotherapy, medication, or both. Talk with the doctor about the best treatment for your child.

Psychotherapy. A type of psychotherapy called "cognitive-behavioral therapy" (CBT) is especially useful as a first-line treatment for panic disorder. CBT teaches you different ways of thinking, behaving, and reacting to the feelings that come on with a panic attack. The attacks can begin to disappear once you learn to react differently to the physical sensations of anxiety and fear that occur during panic attacks.

Medication. Doctors also may prescribe different types of medications to help treat panic disorder:

- Selective serotonin reuptake inhibitors (SSRIs)

- Serotonin-norepinephrine reuptake inhibitors (SNRIs)

- Beta-blockers

- Benzodiazepines

Selective serotonin reuptake inhibitors and SNRIs are commonly used to treat depression, but they are also helpful for the symptoms of panic disorder. They may take several weeks to start working. These medications may also cause side effects, such as headaches, nausea, or difficulty sleeping. These side effects are usually not severe for most, especially if the dose starts off low and is increased slowly over time. Talk to your child's doctor about any side effects that the child may have.

Another type of medication called "beta-blockers" can help control some of the physical symptoms of panic disorder, such as rapid heart rate. Although doctors do not commonly prescribe beta-blockers for panic disorder, they may be helpful in certain situations that precede a panic attack.

Benzodiazepines, which are sedative medications, are powerfully effective in rapidly decreasing panic attack symptoms, but they can cause tolerance and dependence if your child use them continuously. Therefore, their doctor will only prescribe them for brief periods of time if you need them.

Your doctor will work with you to find the best medication and dose for you.

Do not give up on treatment too quickly. Both psychotherapy and medication can take some time to work. A healthy lifestyle can also help combat panic disorder. Make sure that your child get enough sleep and exercise, eat a healthy diet, and turn to family and friends who they trust for support.

Supportive Parenting Can Reduce Child's Anxiety

All kids feel fearful from time to time. The types of fears they experience can change as they age. But if they do not outgrow their fears or if their worries go on for too long, they may have an anxiety disorder. Children with anxiety disorders may act irritable or angry, have trouble sleeping, or experience physical issues, such as headaches or stomach aches. They can have significant problems in social interactions, school, and home life.

The most effective treatment for anxiety disorders is CBT, which teaches people healthy ways to cope with their worries and emotions. But some children will not try the therapy or do not follow the treatment correctly. Of those children who do complete the therapy, only about half respond.

Studies have shown that a parent's involvement in their child's treatment can also help reduce anxiety. Parents are in a unique position to help since their kids naturally rely on them for reassurance and protection. However, while some ways of accommodating a child's fears may lessen their anxiety at the time, they can also prevent the child from learning how to deal with their worries on their own as they get older. For example, a parent might sleep with a child who has separation anxiety or avoid inviting guests over when a child has social phobia.

To determine whether teaching strategies to parents for responding to their child's anxiety works as well as CBT, a team led by Dr. Eli Lebowitz at the Yale Child Study Center tested a program called "Supportive Parenting for Anxious Childhood Emotions" (SPACE). SPACE helps parents identify which accommodating behaviors they can reduce and teaches them new ways to respond. The research was supported by the National Institutes of Health's (NIH) National Institute of Mental Health (NIMH) and the National Center for the Advancement of Translational Science (NCATS). Results were published online in the *Journal of the American Academy of Child and Adolescent Psychiatry*.

Researchers randomly assigned 124 children, aged 7 to 14, who had been diagnosed with an anxiety disorder to either the standard CBT or assigned their parents to the SPACE program. Each treatment program consisted of 12 weekly 60-minute sessions with a therapist.

Parents assigned to the SPACE program learned supportive ways to respond to their child's anxiety and communicate their confidence in their ability to cope with their feelings. They worked with the counselor to identify which accommodations to reduce for the child and to create a plan for doing so. Parents were also given problem-solving strategies for responding to their child's reactions to the changes.

Children assigned to the CBT cohort received standard treatment from a counselor to learn about anxiety and strategies they could use to cope with their worries. Their parents were only given information about the therapy the child was receiving.

Both treatments reduced the children's level of anxiety and anxiety-related emotional disorders to a similar degree. Parents of both groups experienced drops in parenting-related stress. The findings suggest that both approaches work equally well to reduce childhood anxiety.

"There are currently two evidence-based treatments for anxiety—medication and CBT," Lebowitz says. "Yet only half the children respond to these therapies, so there is a great need for alternate treatments."

Section 35.2

Bipolar Disorder

This section includes text excerpted from "Bipolar Disorder in Children and Teens," National Institute of Mental Health (NIMH), 2015. Reviewed September 2019.

What Is Bipolar Disorder?

Bipolar disorder is a serious brain illness. It is also called "manic-depressive illness" or "manic depression." Children with bipolar disorder go through unusual mood changes. Sometimes they feel very happy or "up," and are much more energetic and active than usual, or than other kids their age. This is called a "manic episode." Sometimes children with bipolar disorder feel very sad and "down," and are much less active than usual. This is called "depression" or a "depressive episode."

Bipolar disorder is not the same as the normal ups and downs every kid goes through. Bipolar symptoms are more powerful than that. The mood swings are more extreme and are accompanied by changes in sleep, energy level, and the ability to think clearly. Bipolar symptoms are so strong, they can make it hard for a child to do well in school or get along with friends and family members. The illness can also be dangerous. Some young people with bipolar disorder try to hurt themselves or attempt suicide.

Children with bipolar disorder should get treatment. With help, they can manage their symptoms and lead successful lives.

Who Develops Bipolar Disorder

Anyone can develop bipolar disorder, including children. However, most people with bipolar disorder develop it in their late-teen or early adult years. The illness usually lasts a lifetime.

Why Does Someone Develop Bipolar Disorder?

Doctors do not know what causes bipolar disorder, but several things may contribute to the illness. Family genes may be one factor because bipolar disorder sometimes runs in families. However, it is important to know that just because someone in your family has bipolar disorder, it does not mean other members of the family will have it as well.

Another factor that may lead to bipolar disorder is the brain structure or the brain function of the person with the disorder. Scientists are finding out more about the disorder by studying it. This research may help doctors do a better job of treating people. Also, this research may help doctors to predict whether a person will get bipolar disorder. One day, doctors may be able to prevent the illness in some people.

What Are the Symptoms of Bipolar Disorder?

Bipolar "mood episodes" include unusual mood changes along with unusual sleep habits, activity levels, thoughts, or behavior. In a child, these mood and activity changes must be very different from their usual behavior and from the behavior of other children. A person with bipolar disorder may have manic episodes, depressive episodes, or "mixed" episodes. A mixed episode has both manic and depressive symptoms. These mood episodes cause symptoms that last a week or two or sometimes longer. During an episode, the symptoms last every day for most of the day.

Children having a manic episode may:

- Feel very happy or act silly in a way that is unusual for them and for other people their age

- Have a very short temper

- Talk really fast about a lot of different things

- Have trouble sleeping but not feel tired

733

- Have trouble staying focused
- Talk and think about sex more often
- Do risky things

Children having a depressive episode may:

- Feel very sad
- Complain about pain a lot, such as stomachaches and headaches
- Sleep too little or too much
- Feel guilty and worthless
- Eat too little or too much
- Have little energy and no interest in fun activities
- Think about death or suicide

Can Children with Bipolar Disorder Have Other Problems?

Young people with bipolar disorder can have several problems at the same time. These include:

- **Substance abuse.** Kids with bipolar disorder are at risk of drinking or taking drugs.
- **Attention deficit hyperactivity disorder (ADHD).** Children who have both bipolar disorder and ADHD may have trouble staying focused.
- **Anxiety disorders,** such as separation anxiety.

Sometimes behavior problems go along with mood episodes. Young people may take a lot of risks, such as driving too fast or spending too much money. Some young people with bipolar disorder think about suicide. Watch for any signs of suicidal thinking. Take these signs seriously and call your child's doctor.

How Is Bipolar Disorder Diagnosed?

An experienced doctor will carefully examine your child. There are no blood tests or brain scans that can diagnose bipolar disorder. Instead, the doctor will ask questions about your child's mood and sleeping patterns. The doctor will also ask about your child's energy and behavior. Sometimes doctors need to know about medical problems in your family, such as depression or alcoholism. The doctor may use tests to see if something other than bipolar disorder is causing your child's symptoms.

How Is Bipolar Disorder Treated?

Right now, there is no cure for bipolar disorder. Doctors often treat children who have the illness in much the same way they treat adults. Treatment can help control symptoms. Steady, dependable treatment works better than treatment that starts and stops. Treatment options include:

- **Medication.** There are several types of medication that can help. Children respond to medications in different ways, so the right type of medication depends on the child. Some children may need more than one type of medication because their symptoms are so complex. Sometimes they need to try different types of medicine to see which are best for them. Children should take the fewest number of medications and the smallest doses possible to help their symptoms. A good way to remember this is "start low, go slow." Medications can cause side effects. Always tell your child's doctor about any problems with side effects. Do not stop giving your child medication without a doctor's help. Stopping medication suddenly can be dangerous, and it can make bipolar symptoms worse.

- **Therapy.** Different kinds of psychotherapy, or "talk" therapy, can help children with bipolar disorder. Therapy can help children change their behavior and manage their routines. It can also help young people get along better with family and friends. Sometimes therapy includes family members.

What Can Children Expect from Treatment?

With treatment, children with bipolar disorder can get better over time. It helps when doctors, parents, and young people work together.

Sometimes a child's bipolar disorder changes. When this happens, treatment needs to change too. For example, your child may need to try a different medication. The doctor may also recommend other treatment changes. Symptoms may come back after a while, and more adjustments may be needed. Treatment can take time, but sticking with it helps many children have fewer bipolar symptoms.

You can help treatment be more effective. Try keeping a chart of your child's moods, behaviors, and sleep patterns. This is called a "daily life chart" or "mood chart." It can help you and your child understand and track the illness. A chart can also help the doctor see whether treatment is working.

How You Can Help Your Child with Bipolar Disorder

Help begins with the right diagnosis and treatment. If you think your child may have bipolar disorder, make an appointment with your family doctor to talk about the symptoms you notice.

If your child has bipolar disorder, here are some basic things you can do:

- Be patient.

- Encourage your child to talk, and listen to your child carefully.

- Be understanding about mood episodes.

- Help your child have fun.

- Help your child understand that treatment can make life better.

How Does Bipolar Disorder Affect Parents and Family?

Taking care of a child with bipolar disorder can be stressful for you, too. You have to cope with the mood swings and other problems, such as short tempers and risky activities. This can challenge any parent. Sometimes the stress can strain your relationships with other people, and you may miss work or lose free time.

If you are taking care of a child with bipolar disorder, take care of yourself too. Find someone you can talk to about your feelings. Talk with the doctor about support groups for caregivers. If you keep your stress level down, you will do a better job. It might help your child get better too.

Section 35.3

Depression

This section includes text excerpted from "Anxiety and Depression in Children," Centers for Disease Control and Prevention (CDC), April 15, 2019.

Many children have fears and worries, and may feel sad and hopeless from time to time. Strong fears may appear at different times during development. For example, toddlers are often very distressed about being away from their parents, even if they are safe and cared for. Although fears and worries are typical in children, persistent or extreme forms of fear and sadness could be due to anxiety or depression. Because the symptoms primarily involve thoughts and feelings, they are called "internalizing disorders."

Occasionally being sad or feeling hopeless is a part of every child's life. However, some children feel sad or uninterested in things that they used to enjoy, or feel helpless or hopeless in situations they are able to change. When children feel persistent sadness and hopelessness, they may be diagnosed with depression.

Examples of behaviors often seen in children with depression include:

- Feeling sad, hopeless, or irritable a lot of the time

- Not wanting to do or enjoy doing fun things

- Showing changes in eating patterns—eating a lot more or a lot less than usual

- Showing changes in sleep patterns—sleeping a lot more or a lot less than normal

- Showing changes in energy—being tired and sluggish or tense and restless a lot of the time

- Having a hard time paying attention

- Feeling worthless, useless, or guilty

- Showing self-injury and self-destructive behavior

Extreme depression can lead a child to think about suicide or plan for suicide. For youth ages 10 to 24 years, suicide is among the leading causes of death.

Some children may not talk about their helpless and hopeless thoughts, and may not appear sad. Depression might also cause a child to make trouble or act unmotivated, causing others not to notice that the child is depressed or to incorrectly label the child as a trouble-maker or lazy.

Treatment of Depression

The first step to treatment is to talk with a healthcare provider such as your child's primary care provider, or a mental-health specialist, about getting an evaluation. The American Academy of Child and Adolescent Psychiatry (AACAP) recommends that healthcare providers routinely screen children for behavioral and mental-health concerns.

Some of the signs and symptoms of anxiety or depression in children could be caused by other conditions, such as trauma. Specific symptoms such as having a hard time focusing could be a sign of attention-deficit hyperactivity disorder (ADHD). It is important to get a careful evaluation to get the best diagnosis and treatment. Consultation with a health provider can help determine if medication should be part of the treatment. A mental-health professional can develop a therapy plan that works best for the child and family. Behavior therapy includes child therapy, family therapy, or a combination of both. The school can also be included in the treatment plan. For very young children, involving parents in treatment is key. Cognitive-behavioral therapy (CBT) is one form of therapy that is used to treat anxiety or depression, particularly in older children. It helps the child change negative thoughts into more positive, effective ways of thinking, leading to more effective behavior. Behavior therapy for anxiety may involve helping children cope with and manage anxiety symptoms while gradually exposing them to their fears so as to help them learn that bad things do not occur.

Treatments can also include a variety of ways to help the child feel less stressed and be healthier such as nutritious food, physical activity, sufficient sleep, predictable routines, and social support.

Managing Depression Symptoms

Being healthy is important for all children and can be especially important for children with depression. In addition to getting the right treatment, leading a healthy lifestyle can play a role in managing symptoms of depression. Here are some healthy behaviors that may help:

- Having a healthy-eating plan centered on fruits, vegetables, whole grains, legumes (for example, beans, peas, and lentils), lean protein sources, and nuts and seeds

- Participating in physical activity for at least 60 minutes each day

- Getting the recommended amount of sleep each night based on age

- Practicing mindfulness or relaxation techniques

Prevention of Depression

It is not known exactly why some children develop depression. Many factors may play a role, including biology and temperament. But it is also known that some children are more likely to develop depression when they experience trauma or stress, when they are maltreated, when they are bullied or rejected by other children, or when their own parents have depression.

Although these factors appear to increase the risk for anxiety or depression, there are ways to decrease the chance that children experience them.

Section 35.4

Obsessive-Compulsive Disorder

This section includes text excerpted from "Obsessive-Compulsive Disorder in Children," Centers for Disease Control and Prevention (CDC), March 12, 2019.

Many children occasionally have thoughts that bother them, and they might feel like they have to do something about those thoughts, even if their actions do not actually make sense. For example, they might worry about having bad luck if they do not wear a favorite piece of clothing. For some children, the thoughts and the urges to perform certain actions persist, even if they try to ignore them or make them go away. Children may have an obsessive-compulsive disorder (OCD) when unwanted thoughts, and the behaviors they feel they must do because of the thoughts, happen frequently, take up a lot of time (more than an hour a day), interfere with their activities, or make them very upset. The thoughts are called "obsessions." The behaviors are called "compulsions."

Symptoms of Obsessive-Compulsive Disorder

Having obsessive-compulsive disorder means having obsessions, compulsions, or both.

Examples of obsessive or compulsive behaviors include:

• Having unwanted thoughts, impulses, or images that occur over and over and which cause anxiety or distress

• Having to think about or say something over and over (for example, counting, or repeating words over and over silently or out loud)

• Having to do something over and over (for example, handwashing, placing things in a specific order, or checking the same things over and over, such as whether a door is locked)

• Having to do something over and over according to certain rules that must be followed exactly in order to make an obsession go away

Children do these behaviors because they have the feeling that the behaviors will prevent bad things from happening or will make them feel better. However, the behavior is not typically connected to the actual danger of something bad happening, or the behavior is extreme, such as washing hands multiple times per hour.

A common myth is that OCD means being really neat and orderly. Sometimes, OCD behaviors may involve cleaning, but many times someone with OCD is too focused on one thing that must be done over and over, rather than on being organized. Obsessions and compulsions can also change over time.

Treatment of Obsessive-Compulsive Disorder

The first step to treatment is to talk with a healthcare provider to arrange an evaluation. A comprehensive evaluation by a mental-health professional will determine if the anxiety or distress involves memories of a traumatic event that actually happened, or if the fears are based on other thoughts or beliefs. The mental-health professional should also determine whether someone with OCD has a current or past tic disorder. Anxiety or depression and disruptive behaviors may also occur with OCD.

Treatments can include behavior therapy and medication. Behavior therapy, specifically cognitive-behavioral therapy (CBT), helps the child change negative thoughts into more positive, effective ways of thinking, leading to more effective behavior. Behavior therapy for OCD can involve gradually exposing children to their fears in a safe setting; this helps them learn that bad things do not really occur when they do not do the behavior, which eventually decreases their anxiety. Behavior therapy alone can be effective, but some children are treated with a combination of behavior therapy and medication. Families and schools can help children manage stress by being part of the therapy process and learning how to respond supportively without accidentally making obsessions or compulsions more likely to happen again.

Prevention of Obsessive-Compulsive Disorder

It is not known exactly why some children develop OCD. There is likely to be a biological and neurological component, and some children with OCD also have Tourette syndrome or other tic disorders. There are some studies that suggest that health problems during pregnancy and birth may make OCD more likely, which is one of many important reasons to support the health of women during pregnancy.

Part Five

Additional Help and Information

Chapter 36

Glossary of Terms Related to Childhood Diseases and Disorders

acute otitis media: Ear infection, usually caused by bacteria; when the middle ear becomes infected and swollen, trapping fluid and mucus behind the eardrum.

adenoid: Small pad of infection-fighting tissue located near the eustachian tube.

adenovirus: A member of a family of viruses that can cause infections in the respiratory tract, eye, and gastrointestinal tract. Forms of adenoviruses that do not cause disease are used in gene therapy.

adrenal gland: A small gland that makes steroid hormones, adrenaline, and noradrenaline. These hormones help control heart rate, blood pressure, and other important body functions. There are two adrenal glands, one on top of each kidney. Also called suprarenal gland.

allergy: A condition in which the body has an exaggerated response to a substance (e.g., food or drug). Also known as hypersensitivity.

antibody: A protein found in the blood that is produced in response to foreign substances (e.g., bacteria or viruses) invading the body.

This glossary contains terms excerpted from documents produced by several sources deemed reliable.

Antibodies protect the body from disease by binding to these organisms and destroying them.

anticholinergics: This type of medicine relaxes the muscle bands that tighten around the airways. This action opens the airways, letting more air out of the lungs to improve breathing. Anticholinergics also help clear mucus from the lungs.

arthritis: A disease that causes inflammation and pain in the joints.

asthma: A chronic medical condition where the bronchial tubes (in the lungs) become easily irritated. This leads to constriction of the airways resulting in wheezing, coughing, difficulty breathing, and production of thick mucus.

autism: A chronic developmental disorder usually diagnosed between 18 and 30 months of age.

autosomal: Describes genetic material (chromosomes or genes) that are not gender-related.

bacteria: Tiny one-celled organisms present throughout the environment that require a microscope to be seen. While not all bacteria are harmful, some cause disease.

biopsy: The removal of cells or tissues for examination by a pathologist. The pathologist may study the tissue under a microscope or perform other tests on the cells or tissue. There are many different types of biopsy procedures. The most common types include: (1) incisional biopsy, in which only a sample of tissue is removed; (2) excisional biopsy, in which an entire lump or suspicious area is removed; and (3) needle biopsy, in which a sample of tissue or fluid is removed with a needle.

breathing pattern: A general term designating the characteristics of the ventilatory activity, e.g., frequency of breathing.

bronchitis: Inflammation of the main air passages to your lungs. It causes cough, shortness of breath, and chest tightness.

bronchodilator: A medicine that relaxes the smooth muscles of the airways. This allows the airway to open up (to dilate) since the muscles are not squeezing it shut.

carrier: A person who has a mutated (changed) copy of a gene. This change may cause a disease in that person or in her or his children.

cholesteatoma: Accumulation of dead cells in the middle ear, caused by repeated middle ear infections.

chromosome: Part of a cell that contains genetic information. Except for sperm and eggs, all human cells contain 46 chromosomes.

chronic otitis media with effusion (COME): Repeated occurrences of otitis media with effusion (ear infection), in which fluid remains in the middle ear after the infection is gone.

cognition: Thinking skills that include perception, memory, awareness, reasoning, judgment, intellect, and imagination.

computerized tomography (CT) scan: A series of detailed pictures of areas inside the body taken from different angles. The pictures are created by a computer linked to an X-ray machine.

Crohn disease: A chronic medical condition characterized by inflammation of the bowel.

deep vein thrombosis: A blood clot that forms in a vein deep in the body.

cystic fibrosis: A common hereditary disease in which exocrine (secretory) glands produce abnormally thick mucus. This mucus can cause problems in digestion, breathing, and body cooling.

diabetes: A chronic health condition where the body is unable to produce insulin and properly break down sugar (glucose) in the blood.

dysarthria: Group of speech disorders caused by disturbances in the strength or coordination of the muscles of the speech mechanism as a result of damage to the brain or nerves.

dysphagia: Any impairment of the voice or speaking ability.

encephalopathy: A general term describing brain dysfunction.

endocrine system: A system of glands and cells that make hormones that are released directly into the blood and travel to tissues and organs all over the body. The endocrine system controls growth, sexual development, sleep, hunger, and the way the body uses food.

epilepsy: A group of disorders marked by problems in the normal functioning of the brain. These problems can produce seizures, unusual body movements, a loss of consciousness or changes in consciousness, as well as mental problems or problems with the senses.

exposure: Contact with infectious agents (bacteria or viruses) in a manner that promotes transmission and increases the likelihood of disease.

fever: An increase in body temperature above normal (98.6° F), usually caused by disease.

gastric reflux: The backward flow of stomach acid contents into the esophagus (the tube that connects the mouth to the stomach). Also called esophageal reflux and gastroesophageal reflux.

genetic counseling: A communication process between a specially trained health professional and a person concerned about the genetic risk of disease. The person's family and personal medical history may be discussed, and counseling may lead to genetic testing.

Haemophilus influenzae type b: A bacterial infection that may result in severe respiratory infections, including pneumonia, and other diseases such as meningitis.

hepatitis: Disease of the liver causing inflammation. Symptoms include an enlarged liver, fever, nausea, vomiting, abdominal pain, and dark urine.

hereditary: Transmitted from parent to child by information contained in the genes.

immune system: The complex system in the body responsible for fighting disease. Its primary function is to identify foreign substances in the body (bacteria, viruses, fungi, or parasites) and develop a defense against them.

incubation period: The time from contact with infectious agents (bacteria or viruses) to onset of disease.

infection: Invasion and multiplication of germs in the body. Infections can occur in any part of the body and can spread throughout the body. The germs may be bacteria, viruses, yeast, or fungi.

inflammatory bowel disease (IBD): A general term for any disease characterized by inflammation of the bowel. Examples include colitis and Crohn disease.

inflammation: Used to describe an area on the body that is swollen, red, hot, and in pain.

influenza: A highly contagious viral infection characterized by sudden onset of fever, severe aches and pains, and inflammation of the mucous membrane.

Kallmann syndrome: Disorder that can include several characteristics such as absence of the sense of smell and decreased functional activity of the gonads (organs that produce sex cells), affecting growth and sexual development.

magnetic resonance imaging (MRI): A procedure in which radio waves and a powerful magnet linked to a computer are used to create detailed pictures of areas inside the body. These pictures can show the difference between normal and diseased tissue.

otitis media: A viral or bacterial infection that leads to inflammation of the middle ear. This condition usually occurs along with an upper respiratory infection.

otoscope: Ear infection in which fluid remains trapped behind the eardrum inside the middle ear after the infection is over.

parasitic: Having to do with or being a parasite (an animal or plant that gets nutrients by living on or in an organism of another species).

pathogens: Organisms (e.g., bacteria, viruses, parasites, and fungi) that cause disease in human beings.

pertussis (whooping cough): Bacterial infectious disease marked by a convulsive spasmodic cough, sometimes followed by a crowing intake of breath.

pinkeye: A condition in which the conjunctiva (membranes lining the eyelids and covering the white part of the eye) become inflamed or infected. Also called conjunctivitis.

pneumonia: Inflammation of the lungs characterized by fever, chills, muscle stiffness, chest pain, cough, shortness of breath, rapid heart rate, and difficulty breathing.

prosody: The rhythm, speed, pitch, and tone of spoken language.

Reye syndrome: Encephalopathy (general brain disorder) in children following an acute illness such as influenza or chickenpox. This condition may result in coma or death.

sarcoma: A cancer of the bone, cartilage, fat, muscle, blood vessels, or other connective or supportive tissue.

seizure: Sudden, uncontrolled body movements and changes in behavior that occur because of abnormal electrical activity in the brain.

spasmodic dysphonia: Momentary disruption of voice caused by involuntary movements of one or more muscles of the larynx or voice box.

stuttering: Frequent repetition of words or parts of words that disrupts the smooth flow of speech.

tinnitus: Sensation of a ringing, roaring, or buzzing sound in the ears or head. It is often associated with many forms of hearing impairment and noise exposure.

tumor: An abnormal mass of tissue that results when cells divide more than they should or do not die when they should. Tumors may be benign (not cancer) or malignant (cancer). Also called neoplasm.

ultrasound: A procedure in which high-energy sound waves are bounced off internal tissues or organs and make echoes. The echo patterns are shown on the screen of an ultrasound machine, forming a picture of body tissues called a sonogram. Also called ultrasonography.

upper respiratory tract: Area of the body that includes the nasal passages, mouth, and throat.

Usher syndrome: Hereditary disease that affects hearing and vision and sometimes balance.

vaccine: A product made from very small amounts of weak or dead germs that can cause diseases—for example, viruses, bacteria, or toxins. It prepares your body to fight the disease faster and more effectively so you won't get sick. Vaccines are administered through needle injections, by mouth, and by aerosol.

virus: A tiny organism that multiplies within cells and causes disease such as chickenpox, measles, mumps, rubella, pertussis, and hepatitis. Viruses are not affected by antibiotics, the drugs used to kill bacteria.

wheezing: Breathing with difficulty, with a whistling noise. Wheezing is a symptom of asthma.

x-ray: A type of high-energy radiation. In low doses, x-rays are used to diagnose diseases by making pictures of the inside of the body.

Chapter 37

Resource List for Parents and Caregivers

Government Agencies That Provide Information about Childhood Diseases and Disorders

Center for Food Safety and Applied Nutrition (CFSAN)
U.S. Food and Drug Administration (FDA)
5001 Campus Dr., HFS-009
College Park, MD 20740-3835
Toll-Free: 888-SAFEFOOD
(888-723-3366)
Website: www.fda.gov/
about-fda/center-food-safety-
and-applied-nutrition-cfsan/
contact-cfsan

Centers for Disease Control and Prevention (CDC)
1600 Clifton Rd.
Atlanta, GA 30329-4027
Toll-Free: 800-CDC-INFO
(800-232-4636)
Toll-Free TTY: 888-232-6348
Website: www.cdc.gov

Resources in this chapter were compiled from several sources deemed reliable; all contact information was verified and updated in September 2019.

Eunice Kennedy Shriver
National Institute of Child
Health and Development
(NICHD)
Information Resource Center
(IRC)
P.O. Box 3006
Rockville, MD 20847
Toll-Free: 800-370-2943
Toll-Free Fax: 866-760-5947
Website: www.nichd.nih.gov
E-mail: NICHDInformation
ResourceCenter@mail.nih.gov

National Cancer Institute
(NCI)
9609 Medical Center Dr.
BG 9609, MSC 9760
Bethesda, MD 20892-9760
Toll-Free: 800-4-CANCER
(800-422-6237)
Website: www.cancer.gov
E-mail: NCIinfo@nih.gov

National Diabetes Education
Program (NDEP)
National Institute of Diabetes
and Digestive and Kidney
Diseases (NIDDK) Health
Information Center (HIC)
Website: www.niddk.nih.
gov/health-information/
communication-programs/
ndep/about-national-diabetes-
education-program
E-mail: healthinfo@niddk.nih.
gov

National Diabetes
Information Clearinghouse
(NDIC)
National Institute of Diabetes
and Digestive and Kidney
Diseases (NIDDK) Health
Information Center (HIC)
Website: www.niddk.nih.gov/
health-information/diabetes
E-mail: healthinfo@niddk.nih.
gov

National Eye Institute (NEI)
Information Office
31 Centers Dr., MSC 2510
Bethesda, MD 20892-2510
Phone: 301-496-5248
Website: www.nei.nih.gov
E-mail: 2020@nei.nih.gov

National Heart, Lung, and
Blood Institute (NHLBI)
NHLBI Center for Health
Information
P.O. Box 30105
Bethesda, MD 20824-0105
Phone: 301-592-8573
Website: www.nhlbi.nih.gov
E-mail: nhlbiinfo@nhlbi.nih.gov

National Institute of Allergy and Infectious Diseases (NIAID)
Office of Communications and Government Relations (OCGR)
5601 Fishers Ln.
MSC 9806
Bethesda, MD 20892-9806
Toll-Free: 866-284-4107
Phone: 301-496-5717
Toll-Free TDD: 800-877-8339
Fax: 301-402-3573
Website: www.niaid.nih.gov
E-mail: ocpostoffice@niaid.nih.gov

National Institute of Arthritis and Musculoskeletal and Skin Diseases (NIAMS)
Information Clearinghouse, National Institutes of Health (NIH)
One AMS Cir.
Bethesda, MD 20892-3675
Toll-Free: 877-22-NIAMS (877-226-4267)
Phone: 301-495-4484
TTY: 301-565-2966
Fax: 301-718-6366
Website: www.niams.nih.gov
E-mail: NIAMSinfo@mail.nih.gov

National Institute of Diabetes and Digestive and Kidney Diseases (NIDDK)
Health Information Center
Toll-Free: 800-860-8747
Toll-Free TTY: 866-569-1162
Website: www.niddk.nih.gov
E-mail: healthinfo@niddk.nih.gov

National Institute of Mental Health (NIMH)
Office of Science Policy, Planning, and Communications (OSPPC)
6001 Executive Blvd.
Rm. 6200, MSC 9663
Bethesda, MD 20892-9663
Toll-Free: 866-615-NIMH (866-615-6464)
TTY: 301-443-8431
Toll-Free TTY: 866-415-8051
Fax: 301-443-4279
Website: www.nimh.nih.gov
E-mail: nimhinfo@nih.gov

National Institute on Deafness and Other Communication Disorders (NIDCD)
Office of Health Communication and Public Liaison
31 Center Dr.
MSC 2320
Bethesda, MD 20892-2320
Toll-Free: 800-241-1044
Phone: 301-827-8183
Toll-Free TTY: 800-241-1055
Website: www.nidcd.nih.gov
E-mail: nidcdinfo@nidcd.nih.gov

U.S. Department of Agriculture (USDA)
1400 Independence Ave., S.W.
Washington, DC 20250
Phone: 202-720-2791
Website: www.usda.gov

U.S. Department of Health and Human Services (HHS)
200 Independence Ave., S.W.
Hubert H. Humphrey Bldg.
Washington, DC 20201
Toll-Free: 877-696-6775
Website: www.hhs.gov

U.S. Environmental Protection Agency (EPA)
1200 Pennsylvania Ave., N.W.
Washington, DC 20460
Phone: 202-564-4700
Website: www.epa.gov

U.S. Food and Drug Administration (FDA)
10903 New Hampshire Ave.
Silver Spring, MD 20993-0002
Toll-Free: 888-INFO-FDA
(888-463-6332)
Website: www.fda.gov

Weight-Control Information Network (WIN)
National Institute of Diabetes and Digestive and Kidney Diseases (NIDDK) Health Information Center (HIC)
Website: www.niddk.nih.gov/health-information/communication-programs/win/about
E-mail: healthinfo@niddk.nih.gov

Private Agencies That Provide Information about Childhood Diseases and Disorders

Alpha-1 Foundation
3300 Ponce de Leon Blvd.
Coral Gables, FL 33134
Toll-Free: 877-2-CURE-A1
(877-228-7321)
Phone: 305-567-9888
Fax: 305-567-1317
Website: www.alpha1.org
E-mail: info@alpha-1foundation.org

American Academy of Child and Adolescent Psychiatry (AACAP)
3615 Wisconsin Ave., N.W.
Washington, DC 20016-3007
Phone: 202-966-7300
Fax: 202-464-0131
Website: www.aacap.org
E-mail: communications@aacap.org

American Academy of Dermatology (AAD)
P.O. Box 1968
Des Plaines, IL 60017
Toll-Free: 888-462-DERM
(888-462-3376)
Phone: 847-240-1280
Fax: 847-240-1859
Website: www.aad.org
E-mail: MRC@aad.org

American Academy of Pediatrics (AAP)
National Headquarters
345 Park Blvd.
Itasca, IL 60143
Toll-Free: 800-433-9016
Fax: 847-434-8000
Website: www.aap.org
E-mail: csc@aap.org

American Association for the Study of Liver Diseases (AASLD)
1001 N. Fairfax St., Fourth Fl.
Alexandria, VA 22314
Phone: 703-299-9766
Fax: 703-299-9622
Website: www.aasld.org
E-mail: aasld@aasld.org

American Cancer Society (ACS)
250 Williams St., N.W.
Atlanta, GA 30303
Toll-Free: 800-ACS-2345
(800-227-2345)
Toll-Free TTY: 866-228-4327
Website: www.cancer.org

American College of Gastroenterology (ACG)
6400 Goldsboro Rd.
Bethesda, MD 20817
Phone: 301-263-9000
Website: www.gi.org

American College of Rheumatology (ACR)
Association of Rheumatology
Professionals (ARP),
Rheumatology Research
Foundation
2200 Lake Blvd., N.E.
Atlanta, GA 30319
Phone: 404-633-3777
Fax: 404-633-1870
Website: www.rheumatology.org

American Diabetes Association (ADA)
2451 Crystal Dr.
Ste. 900
Arlington, VA 22202
Toll-Free: 800-DIABETES
(800-342-2383)
Website: www.diabetes.org
E-mail: askada@diabetes.org

American Gastroenterological Association (AGA)
4930 Del Ray Ave.
Bethesda, MD 20814
Phone: 301-654-2055
Fax: 301-654-5920
Website: www.gastro.org
E-mail: member@gastro.org

American Heart Association (AHA)
National Center
7272 Greenville Ave.
Dallas, TX 75231
Toll-Free: 800-AHA-USA-1
(800-242-8721)
Website: www.heart.org

American Liver Foundation (ALF)
National Office
39 Broadway
Ste. 2700
New York, NY 10006
Toll-Free: 800-GO-LIVER
(800-465-4837)
Phone: 212-668-1000
Fax: 212-483-8179
Website: www.liverfoundation.org
E-mail: info@liverfoundation.org

American Society of Pediatric Nephrology (ASPN)
6728 Old McLean Village Dr.
McLean, VA, 22101
Phone: 703-556-9222
Fax: 703-556-8729
Website: www.aspneph.com
E-mail: info@aspneph.com

American Urological Association Foundation (AUA)
1000 Corporate Blvd.
Linthicum, MD 21090
Toll-Free: 800-828-7866
Phone: 410-689-3700
Fax: 410-689-3800
Website: www.auanet.org
E-mail: aua@AUAnet.org

Arthritis Foundation (AF)
National Office
1355 Peachtree St., N.E., Ste. 600
Atlanta, GA 30309
Toll-Free: 844-571-4357
Phone: 404-872-7100
Website: www.arthritis.org

Asthma and Allergy Foundation of America (AAFA)
1235 S. Clark St., Ste. 305
Arlington, VA 22202
Toll-Free: 800-7-ASTHMA
(800-727-8462)
Website: www.aafa.org
E-mail: info@aafa.org

Attention Deficit Disorder Association (ADDA)
Toll-Free: 800-939-1019
Website: www.add.org

Autism Society of America (ASA)
4340 East-West Hwy
Ste. 350
Bethesda, MD 20814
Toll-Free: 800-3-AUTISM
(800-328-8476)
Website: www.autism-society.org
E-mail: info@autism-society.org

Autism Speaks
One E. 33rd St., Fourth Fl.
New York, NY 10016
Phone: 646-385-8500
Fax: 212-252-8676
Website: www.autismspeaks.org
E-mail: contactus@autismspeaks.org

Celiac Disease Foundation (CDF)
20350 Ventura Blvd.
Ste. 240
Woodland Hills, CA 91364
Phone: 818-716-1513
Fax: 818-267-5577
Website: www.celiac.org

Charlie Foundation for Ketogenic Therapies
515 Ocean Ave.
Ste. 602N
Santa Monica, CA 90402
Phone: 310-393-2347
Website: www.charliefoundation.org

Cleveland Clinic
9500 Euclid Ave.
Cleveland, OH 44195
Toll-Free: 800-223-2273
Phone: 216-444-2200
Website: www.my.clevelandclinic.org

Crohn's & Colitis Foundation
733 Third Ave.
Ste. 510
New York, NY 10017
Toll-Free: 800-932-2423
Website: www.crohnscolitisfoundation.org
E-mail: info@crohnscolitisfoundation.org

Cyclic Vomiting Syndrome Association (CVSA)
P.O. Box 270341
Milwaukee, WI 53227
Phone: 414-342-7880
Website: www.cvsaonline.org
E-mail: cvsaonline@gmail.com

Digestive Disease National Coalition (DDNC)
507 Capitol Ct., N.E.
Ste. 200
Washington, DC 20002
Phone: 202-544-7497
Fax: 202-546-7105
Website: www.ddnc.org
E-mail: herzog@hmcw.org

Epilepsy Foundation
8301 Professional Pl., W.
Landover, MD 20785-2356
Toll-Free: 800-EFA-1000
(800-332-1000)
Phone: 301-459-3700
Fax: 301-577-2684
Website: www.epilepsy.com
E-mail: ContactUs@efa.org

Food Allergy Research and Education (FARE)
7901 Jones Branch Dr.
Ste. 240
McLean, VA 22102
Toll-Free: 800-929-4040
Phone: 703-691-3179
Fax: 703-691-2713
Website: www.fare.foodallergy.org

Hepatitis Foundation International (HFI)
8121 Georgia Ave.
Ste. 350
Silver Spring, MD 20910
Toll-Free: 800-891-0707
Phone: 301-565-9410
Website: www.
hepatitisfoundation.org
E-mail: info@
hepatitisfoundation.org

Human Growth Foundation (HGF)
997 Glen Cove Ave.
Ste. 5
Glen Head, NY 11545
Toll-Free: 800-451-6434
Fax: 516-671-4055
Website: www.hgfound.org
E-mail: hgf1@hgfound.org

International Foundation for Functional Gastrointestinal Disorders (IFFGD)
P.O. Box 170864
Milwaukee, WI 53217
Phone: 414-964-1799
Website: www.iffgd.org

Juvenile Diabetes Research Foundation International (JDRF)
26 Broadway
14th Fl.
New York, NY 10004
Toll-Free: 800-533-CURE
(800-533-2873)
Fax: 212-785-9595
Website: www.jdrf.org
E-mail: info@jdrf.org

Learning Disabilities Association of America (LDA)
P.O. Box 10369
Pittsburgh, PA 15234-1349
Phone: 412-341-1515
Fax: 412-344-0224
Website: www.ldaamerica.org
E-mail: info@LDAAmerica.org

The Leukemia & Lymphoma Society (LLS)
Three International Dr.
Ste. 200
Rye Brook, NY 10573
Toll-Free: 888-557-7177
Website: www.lls.org

Lighthouse Guild
250 W. 64th St.
New York, NY 10023
Toll-Free: 800-284-4422
Toll-Free TTY: 800-284-4711
Website: www.lighthouseguild.
org

MAGIC Foundation
4200 Cantera Dr.
Ste. 106
Warrenville, IL 60555
Toll-Free: 800-362-4423
Phone: 630-836-8200
Fax: 630-836-8181
Website: www.magicfoundation.
org
E-mail: contactus@
magicfoundation.org

Mental Health America (MHA)
500 Montgomery St.
Ste. 820
Alexandria, VA 22314
Toll-Free: 800-969-6642
Phone: 703-684-7722
Fax: 703-684-5968
Website: www.mentalhealthamerica.net

Muscular Dystrophy Association (MDA)
National Office
161 N. Clark
Ste. 3550
Chicago, IL 60601
Toll-Free: 800-572-1717
Website: www.mda.org
E-mail: resourcecenter@mdausa.org

National Association for Children's Behavioral Health (NACBH)
Website: nacbh.memberclicks.net

National Association for Continence (NAFC)
P.O. Box 1019
Charleston, SC 29402
Toll-Free: 800-BLADDER
(800-252-3337)
Website: www.nafc.org

National Celiac Association (NCA)
20 Pickering St.
Needham, MA 02492
Toll-Free: 888-4-CELIAC
(888-423-5422)
Phone: 617-262-5422
Website: www.nationalceliac.org
E-mail: info@nationalceliac.org

National Center for Learning Disabilities (NCLD)
One Thomas Circle N.W.
Ste. 700
Washington, DC 20005
Phone: 212-545-7510
Website: www.ncld.org

The National Children's Cancer Society (NCCS)
500 N. Broadway
Ste. 1850
St. Louis, MO 63102
Toll-Free: 800-5FAMILY
(800-532-6459)
Phone: 314-241-1600
Fax: 314-241-1996
Website: www.thenccs.org

National Federation of Families for Children's Mental Health (FFCMH)
15800 Crabbs Branch Way
Ste. 300
Rockville, MD 20855
Phone: 240-403-1901
Website: www.ffcmh.org
E-mail: ffcmh@ffcmh.org

National Hemophilia Foundation (NHF)
Seven Penn Plaza
Ste. 1204
New York, NY 10001
Phone: 212-328-3700
Fax: 212-328-3777
Website: www.hemophilia.org

National Organization for Rare Disorders (NORD)
55 Kenosia Ave.
Danbury, CT 06810
Phone: 203-744-0100
Fax: 203-263-9938
Website: www.rarediseases.org

National Scoliosis Foundation (NSF)
5 Cabot Pl.
Stoughton, MA 02072
Toll-Free: 800-NSF-MYBACK
(800-673-6922)
Fax: 781-341-8333
Website: www.scoliosis.org
E-mail: nsf@scoliosis.org

The Nemours Foundation / KidsHealth®
Website: www.kidshealth.org

North American Society for Pediatric Gastroenterology, Hepatology, and Nutrition (NASPGHAN)
714 N. Bethlehem Pike
Ste. 300
Ambler, PA 19002
Phone: 215-641-9800
Fax: 215-641-1995
Website: www.naspghan.org
E-mail: naspghan@naspghan.org

Pediatric Brain Foundation (PBF)
2144 E. Republic Rd., Bldg. B.
Ste. 201
Springfield, MO 65804
Phone: 417-887-4242
Website: www.
pediatricbrainfoundation.org
E-mail: madison@
pediatricbrainfoundation.org

Pediatric Brain Tumor Foundation (PBTF)
302 Ridgefield Ct.
Asheville, NC 28806
Toll-Free: 800-253-6530
Fax: 828-665-6894
Website: www.curethekids.org
E-mail: info@curethekids.org

Safe Kids Worldwide
1255 23rd St., N.W.
Ste. 400
Washington, DC 20037-1151
Phone: 202-662-0600
Fax: 202-393-2072
Website: www.safekids.org

Urology Care Foundation
1000 Corporate Blvd.
Linthicum, MD 21090
Toll-Free: 800-828-7866
Phone: 410-689-3700
Fax: 410-689-3800
Website: www.urologyhealth.org
E-mail: info@
UrologyCareFoundation.org

Index

Index

791